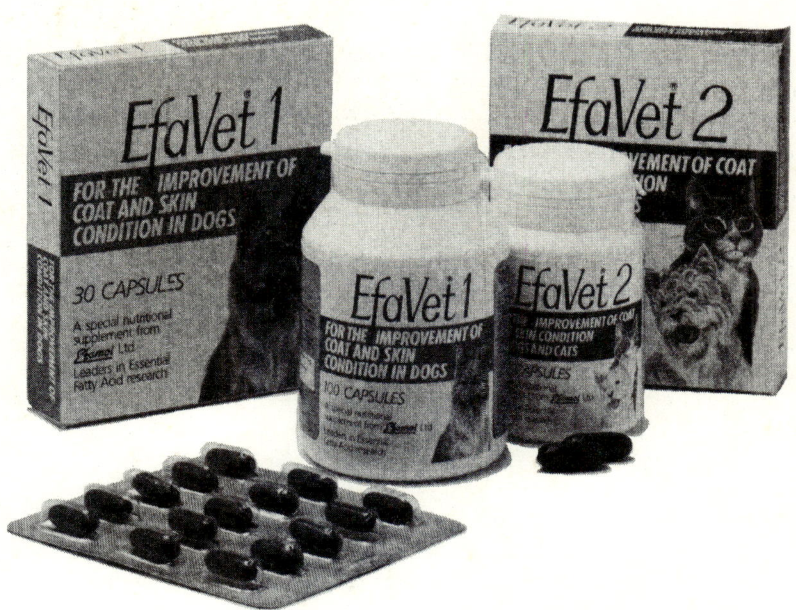

100 CAPSULE PACK AND 30 CAPSULE PACK

EfaVet® CAPSULES

A UNIQUE DIETARY SUPPLEMENT FOR IMPROVEMENT OF SKIN AND COAT CONDITION

FROM

Efamol Vet

LEADERS IN ESSENTIAL FATTY ACID RESEARCH

Further information is available from:
FREEPOST EFAMOL VET, WOODBRIDGE MEADOWS, GUILDFORD, SURREY, GU1 1BR
TELEPHONE: (0483) 578060

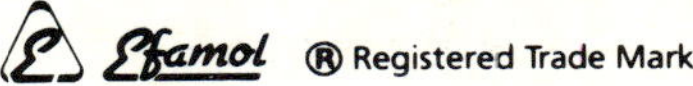 Efamol ® Registered Trade Mark

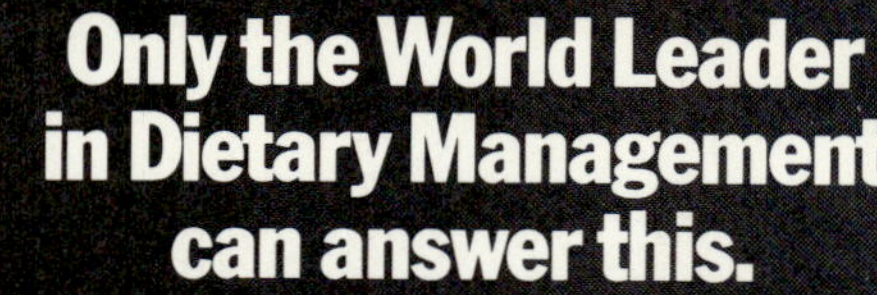

Only the World Leader
in Dietary Management
can answer this.

Hill's
World Leaders in Dietary Management

**The Veterinary Annual

Editors

C. S. G. Grunsell CBE, PhD, FRCVS
Mary-Elizabeth Raw BVSc, FRCVS, DVR
F. W. G. Hill BVetMed, PhD, MRCVS, MACVSc

THE VETERINARY ANNUAL

Twenty-ninth issue

Wright

London   **Boston**   **Singapore**   **Sydney**   **Toronto**   **Wellington**

British Library Cataloguing in Publication Data
The veterinary annual. – 29th issue.
   1. Veterinary medicine, – Serials
   636.089'05

ISBN 0–407–01767–4

Typeset by TecSet Ltd, Lavender Vale, Wallington, Surrey SM6 9RU
Printed and bound in Great Britain by Butler and Tanner, Frome, Somerset

Preface

This year there are a few innovations in the *Veterinary Annual*. For many years now we have had regular reviews on reproduction and husbandry from Dr F. L. M. Dawson and Professor T. K. Ewar, respectively. They have both now retired from this task and we would like to thank them for their valuable contributions over the years.

It is very pleasing to be able to have some figures in colour for the first time. This has been made possible by the generosity of Keymed Ltd and we are very grateful to them.

We would like to thank the publishers, especially the Managing Editor, Ms Diane Cogan, for their support over the year.

C. S. G. Grunsell
Mary-Elizabeth Raw
F. W. G. Hill

Contents

The Contributors

D. P. Attenburrow BVSc, FRCVS St David's Veterinary Hospital, 43 St David's Hill, Exeter, Devon
The application of radioisotope scanning and imaging in general veterinary practice (jointly), 15

D. M. Broom MA, PhD Colleen MacLeod Professor of Animal Welfare, Department of Clinical Veterinary Medicine, University of Cambridge, Madingley Road, Cambridge CB3 0ES
Animal Welfare, 9

Serena Brownlie BVM&S, PhD, MRCVS Department of Veterinary Medicine, Royal Veterinary College Field Station, Hawkshead House, Hawkshead Lane, North Mymms, Hatfield, Herts AL9 7JA
The primary treatment of heart conditions, 217

M. Dawson BVetMed, MRCVS Central Veterinary Laboratory, New Haw, Weybridge, Surrey KT15 3NB
The caprine arthritis encephalitis syndrome, 98

Ruth Dennis MA, VetMB, MRCVS, DVR Department of Clinical Veterinary Medicine, Madingley Road, Cambridge CB3 0ES
Radiology of metabolic bone disease, 195

T. K. Dunn BVM&S, MVetSci, MRCVS Department of Clinical Veterinary Medicine, Madingley Road, Cambridge CB3 0ES
Canine hypothyroidism, 232

M. Eysker DVM Department of Infectious Diseases and Immunology, University of Utrecht, Yaklaan 1, Utrecht, The Netherlands
The epidemiology of lungworm infection in cattle, 69

Christine Gibbs BVSc, PhD, MRCVS, DVR Department of Veterinary Medicine, University of Bristol School of Veterinary Science, Langford House, Langford, Bristol BS18 7DU
The radiographic evaluation of pleural and mediastinal disease in the horse (jointly), 136

T. J. Gruffydd-Jones BVetMed, PhD, MRCVS Department of Veterinary Medicine, University of Bristol School of Veterinary Science, Langford House, Langford, Bristol BS18 7DU
Episodic collapse and weakness in cats (jointly), 261

H. J. Guise BSc Cambac, JMA Research Ltd, 1 Castle Street, Wallingford, Oxon OX10 10DL
Boar usage and wastage: results of a twenty-six herd survey and limited literature review (jointly), 115

Edward Hall MA, VetMB, PhD, MRCVS The University of Liverpool, Department of Veterinary Pathology, PO Box 147 Prescot Street, Liverpool L69 3BX
Primary treatment of small intestinal diseases, 226

D. A. Harbour BSc, PhD Department of Veterinary Medicine, University of Bristol School of Veterinary Science, Langford House, Langford, Bristol BS18 7DU
Feline T-lymphotrophic lentivirus infection — a new disease (jointly), 278

F. W. G. Hill BVetMed, PhD, MRCVS, MACVSc Faculty of Veterinary Science, University of Zimbabwe, PO Box 167, Mount Pleasant, Harare, Zimbabwe
Entrapment of the left colon over the nephro-splenic ligament in the horse: a review of the clinical features and treatment (jointly), 161

J. R. Holmes MVSc, PhD, MRCVS Department of Veterinary Medicine, University of Bristol School of Veterinary Science, Langford House, Langford, Bristol BS18 7DU
Circulatory causes of collapse in the horse, 156

C. D. Hopper BSc, BVSc, MRCVS Department of Veterinary Medicine, University of Bristol School of Veterinary Science, Langford House, Langford, Bristol BS18 7DU
Feline T-lymphotropic lentivirus infection - a new disease (jointly), 278

B. O. Hosie BVM&S, MSc, MRCVS St Boswells VI Centre, Greyoak, St Boswells, Roxburgh TO6 0EU
Infectious keratoconjunctivitis in sheep and goats, 93

R. S. Jones MVSc, DrMedVet, FRCVS, DVA, FIBiol Department of Anaesthesia, Royal Liverpool Hospital, Prescot Street, PO Box 147, Liverpool L69 3BX
The use of detomidine as a premedicant and sedative in horses, 175

S. Jones BSc Department of Zoology, University of Bristol, Woodland Road, Bristol BS8 1UG
Precepts for the successful husbandry of lizards and snakes: how best to avoid disease (jointly), 295

F. D. Kirby BVM&S, MSc, MRCVS Veterinary Investigation Centre, Y Buarth, Aberystwyth, Dyfed SY23 1ND
Some changes in infectious diseases of British farm livestock in the last two decades, 29

D. C. Knottenbelt BVM&S, MRCVS Faculty of Veterinary Science, University of Zimbabwe, PO Box 167, Mount Pleasant, Harare, Zimbabwe
Entrapment of the left colon over the nephro-splenic ligament in the horse: a review of the clinical features and treatment (jointly), 161

C. R. Lamb MA, VetMB, MRCVS Tufts University School of Veterinary Medicine, 200 Westboro Road, North Grafton, MA 01536, USA
Aspects of diagnostic imaging in equine pulmonary disease, 127

J. G. Lane BVetMed, FRCVS Department of Veterinary Surgery, University of Bristol School of Veterinary Science, Langford House, Langford, Bristol BS18 7DU
Endoscopy of the equine upper respiratory tract - achievements and challenges, 147

P. Lievesley BVMS, MRCVS Department of Veterinary Medicine, University of Bristol School of Veterinary Science, Langford House, Langford, Bristol BS18 7DU
Episodic collapse and weakness in cats (jointly), 261

K. A. Linklater BVMS, PhD, FRCVS Veterinary Investigation Service, Oakbank Road, Penrith PH1 1HP
Watery mouth in lambs, 88

C. J. L. Little BVMS, MRCVS Department of Veterinary Surgery, University of Glasgow, Bearsden Road, Bearsden, Glasgow G61 1QH
Otitis media in the dog: a review, 183

P. J. Llewellyn Department of Biological Sciences, University of Swansea, Singleton Park, Swansea SA2 8PP
Precepts for the successful husbandry of lizards and snakes: how best to avoid disease (jointly), 294

J. Adrian Longstaffe BVetMed, PhD, MRCVS Department of Comparative Pathology, University of Bristol School of Veterinary Science, Langford House, Langford, Bristol BS18 7DU
Pruritus, pyrexia and haemorrhage syndrome in cattle, 64

E. Gregory MacEwen VMD School of Veterinary Medicine, University of Wisconsin – Madison, WI 53706 USA
Therapy prognosis for canine multiple myeloma, 178

T. S. Mair BVSc, PhD, MRCVS Department of Veterinary Surgery, University of1Bristol School of Veterinary Science, Langford House, Langford, Bristol BS18 7DU
The radiographic evaluation of pleural and mediastinal disease in the horse (jointly), 136

Christopher May MA, VetMB, MRCVS Small Animal Hospital, University of Liverpool, Crown Street, Liverpool L7 7EX
Osteochondrosis in the dog: a review, 207

A. R. Michell BSc, BVetMed, PhD, MRCVS Department of Veterinary Medicine, Royal Veterinary College, Hawkshead House, Hawkshead Lane, North Mymms, Hatfield, Herts AL9 7TA
Shock in companion animals, 48

E. M. Milne BVM&D, PhD, MRCVS Department of Veterinary Medicine, Veterinary Field Station, Easter Bush, N. Roslin, Midlothian
Insulinoma in the dog, 251

P.Msolla Department of Veterinary Medicine and Public Health, Sokoine University of Agriculture, PO Box 3021, Morogoro, Tanzania
Bovine parasitic otitis: an up-to-date review, 73

M. R. Muirhead BVM&S, FRCVS, DPM, Willowgarth, Beeford, Driffield YO25 8AY
Factors affecting efficient growth rate in the feeding pig, 103

G. O. Odiawo BVetMed, MSc Faculty of Veterinary Sciences, University of Zimbabwe, PO Box 167, Mount Pleasant, Harare, Zimbabwe
Mucormycosis infection in cattle, 78

Phillippa Paton BVM&S, MRCVS 10/12 Effick Road, Edinburgh, Midlothian EH10 5BJ
Ethylene glycol poisoning in small animals, 189

R. H. C. Penny DVSc, PhD, FRCVS, DPM Nether End, Austrey, Nr Atherstone, Warwickshire CV9 3EJ
Boar usage and wastage: results of a twenty-six herd survey and limited literature review (jointly), 115

B. D. Perry BVM&S, MSc, DTVM, MRCVS International Laboratory for Research on Animal Diseases, P.O. Box 30709, Nairobi, Kenya
The oral immunization of animals against rabies, 37

P. J. N. Pinsent BVSc, FRCVS Saxon Place, Langford, Bristol
Grass sickness of horses (grass disease: equine dysautonomia), 169

Mary-Elizabeth Raw BVSc, FRCVS, DVR 40 Milton Green, Weston-super-Mare, BS22 8EP
Episodic weakness, 255

D. H. Roberts BVMS, DVM, MTech, MRCPath, Dip.Bact., MRCVS Virology Department, Central Veterinary Laboratory, Weybridge, Surrey KT15 3HB
Pigs and influenza, 110

Polly M. Taylor MA, VetMB, PhD, MRCVS, DVA Animal Health Trust, Newmarket, Suffolk CB8 7DW
Intensive care of small animals, 241

A. H. M. van den Broek BVSC, FRCVS, DVR Edinburgh University Field Station, Easter Bush, Nr Roslin, Midlothian
Cutaneous hypersensitivity (allergy) in dogs, 245

W. Vennart BSc, PhD, CPhys Physics Department, University of Exeter, Devon.
The application of radioisotope scanning and imaging in general veterinary practice (jointly), 15

A. J. F. Webster MA, VetMB, PhD, MRCVS Department of Animal Husbandry, University of Bristol School of Veterinary Science, Langford House, Langford, Bristol BS18 7DU
Animal housing as perceived by the animal, 1

G. A. H. Wells BVetMed, MRCVS Central Veterinary Laboratory, New Haw, Weybridge, Surrey KT15 3HB
Bovine spongiform encephalopathy, 59

Simon J. Wheeler BVSc, PhD, MRCVS, CertVR Department of Companion Animal and Special Species, College of Veterinary Medicine, North Carolina State University, 4700 Hillsborough Street, Raleigh, North Carolina 27606, USA
Spinal tumours in cats, 270

D. Whittaker BVM&S, MRCVS, Cert LAS ICI Pharmaceutical Division, Mereside, Alderley Park, Macclesfield, Cheshire SK10 4TG
Pasteurellosis in the laboratory rabbit - a review, 285

Susan Yeo BVetMed, PhD, MRCVS Department of Veterinary Medicine, University of Bristol School of Veterinary Science, Langford House, Langford, Bristol BS18 7DU
Bovine neonatology, 83

A. J. F. WEBSTER

Animal housing as perceived by the animal

INTRODUCTION

THE DESIGN and management of animal housing inevitably involves compromise between the needs of the animals and those of their owners. Until recently, trends in livestock housing, particularly in intensive units, have been governed almost entirely by the requirements of the owner for low cost and efficiency of operation and it has been tacitly assumed that optimal production efficiency and optimal welfare are synonymous. This assumption is increasingly being called to question by those whose concern is primarily for animal welfare. Unfortunately, the protagonists on opposing sides in this debate tend to speak a different language. Producers argue from statistics for growth rate and mortality whereas the welfare protagonists offer concepts such as stress and freedom. Clearly neither language is, by itself, adequate to describe the impact of the housing environment on the animal, nor what we should do about it.

Several years ago I proposed that any animal in the care of man should ideally be permitted a basic five freedoms (Webster, 1984). These are:
1. Freedom from malnutrition.
2. Freedom from thermal and physical discomfort.
3. Freedom from injury and disease.
4. Freedom to express most normal patterns of behaviour.
5. Freedom from fear and stress.

The expression 'Five freedoms', as applied to animals, was originally coined by the Brambell Committee (1965) but their definition, in my opinion, was an inadequate description of adequate welfare because it related only to behaviour (standing up, lying down, turning round, grooming and stretching limbs). My broader concept of the five freedoms is intended as more than a series of pious hopes. It is a logical matrix by which alternative systems of housing and husbandry may be assessed. Points 2 and 5 are all highly influenced by housing design. Table 1 illustrates, for example, how the matrix can be used to compare housing systems for dry sows.

Each item merits more explanation than appears in the table. However, the use of all five freedoms to assess a particular husbandry system avoids the trap of thinking that livestock systems can be assessed in terms of productivity alone (which may be the view of some producers), or in terms of behaviour alone (which may be the view of some consumers). It also reveals that it is extremely difficult to devise an ideal system. The concept presents a set of unchanging standards to evaluate the

Table 1 EVALUATION OF ALTERNATIVE ACCOMMODATION FOR DRY SOWS

	Paddocks and arks	Individual stalls (no bedding)	Covered straw yards
Thermal comfort	very variable	fair to poor	good
Physical comfort	variable	bad	good
Injury	slight	feet, 'bed sores'	fighting
Hygiene	fair to poor	usually good	fair to poor
Disease	some parasitism; control difficult	usually good	parasitism control easy
Abnormal behaviour	slight	severe	slight

consequences of continual change in livestock genetics, nutrition and housing. It also encourages changes in the consumer's perception of the way in which they wish their food to be produced.

HOUSING TO MEET THE FIVE FREEDOMS

BEDDING

The surface upon which an animal lies is potentially a source of thermal and physical discomfort, injury and infectious disease. The ideal bed needs therefore to be hygienic, dry, resilient and reasonably warm. The relative importance of these four criteria differs markedly for the different species and classes of farm animals. The chicken is very light and can sleep while holding on to a perch so does not need a bed on which to rest. Her motivation to lay eggs in a nest is a separate issue which will be considered later. Wire floors are hygienic, thermally comfortable and probably less likely to injure the skin of the legs than poorly maintained litter. However, the feet of laying hens kept permanently on wire floors do become distorted and this can be prevented at little cost by proving sufficient perching space for each bird (Moss, 1980).

Deep, clean, dry straw provides an ideal bed for weaner and grower pigs, because it is warm, dry, hygienic, resilient and a constant source of interest. However, an inadequate bed of wet, filthy straw fails on all accounts. Perforated or slatted floors for young pigs are not ideal but almost certain to be drier, warmer and more hygienic than solid floors with minimal bedding.

The requirements of the dry, pregnant sow are different. She is heavy and her food intake is severely restricted. When lying on concrete she is prone to excessive heat loss, foot lameness and severe skin abrasions, hunger and boredom. Moreover, abnormal 'dog-sitting' can predispose to acute nephritis. A resilient, insulated, sow-proof mat in a sow stall will improve thermal and physical comfort but not affect hunger or boredom or reduce the incidence of lameness associated with prolonged, extreme inactivity. One promising solution to this problem is to house sows in straw yards with access to a computer-controlled feeding station where they can obtain their proper ration when they want and without interference from other pigs.

For growing beef cattle the two main problems are their large size and the risk of pneumonia. Slatted floors for beef cattle are not ideal but cause relatively few foot and leg problems. However, a high stocking density is essential in order to keep the slats clean and dry and this can greatly increase the risk of pneumonia in young animals.

The modern Holstein-type dairy cow is an extremely heavy ($\approx$ 700 kg), large-jointed, raw-boned, awkward animal with a large, pendulous udder. For her, the three most important criteria for a satisfactory bed are that it should be resilient, hygienic and non-slip. These can be achieved in a cubicle or free stall by, for example, a suitable rubber mat or perhaps a little dry bedding such as chopped straw or a sufficient depth of clean sand. Any bedding that becomes contaminated with slurry, usually carried into the stall on the cow's feet, increase the risk of environmental mastitis.

HYGIENE AND DISEASE

The close confinement of large numbers of animals in an enclosed space, whatever its advantages, undoubtedly increases the risk of infectious disease. Infection is transmitted by contagion (e.g. animal to animal via excreta or the stockman) or by the airborne route. Spread by contagion can usually be controlled reasonably effectively by isolation, floors that minimize build-up of excreta and disinfection of all surfaces between batches of animals.

The control of air hygiene is inherently more difficult. It is important to distinguish between effects of environmental design on

1. The spread of primary pathogens.
2. The spread of airborne pollutants which, although not themselves primary pathogens, may compromise the defence mechanisms of the respiratory tract.

It is often assumed that respiratory pathogens of housed farm animals are primarily transmitted through the air and the enteropathogens are transmitted by contagion. This generalization is untenable because the survival time of many respiratory pathogens in air is much shorter than that of the main enteropathogens (Donaldson, 1978). Furthermore, Wathes (1988) has recently demonstrated airborne infection of pigs and calves with *E. coli* and *Salmonella typhimurium*, respectively.

In pig and poultry units the primary pathogens responsible for the major respiratory diseases can be controlled by eradication or vaccination. In these circumstances animals can exist in seriously polluted environments without succumbing to respiratory infections. The structure of the calf industry is such that the eradication of primary respiratory pathogens is impossible. Moreover, vaccination has only been partially successful. Control of respiratory disease in calves must therefore seek to minimize the concentration of pollutants which may compromise the defences of the respiratory tract.

The concentration (C_b in n cm^{-3}) of particles, or any pollutant, in the air of a livestock building is determined by its rate of release (R, n in cm^3 h^{-1}), entry from incoming air (C_i, q_v) and clearance (q in h^{-1}) by pathways such as ventilation (q_v), death *in situ* etc. (q_d). At equilibrium

$$C_b = 1/q \;\; (R + C_i \, q_v)$$

Most bacteria and viruses arise from the animals themselves. Other major elements of respirable dust, such as fungal spores, and most gaseous pollutants arise primarily from feed, bedding or excreta. Spores, inert respirable particles less than 5 μm in aerodynamic diameter, and gaseous pollutants are primarily cleared by ventilation. Figure 1 illustrates effects of varying R and q_v on the concentration of respirable particles (mainly fungal spores) in an equine stable. Ventilation improves the 'cleanness' of the air in linear fashion. The 'dirtiness' of the air (C_b) is proportional to $1/q_v$ so increases very rapidly as q_v declines below 4 h^{-1}.

Chronic pulmonary disease in horses is a response to allergic substances in fungal spores, whether dead or alive. It should be apparent from Figure 1 that control is achieved more effectively by minimizing release from bedding or, especially, mouldy fodder than by increasing ventilation, once a minimal acceptable standard of 4 air changes h^{-1} has been achieved.

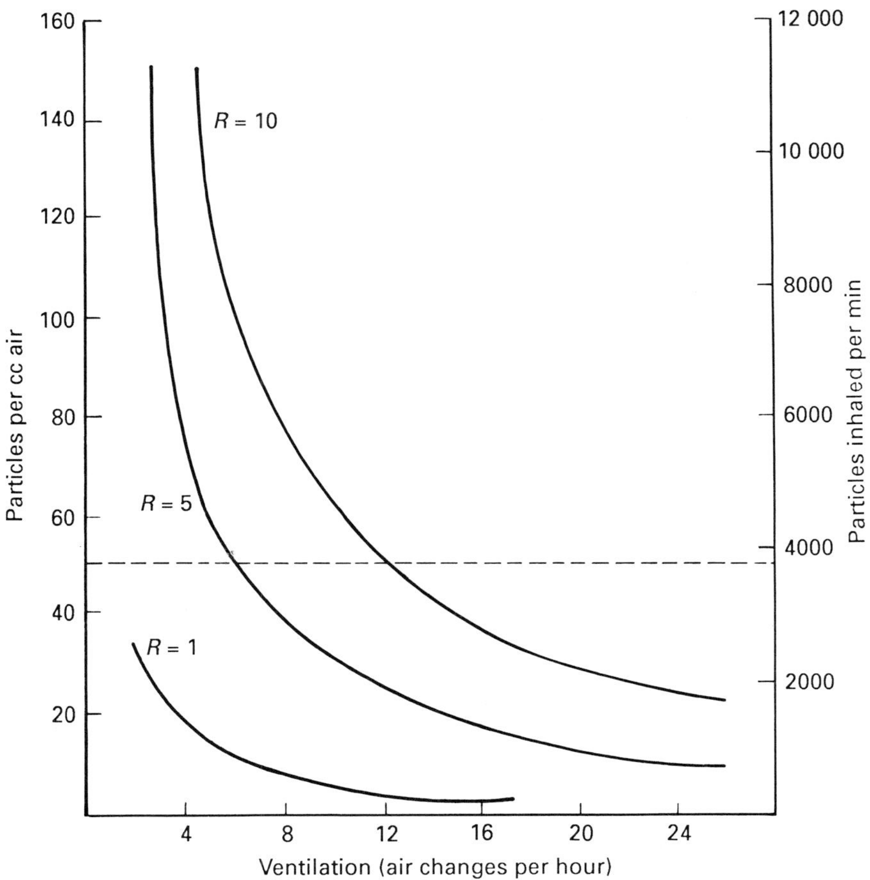

Fig. 1. Effect of release rates (air numbers/cc air min^{-1}) and ventilation rates (air changes h^{-1}) on the concentration of particles in stable air and inhaled by horses. The dotted line may be taken as the 'danger' threshold. (Figure from Webster *et al.*, 1987).

The role of ventilation in the control of infectious respiratory disease is less straightforward. Most viruses and bacteria recognized as primary pathogens of the respiratory tract die within a few seconds of exposure to air (Donaldson, 1978). Where q_d greatly exceeds q_v ventilation has relatively little direct effect on C_b. Thus:

1. The overwhelming majority of organisms recovered from the air are not primary pathogens.
2. The usual source of primary pathogens is infected animals and their survival time following release is usually very brief.

It follows that the challenge from primary pathogens increases in direct proportion to stocking density but is relatively unaffected by ventilation rate (Figure 2). The main effect of ventilation on air hygiene is to clear fungal spores, noxious gases and other pollutants which may compromise the defence mechanisms of the respiratory tract.

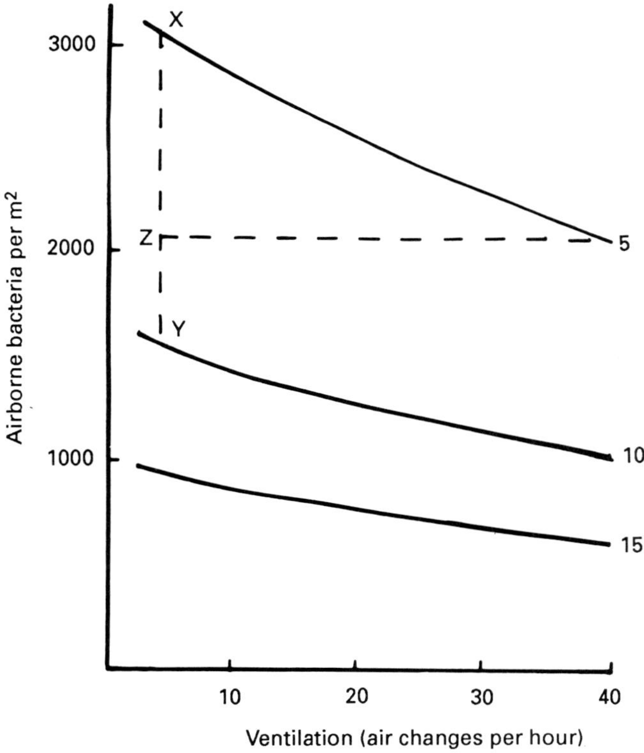

Fig. 2. Effects of space allowance (m³ per calf) and ventilation rate (air changes h⁻¹) on the concentration of airborne bacteria in a calf house when q_d accounts for 90% of total clearance. The intervals XY and XZ indicate effects of increasing space allowance from 5 to 10 m³ per calf (XY) and increasing ventilation rate from 4 to 40 air changes h⁻¹ (XZ), respectively. (Figure from Webster 1984).

Effects of environmental stresses such as heat, cold and exercise on the systemic immune responses of farm animals are complex and hard to incorporate into a model for the pathogenesis of multifactorial infectious disease (Kelley, 1982). However, most experiments that have succeeded in altering the immune response have involved thermal or other environmental stresses of a severity that is unlikely to be encountered by housed animals. It is reasonable to assume that the immune mechanisms of the respiratory tract of housed animals are less likely to be compromised by thermal stresses than by inhaled pollutants (Curtis, 1983). Ian Gilmour (1988) recently exposed mice for 2 and 4 weeks to 2 and 20 mg m^{-3} of an inert dust, titanium dioxide, then exposed them to a standard aerosol challenge with *Pasteurella haemolytica*. There was a clear dose and time effect of dust burden on the ability of *P.haemolytica* to multiply in the lung, on the immune response in local lymphocytes and on the capacity of the mice to manufacture systemic antibody. This elegant study reinforces the conclusion that the main reason why respirable dust and other pollutants in animal houses increase the incidence and severity of diseases such as calf pneumonia or *Haemophilus* pneumonia in pigs is not through any effect on the primary pathogen but by compromising the mechanical and immunological defence mechanisms of the animal to the point where it cannot clear a primary challenge that would be insufficient to cause clinical disease in otherwise fresh air. Whereas ventilation may have little effect on the magnitude of the challenge from primary pathogens, it can do much to maintain the capacity of the animal to resist that challenge.

BEHAVIOURAL FREEDOM

The question of behavioural freedom for farm animals is one which generates the greatest conflict between the producer and the welfare lobby. This conflict characteristically generates more heat than light because both parties hold strong opinions but neither can fully understand the problem. Logically, the best approach to the question 'What are an animal's needs?' is to ask the animal itself. Marian Dawkins (1980) has developed a scientific approach to the evaluation of a chicken's perception of its own needs by applying the basic economic laws of the market. A commodity such as coffee is price inelastic for man, i.e. consumption remains almost constant when the price increases. It is, for us, a high-priority 'need'. Conversely, apples are price elastic. We buy them if they are cheap; they are a relative luxury. Experimental environments can be set up in which farm animals can 'purchase' desirable features of their environment *at a price*. For example, the laying hen may be offered a nest box and a dust bath. The price of each is then increased by increasing the work she has to do to reach them. Evidence to date suggests that a nest box is price inelastic, i.e. a 'need'; dust baths are price elastic, i.e. a luxury. Well designed research of this sort reveals the motivation of different farm animals to seek, and avoid, various features in their environment and will generate an objective list of priorities for constructively enhancing the environment of farm animals. The extent to which the environment of any farm animal may be enhanced will depend, of course, on what is economic and on consumer pressure to achieve change by legislation. It is the responsibility of scientists and veterinary surgeons to respond to, or anticipate, consumer pressure with sound, objective advice.

We are more likely to generate this objective advice through experiments designed to test animals' perception of their environment than through field studies of alternative husbandry systems based on our own preconceptions of what looks right. It is important that we continue to test novel, apparently more humane alternatives to conventional intensive husbandry systems mainly to ensure that they do not compromise health and efficiency of production.

FEAR AND STRESS

The engineered environment of the intensively housed farm animal may be criticized on several grounds relating to behaviour but it probably provokes less fear and stress than that experienced by animals on free range. Aggressive encounters between animals can be a severe problem in intensive units but are usually controllable. However, if the control involves isolation and extreme confinement (e.g., tethering sows in individual stalls) then the stress imposed by the cure *may* be more severe than the original problem. Stereotyped patterns of behaviour such as 'weaving' in horses and bar-chewing in sows can confidently be attributed to boredom, probably linked to frustration. However, they cannot be offered as evidence for stress because they may be 'coping' behaviours which allow the animal to adapt to a barren environment. It would, subjectively, be better to devise housing that did not generate stereotyped behaviour but we cannot yet decide *how* important this may be relative to, say, the provision of thermal comfort and good hygiene until we can determine by research whether the individual that performs the most stereotyped behaviour in a barren environment is the one most consumed by frustration or the one who has best come to terms with life and developed a satisfactory, if apparently futile, hobby.

CONCLUSIONS

The concept of the five freedoms offers a rational basis for the evaluation of animal housing as perceived by the animal. Each ideal is difficult to attain and tends to conflict with the others. Nevertheless, it may allow farmers and veterinary surgeons to define acceptable housing standards for animals in a way that is not determined solely by the economics of production or by changing, subjective consumer perception of what constitutes animal welfare. There is, however, a central principle that we must accept, namely that the welfare of farm animals cannot be entrusted to the workings of the free market. A set of rules to impose minimal standards of animal welfare, enforced and properly policed within the European Community, would protect not only the animals but also those owners and veterinary surgeons who wish to see their animals treated within the reasonable bounds of humanity, but not bankrupt themselves in the process.

REFERENCES

Brambell, F. W. R. (1965) *Report of the technical committee to enquire into the welfare of animals kept under intensive livestock husbandry systems,* Cmd 2836, HMSO, London

Curtis, S. E. (1983) *Environmental management in animal agriculture*   Iowa State University Press, Iowa, USA

Dawkins, M. (1980) *Animal suffering; the science of animal welfare*   Chapman & Hall, London

Donaldson, A. I. (1978) Factors influencing the dispersal, survival and deposition of airborne pathogens of farm animals *Vet. Bull. 48,* 83–94

Gilmour, M. I. (1988) *Airborne pollutants and respiratory disease in animal houses* Unpublished PhD thesis, University of Bristol, Bristol, UK

Kelley, K. W. (1982) Immunobiology of domestic animals as affected by hot and cold weather. In *Proc. 2nd Int. Livestock Envt. Symp.,* (Ames, Iowa, USA) pp. 470-482

Moss, R. (1980) *The laying hen and its environment* Martinus Nijhoff, Dordrecht

Wathes, C. M. (1988) Airborne transmission of enteric pathogens in farm livestock. In *Proc. 3rd Int. Congress of Animal Hygiene,* (Skara, Sweden) (ed. I.Ekesbo) p. 421

Webster, A. J. F. (1984) *Calf Husbandry, Health and Welfare* Collins, London

Webster, A. J. F., Clarke, A. F., Madelin, T. M. and Wathes, C. M. (1987) Air hygiene in stables. 1. Effects of stable design, ventilation and management on the concentration of respirable dust. *Equine Vet. J.* **19**, 448–453

D. M. BROOM

Animal welfare

THE WELFARE CONCEPT

ANIMALS FREQUENTLY encounter factors which make their lives difficult. They have an array of systems within their bodies which help them to cope with these factors. When there are fluctuations in their environment individuals must respond to change, or predict change, in such a way that the body state is regulated. The term environment refers to anything which can affect the animal. Problems arise if control is not adequate and the state is not kept within the tolerable range. Possible consequences are discomfort, pain, or psychological disturbance. One important category of environmental effects on an animal includes those caused by pathogens or parasites where the immune system plays a major part in the body's responses. Examples of other systems involved in the coping process, each of which has physiological and behavioural components, are the thermoregulatory system, the nutritional system and systems for the avoidance of predation. Given our ability to measure aspects of the functioning of such systems, a definition of welfare is possible. The welfare of an individual is its state with regard to its attempts to cope with its environment (Broom, 1986b).

Individual animals cope with some environmental effects easily with little expenditure of energy. They cope with other environmental effects with difficulty, and fail to cope with others in that they die or are unable to grow or reproduce. Hence, welfare varies on a continuum from good to poor. Both failure to cope and degree of difficulty in coping can be evaluated scientifically so welfare can be measured. Welfare, however good or poor, is a characteristic of the animal and does not refer to any human care for that animal. Its measurement is independent of any moral considerations. The moral decision which must be taken after the measurement is made concerns how poor welfare must be before it is considered unacceptable. Views on where to draw the line between the acceptable and the unacceptable will differ from one person to another. The scientist provides the evidence about welfare but each person adopts a moral position on the basis of that evidence. Laws should be based upon the consensus of opinion about what is unacceptable. There are considerable national differences in attitudes to animal welfare.

WELFARE PROBLEMS

In animals which interact with man, poor welfare can result from disease, adverse housing conditions, operations or other procedures, deliberate ill-treatment or neglect. Examples of some problems are listed briefly below but it is clearly unnecessary to catalogue diseases which have adverse effects on welfare. Some pathogens and parasites have little effect on welfare, in that the animal copes very easily, but the welfare of most diseased animals is poor and disease reduction is a most important part of welfare improvement (Gibson, 1988).

In numerical terms, by far the largest category of animals which are used by man is that of farmed animals. Recent research emphasizes the complexity and sophistication of the behaviour of these animals (Broom, 1981). Modern farming methods result in high stocking densities in systems which can be run with minimal labour input. Housing conditions where welfare can be poor include crates for calves; stalls, tethers and farrowing crates for sows; high density accommodation for early weaned piglets; battery cages for hens and conditions for pigs or poultry which lead to high levels of aggression. Extensive systems in which animals may die of hunger or thirst, be exposed to extremes of temperature, or be subject to predation or other harrassment are clearly causing welfare problems, as indeed are all other situations where animals are neglected. Another kind of farming operation which is known to result in some behavioural abnormalities and hence welfare problems, is the farming of mink, silver foxes and other fur-bearing animals.

All systems which make inspection of individuals difficult or which have inadequate provision for emergencies such as fire or power failure may lead to poor welfare. The handling and transport of farm animals poses serious welfare problems. Conditions at markets and procedures before and during slaughter are also a major cause for concern. In particular, the practice of marketing young animals, such as calves, is undesirable and the cutting of the throat of an animal without adequate prior stunning presumably causes great pain. Operations on farm animals without anaesthetic, for example mulesing, beak-trimming, hot-iron branding, tail-docking, castration, disbudding, dehorning, and ear-punching must also cause pain which may continue over a long period.

Pet animals usually have much human contact. This can include ill-treatment or misguided care, as well as neglect. Some dogs and cats are given inadequate home bases, have insufficient exercise, or are managed in a way which results in poor socialization with their own species or with man. Such deficiencies may result in behaviour problems. Other obvious welfare problems result from failure to treat disease or causing the animal to take part in fights. Some operations on pet animals, like castration or spaying, although ideally avoided, are socially desirable and need not cause pain. Other operations, however, are merely mutilations carried out for cosmetic purposes. These include tail-docking or removal of areas of skin. These procedures may cause much discomfort to the animal and, in the case of tail-docking, deprive it of an important social signalling organ. Many of these welfare problems have not been investigated adequately so their severity is not known. The same must be said for the effects of housing conditions on pets such as rabbits, guinea pigs and budgerigars, whose conditions are often much worse than those of animals in zoos, on farms or in laboratories. The housing of horses needs further investigation as long-term individual stabling can result in high levels of stereotyped behaviour such as crib-biting. Guard dogs are also sometimes ill-treated and kept chained or closely confined for long periods.

The welfare of animals kept in laboratories depends, in part, upon their housing conditions. Because most of their lives are spent in cages, these conditions are especially important. Rodents and primates are sometimes kept in small uninteresting cages. The conditions are generally much better if the animals are kept in social groups rather than in isolation. Environmental variety is desirable. The effects of laboratory procedures on the welfare of animals are sometimes clearly adverse in that there is no doubt that pain and other discomfort are caused.

In the best zoos, animals are well cared for and the conditions for some animals are good. There are many zoos, however, where welfare is poor. For some species such as bears, some small carnivores and a range of other species, behavioural abnormalities are common. For many species the conditions in the average zoo are such that breeding is not successful and life expectancy is short. It is possible to provide better conditions for many zoo animals but for some species, it may be that good welfare is not possible within a zoo. In circuses the confinement of animals in very small cages for long periods and some training procedures must lead to poor welfare. Harsh training procedures may also be a problem for horses used in show jumping and for pet animals which are exhibited at shows. Other exhibitions which result in animal suffering include rodeos and especially bull-fighting.

The welfare of wild animals which are hunted or trapped may also be adversely affected by man. There is no doubt that great suffering is caused by the trapping of animals in leg-hold traps whether for fur, food or by accident. Animals which are shot may carry shot for a long period and die slowly. Animals which are chased using hounds, like foxes or deer, must be very frightened during the hunt and often suffer when they are killed. Pest animals also can suffer. Therefore any killing should be humane.

A general moral point about all kinds of animals with which man interacts is that we should consider the situation from the point of view of the animal. If a rabbit is suffering, it should not matter whether it is regarded by man as a pet, a subject for laboratory work, a source of food or an object of sport and entertainment.

ASSESSING SHORT-TERM WELFARE PROBLEMS

When animals are handled, transported, exposed to a predator or subjected to some operation they show a range of behavioural and physiological changes which have the general effect of helping them to survive the treatment. Measurements of these are indicators of welfare (Broom, 1986b. 1988). Physiological responses to difficult conditions include problems of orientation, variations in regulatory responses and suppression of function including that of the gut, and suppression of preparations for flight or defence. Changes which can be measured include those in heart rate, ventilation rate, adrenal functioning and brain chemistry. Work by Duncan and Filshie (1979) showed that some strains of hens showed a prolonged heart rate response to the close approach of a person but others showed a strong behavioural response. This observation emphasizes that several measurements must be made when assessing welfare. Transport also increases adrenal cortex activity, as seen in the studies of Freeman *et al.* (1984) on chickens and Kent and Ewbank (1983) on calves. This measurement, like heart-rate, provides information about what the animal must do to cope with being transported. When animals are handled and transported their muscle metabolism is altered, so measurements of meat quality and skin blemishes after slaughter provide information about welfare during the pre-slaughter period (Hails, 1978).

Pain results in poor welfare but the assessment of pain in animals is very difficult. Although the basic nociceptive system is similar in different animals there is considerable variation in the extent of behavioural manifestation of pain. As Morton and Griffiths (1985) point out in their review of methods of assessing pain, pain is not obvious in some animals but where extrapolation from other species suggests that pain is likely to be experienced, we should assume that the animal is in pain and act accordingly. Experimental studies of pain include recording from nociceptive nerves and identifying neuromas after beak-trimming in poultry (Gentle, 1986), measuring how long the tail of a rat or pig can be heated before the animal flicks it away (Dantzer *el al.*, 1986) or measuring sound production and duration of abnormal behaviour after castration in piglets (Wemelsfelder and van Putten, 1985).

ASSESSING LONG-TERM WELFARE PROBLEMS

When difficult conditions are encountered for long periods the same responses as those described for short-term problems occur at first. They may cease to occur after some time and be replaced by others. Hence, different measurements are used to measure the effects of long term problems. Methods such as ACTH challenge can give useful information about adrenal enzyme activity and hence previous frequency of adrenal activity (Friend *et al.*, 1977). Frequent adrenal activity may also suppress immune system activity, so poor welfare may be detectable by measurements of immune system function or the effects of disease challenge (Kelley *et al.*, 1982; Siegel, 1987).

There are many behavioural measures which allow some assessment of poor welfare (Wiepkema *et al.*, 1983). A behaviour may be solely a sign of abnormality in the individual showing it. It may also cause injury to other animals. An example of a housing system which leads to abnormal behaviour is the confinement of dry sows in stalls or tethers. Such sows may be inactive and unresponsive (Broom, 1986a) or may show high levels of stereotyped behaviour (Cronin and Wiepkema, 1984). Both responsiveness and duration of stereotyped behaviour can be quantified. These behaviours may be associated with release of analgesic opiate peptides in the brain which allow animals to cope with difficult conditions by self-narcotization. There are many other behavioural indicators of poor welfare, for example abnormalities of lying behaviour on slippery floors (Andreae and Smidt, 1982), misdirected sucking in early weaned mammals, disturbed social behaviour after early isolation (Broom, 1982), misdirected pecking at feathers in hens or biting at tails in pigs, and aggressive behaviour which affects the welfare of those individuals which cannot get away.

Other important welfare indicators which are useful when comparing management systems are measurements of mortality rate, growth rate, production of eggs or milk, and production of offspring. Because we know that animals may survive, grow and reproduce in conditions which they find difficult and, hence, where their welfare is poor, these measurements cannot be used as certain indicators of good welfare. However, we can say that if conditions are such that animals are unable to survive, grow or reproduce given adequate opportunity, then their welfare is poor. It is clear that individuals vary in the methods which they use to cope with adversity, so any single indicator can demonstrate poor welfare.

RECOGNIZING GOOD WELFARE

Our ability to make direct measurements which identify pleasure is extremely limited, but if animals organize their lives efficiently then their preferences should tell us something about what they regarded as an improvement in their welfare. Studies of feral farm animals or pets give some information about how they choose to allocate their time and provide ideas for the design of management systems for such animals. For example, work on pigs in a park environment allowed the design of the family pen system and of other improved pig housing (Stolba, 1982). Experimental preference tests, provided that they show the importance of that preference to the animal, can also be used to change conditions or management in such a way that welfare is improved. Such tests have included preferences for foods in companion and farm animals, (Kilgour and Dalton 1984), flooring (Hughes and Black 1973), material to explore (Wood-Gush and Beilharz, 1983), space (Dawkins 1977) or social companions.

VETERINARY RESPONSIBILITY FOR ANIMAL WELFARE

The treatment of disease usually improves animal welfare, so much veterinary work benefits animals. The veterinary profession is generally regarded by the general public as being sympathetic to the interests of animals. Some veterinary activity, however, benefits owners of pets and farm animals but has adverse effects on the animals. Veterinary inactivity can adversely effect animals in that they remain untreated when they need treatment or remain ill-treated when their conditions should be improved.

Each British veterinary surgeon takes an oath on admission to the Royal College of Veterinary Surgeons which includes the sentence 'That my constant endeavour will be to ensure the welfare of animals committed to my care'. If 'committed to my care' is interpreted in a broad way then the veterinary surgeon should act in the interest of the animals which he or she encounters. Veterinary surgeons need to live up to the trust which society has in them, to acquaint themselves with modern studies on animal welfare, and to combat poor welfare of all kinds whenever they can do so.

REFERENCES

Andreae, U. and Smidt, D. (1982) *Hohenheimer Arbeiten,* **121**, 51–60
Broom, D. M. (1981) *Biology of Behaviour,* Cambridge University Press, Cambridge
Broom, D. M. (1982) *Hohenheimer Arbeiten,* **121**, 42–50
Broom, D. M. (1986a) *Anim. Prod.* **42**, 438–439
Broom, D. M. (1986b) *Br. Vet. J.,* **142**, 524–526
Broom, D. M. (1988) *Appl. Anim. Behav. Sci.,* **20**, (in press)
Cronin, G. M. and Wiepkema, P. R. (1984) *Ann. Rech. Vét.,* **15**, 263–270
Dantzer, R., Bluthé, R-M., and Tazi A. (1986) *Ann. Rech. Vét.,* **17**, 147–151
Dawkins, M. (1977) *Anim. Behav.,* **25**, 1034–1046
Duncan, I. J. H., and Filshie, J.H. (1979) In *A Handbook on Biotelemetry and Radio Tracking* (ed. C. H. Amlaner and D. W. MacDonald) pp. 579–588
Freeman, B. M., Kettlewell, P. J., Manning, A. C. C. and Berry, P. S. (1984) *Vet Rec.,* **114**, 286–287
Friend, T. H., Polan, C. E., Gwazdauskas, F. C., and Heald, C. W. (1977) *J. Dairy Sci.,* **60**, 1958–1963
Gentle, M. J. (1986) *Res. Vet. Sci.,* **43**, 383–385
Gibson, T. E. (ed.) (1988) *Animal Disease – a Welfare Problem?* London, B.V.A. Animal Welfare Foundation, London

Hails, M. R. (1978) *Anim. Regul. Stud.,* **1,** 289–343
Hughes, B. O. and Black, A. J. (1973) *Br. Poult. Sci.,* **14,** 615-619
Kelly, K. W., Greenfield, R. E. Evermann, J. F., Parish, S. M. and Perryman, L. E. (1982) *Amer. J. Vet. Res.,* **43,** 775–779
Kent, J. E. and Ewbank, R. (1983) *Br. Vet. J.,* **139,** 228–235
Kilgour, R. and Dalton, C. (1984) *Livestock Behaviour : a Practical Guide* Granada, London
Morton, D. B. and Griffiths, P. H. M. (1985) *Vet. Rec.,* **116,** 431–436
Siegel, H. S. (1987) *Curr. Top. Vet. Med. Anim. Sci.,* **42,** 39–54
Stolba, A. (1982) *Proc. Symp. Alternatives to Intensive Husbandry Systems* Universities Federation for Animal Welfare, Potters Bar
Wemelsfelder, F. and van Putten, G. (1985) *Behaviour as a Possible Indicator for Pain in Piglets,* Instituut voor Veetelkundig Onderzoek 'Schoonoord' Zeist, 61 pp
Wiepkema, P. R., Broom, D. M., Duncan, I. J. H. and van Putten, G. (1983) *Abnormal Behaviours in Farm Animals* Commission of the European Communities Report, Brussels 16 pp
Wood-Gush, D. G. M. and Beilharz, R. G. (1983) *Appl. Anim. Ethol.* **10,** 209–217

D. P. ATTENBURROW and W. VENNART

The application of radioisotope scanning and imaging in general veterinary practice

INTRODUCTION

THERE ARE a number of techniques in common use in human medicine that have been developed to image organs of the body to demonstrate pathological and physiological processes. Such techniques include X-radiography, X-ray computer tomography and ultrasound, radioisotope and nuclear magnetic resonance imaging.

X-radiography, X-ray computer tomography and ultrasound imaging demonstrate structural change in whole organ function. The main and most useful application of radioisotope imaging is the detection, localization and quantitative assessment of dynamic tissue change or turnover although it is used to a limited extent to monitor whole organ function (e.g. heart blood flow). Radioisotope imaging, therefore, is useful not only as an adjunct to X-radiography to indicate the degree of activity of established anatomical change, but perhaps more importantly, to predict the initiation of structural abnormalities resulting from continuing pathological activity.

X-radiography and ultrasound imaging are well established and widely used in veterinary practice. The use of radioisotope imaging in the horse and other animals has been investigated during the last decade (Tofe *el al.*, 1974; Metcalf, 1985; Ueltschi, 1977; Devous and Twardock, 1984) in academic institutions in several countries. There is, however, no indication in the literature before 1984 (Attenburrow *et al.*, 1984) that this technique has been used in both large and small animals attended in general practice. This is no doubt due, until recently, to the difficulties in obtaining a satisfactory supply of radioisotopes and the relatively high cost of scanning equipment. The development of radiopharmaceuticals and scanning equipment in human medicine have progressed so greatly in the last 10–15 years that the technique has become realistically available to the veterinary profession.

Although it is possible to investigate many organ and tissue functions by radioisotope tracer techniques, the most widely investigated and perhaps the most applicable to veterinary nuclear medicine is the scanning of bone.

TECHNIQUE

The principle of radioisotope imaging and scanning is based on the use of pharmaceuticals which, when introduced into the blood stream concentrate in a particular tissue or organ. The pharmaceutical is first labelled with a suitable gamma-ray emitting radioisotope so that its distribution and concentration within a particular organ can be imaged and quantified. Methylene diphosphonate labelled with technetium-99 m (^{99m}Tc), for instance, is the radiopharmaceutical used for bone scanning and imaging. ^{99m}Tc can be used to label a number of chemicals. It has a relatively short half-life (6 hours) and emits gamma rays of 140 keV. These physical characteristics ensure that the radiation dose to the patient and clinician is well within acceptable limits.

The distribution and concentration of labelled radiopharmaceutical in a particular organ is mapped by using either a gamma camera or hand-held detector. Both types of detector incorporate a single sodium iodide crystal and multiple, in the case of a gamma camera, or single photomultiplier tubes. Gamma rays emitted from the patient are absorbed by the sodium iodide crystal and cause a flash of light to be generated within the crystal as each gamma ray is detected. The photomultipliers convert each light flash to an electrical impulse. Either a computer or display oscilliscope is usually connected to the gamma camera, which converts the electrical impulses to an image of the radiopharmaceutical distribution and concentration. The hand-held detector monitors and displays the amount of gamma ray activity at a particular site on the patient on an analogue meter.

RADIOPHARMACEUTICAL

A number of companies (e.g., Amersham International) supply various pharmaceuticals in powdered form to which ^{99m}Tc in saline (pertechnetate) is added. Most district general hospitals have regular supplies of ^{99m}Tc through a generator which is eluted each day with normal saline to produce pertechnetate. It is possible to obtain pertechnetate under contract from District Health Authorities. Typically the total radiopharmaceutical costs approximately £10 to £20.

For a gamma camera skeletal scan the radiopharmaceutical is administered at the rate of 8 MBq kg^{-1} body mass (this is reduced to 2 MBq kg^{-1} for hand-held probe scanning) usually in a volume less than 5 ml. If the blood supply to a particular skeletal site is to be assessed the imaging or scanning is performed immediately after the introduction of the radiopharmaceutical into the blood stream. To allow clear differentiation between bone and soft tissue skeletal scans are performed 2-3 h after the introduction of the radiopharmaceutical. This period of time is required to allow excretion of radiopharmaceutical distributed in soft tissue via the urinary system. The amount excreted is approximately 70% of the total activity administered.

DETECTORS

Single photomultiplier tube systems

A schematic diagram and photograph of a hand-held detector is illustrated in Figure 1. The collimator provides spatial resolution and the lead casing shields the sodium iodide crystal from radiation other than that entering through the collimator. The high voltage supply for the photomultiplier tube is contained in a small portable back-pack along with electronics to display the number of gamma rays detected per second (i.e. count rate). It has been found useful to have a read-out of the count rate displayed on the analogue meter positioned on top of the detector. A resolution of between 3 and 5 mm can be achieved with the hand-held detector system. A single hand-held detector can be purchased for approximately £1500 (e.g. John Caunt Scientific Ltd., Oxford).

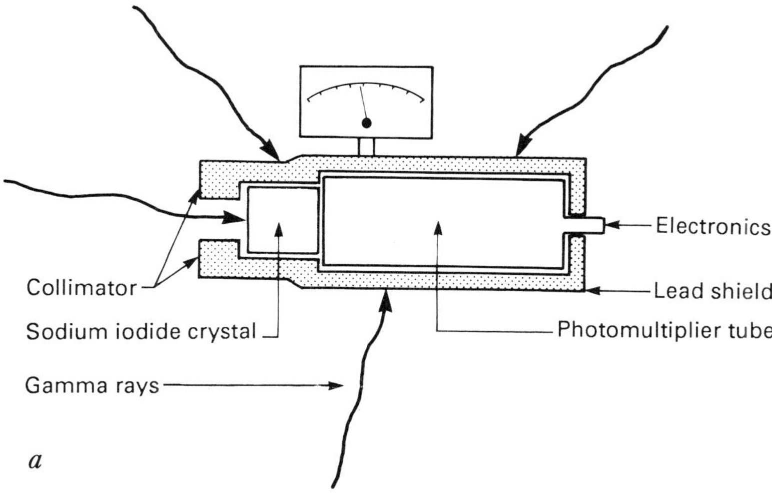

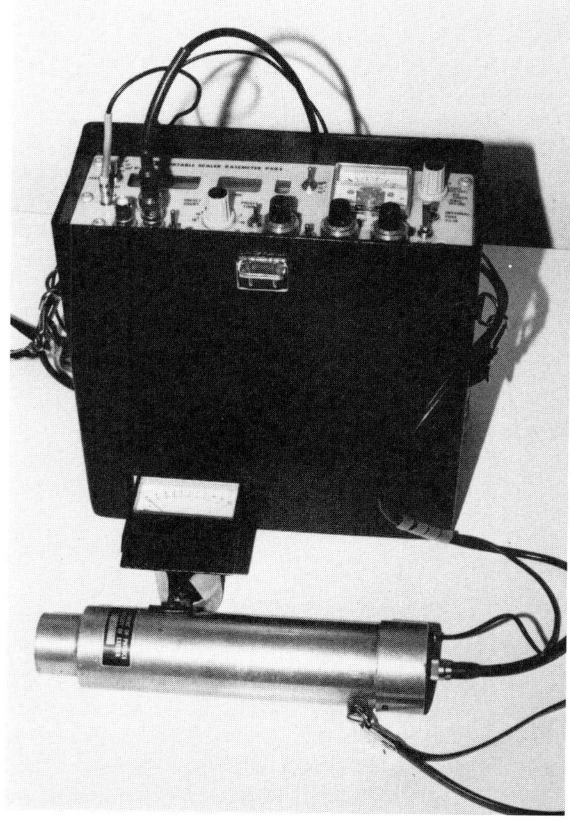

Fig. 1. (a) Schematic diagram of the hand-held detector and (b) photograph of the detector and associated portable electronics. Note the count rate indicator is fixed to the detector itself.

Gamma cameras

A gamma camera incorporates a much larger sodium iodide crystal (200–500 mm diameter) backed by a number of photomultiplier tubes (Figure 2). The system is collimated in order that only gamma rays incident perpendicular on the crystal face will be detected. Each gamma ray absorbed by the crystal produces a light flash whose position can be determined by the relative response of each photomultiplier tube. There are typically 30 to 90 tubes. An electrical pulse is then fed to an image display device such as a computer or cathode ray oscilloscope from which a scintigram, composed of approximately 200 000 events, is generated. Images can be produced in both colour and grey-scale. It is important to note that black and white prints displayed in this publication are obtained from colour images and are included only as a demonstration. To obtain the best results with a gamma camera it is essential that it is linked to a computer system which can control the gathering of image data and its subsequent storage, display and quantification.

The head of the gamma camera is supported in a yoke which can be lifted from ground level to 4 m using a mobile hoist (Sherpa Stackers Ltd). The room housing the gamma camera must be temperature controlled because large variations in ambient temperature could cause the sodium iodide crystal to crack. Further details of the design and construction of a purpose-built building for veterinary nuclear medicine have been published elsewhere (Attenburrow *el al.*, 1988).

As hospitals update their gamma camera systems, useful second-hand cameras become available at reasonable cost. Suitable computer systems can be obtained from a number of companies, either new or second-hand, (e.g. Nodecrest Ltd). Second-hand computers are available for approximately £18 000.

Scanning

Gamma camera scans require the patient to be mildly sedated because each image is captured over a period of 2 to 3 minutes. Large animals are restrained in stocks (Figure 3), while small animals are either imaged on the gamma camera head or on a table (Figure 4). It is not usually necessary to sedate animals for hand-held scanning because the detector is held in place at a particular site for only a few seconds. Figure 5 demonstrates the use of the hand-held detector on a cow in the field and on a dog in the clinic. The count rate at contralateral or adjacent sites and to a standard landmark on the animal (e.g. the withers in the horse) are compared.

Radiation protection

It is a requirement in the United Kingdom that licences for the use and storage of radioactive materials and the disposal of radioactive waste be first obtained from the Department of the Environment, Romney House, 43 Marsham Street, London SW1P 3PY. The protection of personnel involved in radioisotope scanning is required by law and the appropriate radiation levels and exposures are laid down in the Ionizing Radiations Regulations 1985, which form part of the Health and Safety at Work Act. The largest amount of radioactive material is used during gamma camera scanning of the skeletons of horses and cattle. In these cases the radiation dose 1–2 m from the animal is approximately 3 μSv h^{-1}. This represents an exposure

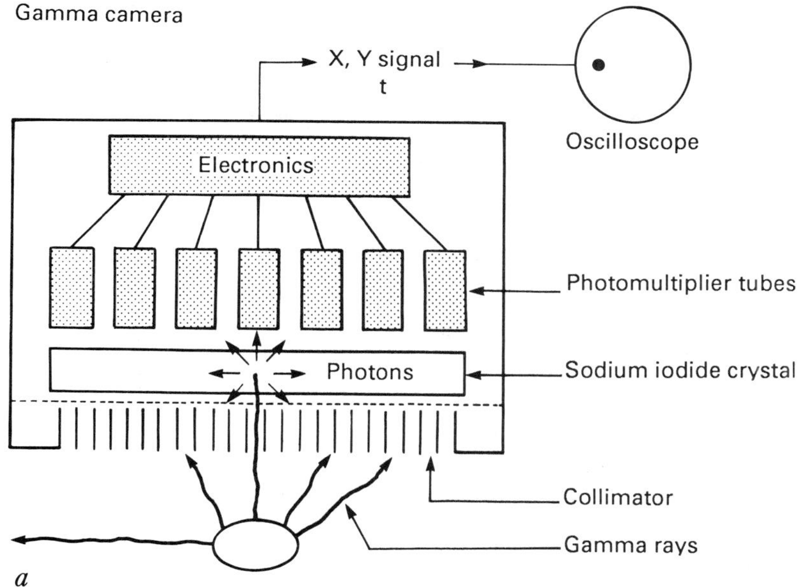

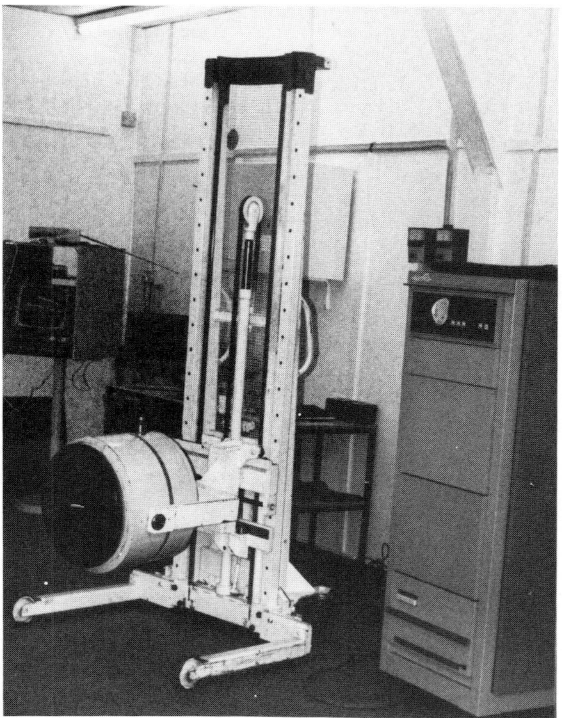

Fig. 2. (a) Schematic diagram of a gamma camera and (b) photograph of the gamma camera supported by a mobile carrier which can be adjusted both vertically and horizontally.

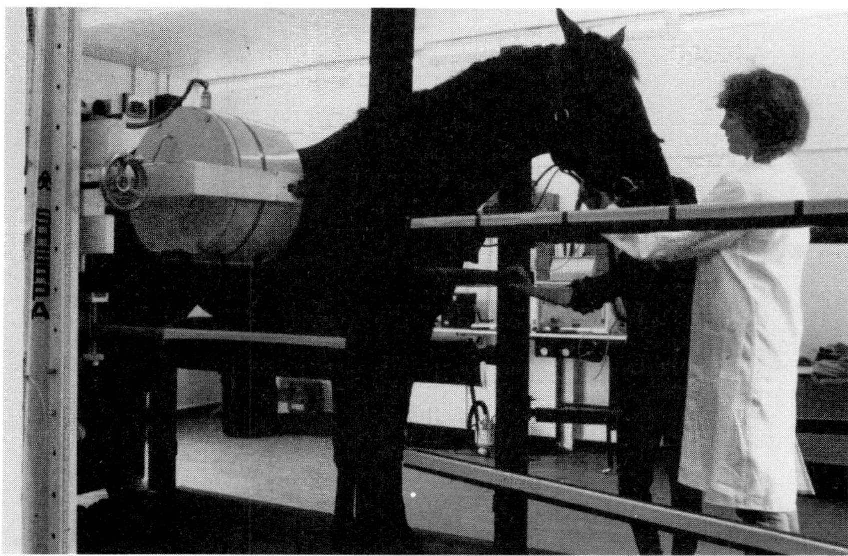

Fig. 3. The gamma camera being used to scan a horse restrained in stocks in the centre of the laboratory.

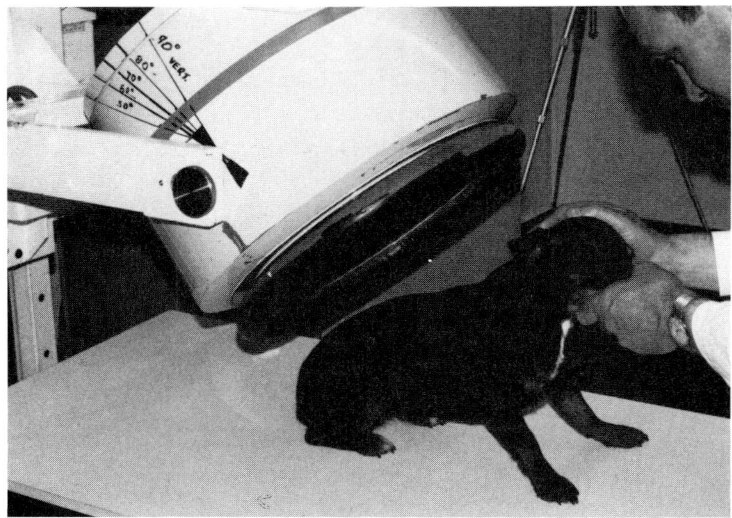

Fig. 4. The use of the gamma camera with small animals.

rate well within the recommended limits for designated radiation workers of 7.5 μSv^{-1} and is comparable to levels routinely encountered in human nuclear medicine. All staff should wear personal monitors and appropriate protective clothing, such as gloves, when dealing with injections. Special care should be taken with soiled bedding

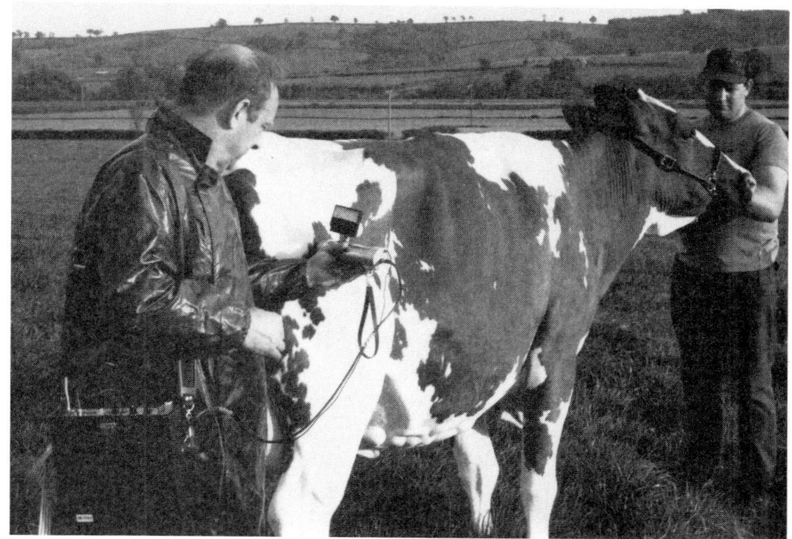

a

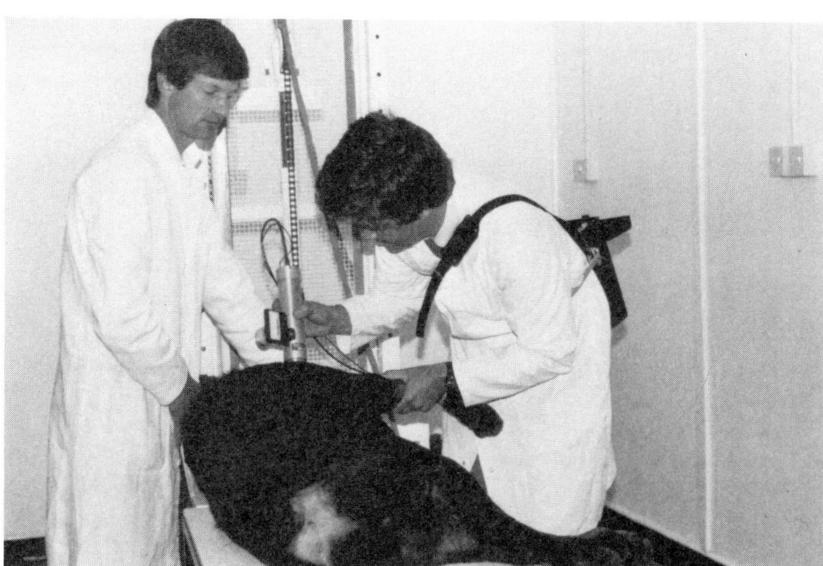

b

Fig. 5.(a) The use of the hand-held detector in the field and (b) the scanning of a large dog in the clinic. In this case profound sedation was necessary.

of animals scanned. In general, animals should be confined to a controlled area, allowing only limited access, for 24–36 h after scanning before being returned to their owners. After this period the area can be cleaned.

APPLICATION

Skeletal changes, brain lesions, kidney function, lung ventilation, ureter patency, lung ventilation and perfusion, space occupying lesions in the liver and function and heart function can all be usefully investigated in both large and small animals by a gamma camera and its associated computer.

The resolution of typical gamma camera imaging systems used in veterinary nuclear medicine significantly limit their use for brain scanning except for large lesions in large and small animals. Ventilation and perfusion imaging of the lung, liver function and cardiac function, although very interesting and holding considerable diagnostic potential, remain within the field of veterinary clinical research.

Kidney function and ureter patency are relatively easily investigated, particularly in the small animal. Figure 6 shows a renogram which demonstrates the clearance, as a function of time, of the radiopharmaceutical from the left and right kidney of a cat. The rate of clearance from the kidneys and the relative contribution of each kidney to renal function, can be obtained from the graphs. Figure 7 shows a radioisotope image of the pelvis of the left kidney and adjacent ureter of an eighteen year old thoroughbred gelding with the body of the kidney shielded by a lead sheet. The obvious concentration of the radiopharmaceutical at the proximal ureter and pelvis indicates constriction of the lumen.

The detection of localized increase or decrease in bone turnover resulting from trauma or disease is perhaps the most useful application of radioisotope imaging and scanning in veterinary practice. The technique is very sensitive. Thus changes in bone activity which occur at the stage of degenerative joint disease where the

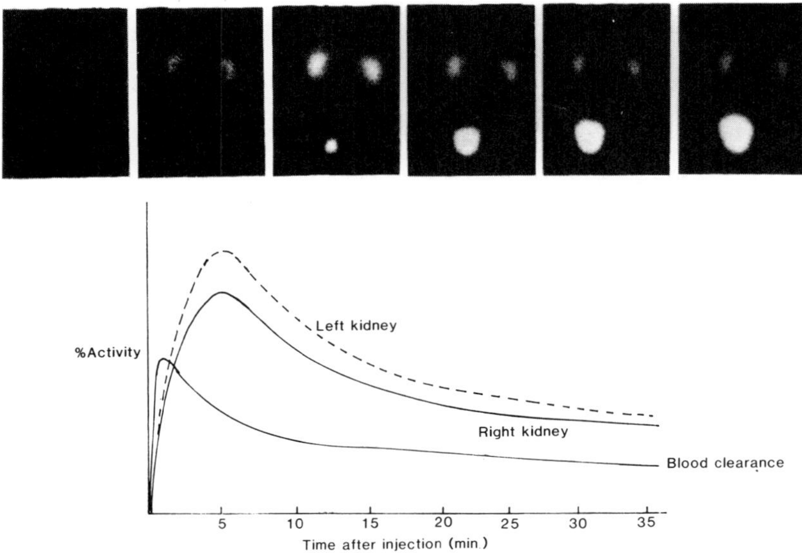

Fig. 6. The uptake and subsequent execretion of radiopharmaceutical by the renal system of a cat. The scintigrams running from left to right are taken at 4 min intervals. The graphs were obtained using the computer to generate activity time graphs from regions of interest over the left and right kidneys and the renal artery.

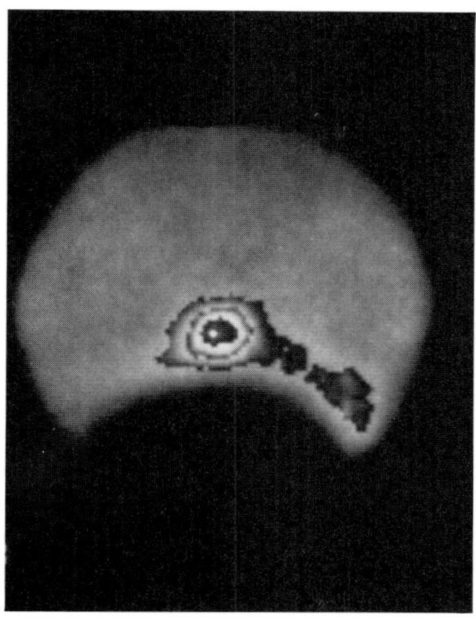

Fig. 7. Scan of the kidney of a horse. There was a marked concentration of radioactivity the pelvis of the right kidney. To demonstrate this more clearly the main body of the kidney was shielded by a lead sheet. This scan demonstrates a constriction of the ureter at the kidney of pathological significance

condition progresses from a degenerative chondritis to an osteoarthritis can be detected, imaged and quantified. In the horse anatomical changes in bone associated with the relatively advanced stages of degenerative joint disease can be predicted as much as a year before such changes are identified by X-radiography in many cases.

Osteosarcoma and osteoarthritic conditions associated with increased bone activity in the small animal are also accurately detected and assessed. Figure 8 shows the radioisotope image of the bones of the hind limb of a dog. The localized increased activity in subchondral bone at the right hock indicates established osteoarthritis.

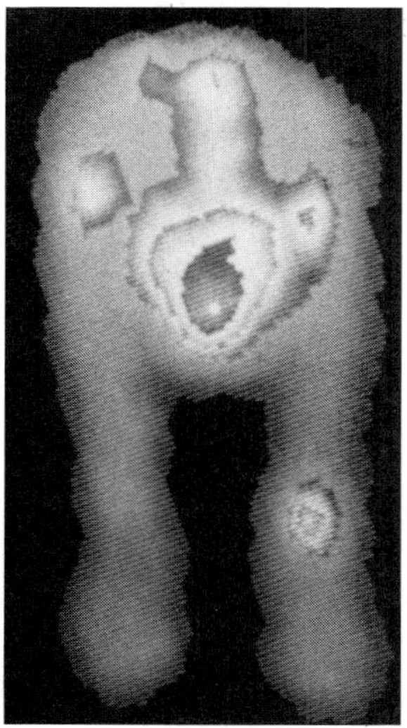

Fig. 8. The image obtained from the hind limbs and pelvis of a dog with the hind limbs extended backwards. The image of the right hock indicates pathological bony activity associated with osteoarthritis. This image clearly demonstrates the value of comparison of images of contralateral sites

This condition has not progressed to anatomical change in the bone and thus was not detected by X-radiography, even though the dog demonstrated signs of severe pain and lameness in the affected limb.

Localized increase in bone activity in the horse initiated by microstress fractures caused by the stress of athletic performance can be clearly delineated and quantified using bone scanning techniques. In most cases, the results of skeletal scanning form the basis of a definitive diagnosis of the seat of pain and bone pathology associated with established lameness.

Figure 9 shows the lateral views of the fetlock joints of the left and right forelimbs of a four year old thoroughbred. The localized increase in subchondral bone activity at the fetlock of the right forelimb clearly indicates that degenerative joint disease (i.e. osteoarthritis) is well established in that joint. Hair-line fractures, which very often escape diagnosis by X-radiography, can be clearly identified by demonstrating localized increase in bone activity associated with the process of healing. The progress of bone healing can also be monitored. Figure 10 shows localized increase in bone activity in the left pedal bone of a seven year old thoroughbred mare. This mare was very lame but no evidence of bone trauma was provided by X-radiography. This radioisotope image demonstrates the post-traumatic healing of the hair-line fracture in the bone. *Figure 11* shows increased bone activity of the sesamoid bone (sesamoiditis) of a nine year old eventer.

Very useful images of the vertebral column of the small animal and the horse can be obtained using a gamma camera. Figure 12 shows a typical image of the body and part of the asociated ribs of three thoracic vertebrae of a horse and the sacro-iliac joint.

Areas of inflammatory and other pathological processes in bone which cause increase in bony activity can be identified. This leads to a precise diagnosis. For example, Figure 13 demonstrates localized increase in bony activity at the roots of a molar in both the right upper and lower jaws of a five year old gelding.

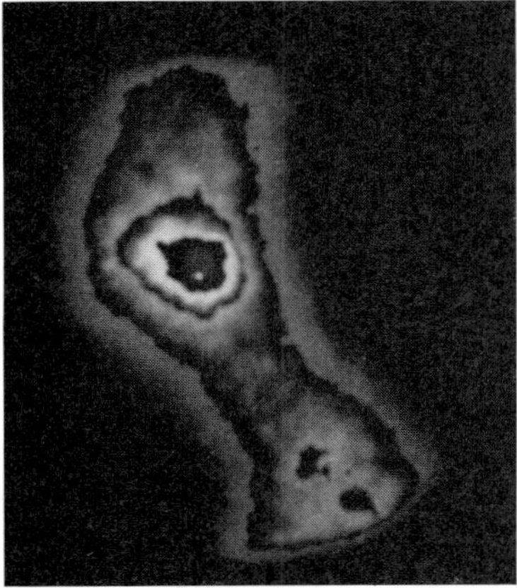 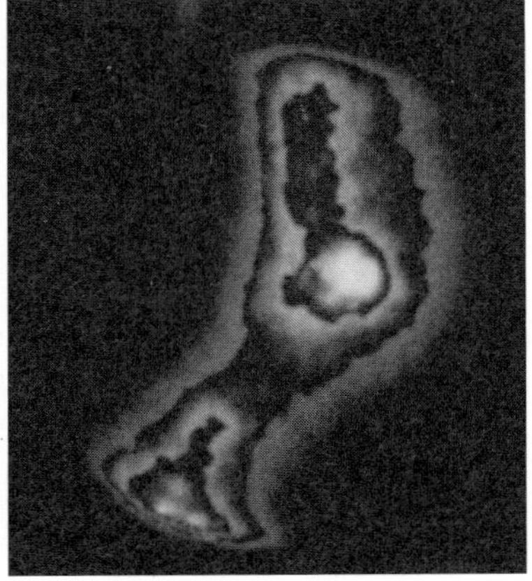

Fig. 9. The fetlock joints of the left and right forelimbs of a four year old thoroughbred imaged from the lateral aspect. The differences in the intensity of bony activity shown in these images clearly indicates established degenerative joint disease. The left image indicates greater activity at the fetlock joint than the right image.

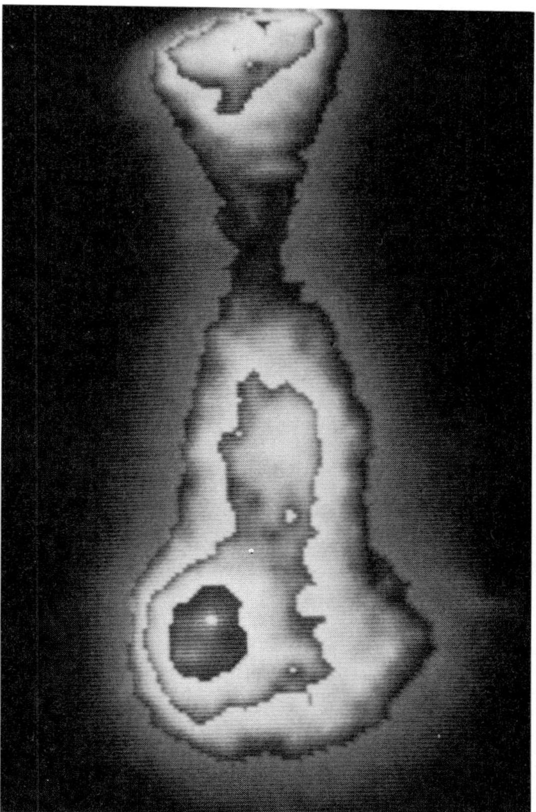

Fig. 10. This image demonstrates the usefulness of skeletal scanning in detecting and demonstrating occult hair-line fractures. There is a marked increase in bony activity associated with a hair-line fracture of the wing of the pedal bone of a forelimb of thoroughbred mare.

CONCLUSION

The establishment of gamma camera imaging units for use in veterinary nuclear medicine is not likely to be commonplace in general practice because of financial limitations. It is hoped, however, that these diagnostic procedures will be established at several referal centres and thus become indirectly available to the general practitioner. Scanning by hand-held single photomultiplier detectors presents no serious financial burden because the capital cost is less than that required for X-radiography units commonly used in general practice. The availability of radioisotope could be a limiting factor. However, most District General Hospitals are regularly supplied with ^{99m}Tc generators and no difficulties have yet been found in obtaining supplies. The amount of ^{99m}Tc used for hand-held probe scanning is similar to that used for gamma camera bone scans in humans. Thus this quantity can easily be supplied on request without the use of larger generators. This would not be the case if regular gamma camera bone imaging of large animals is to be undertaken.

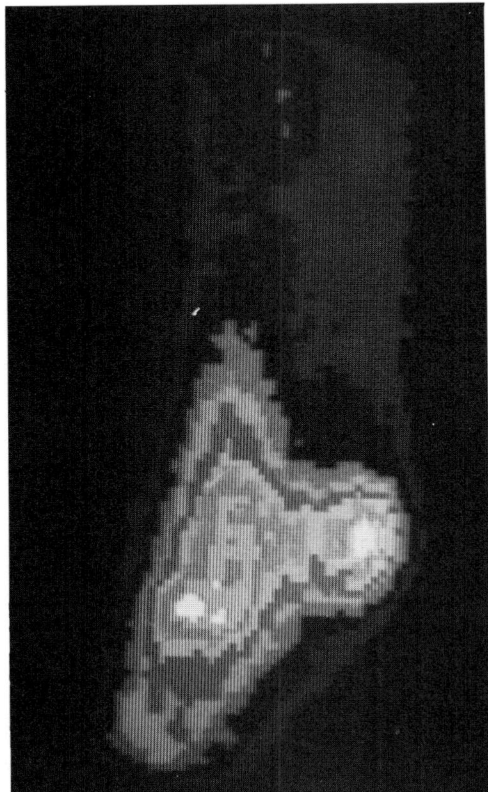

Fig. 11. The definitive diagnosis of sesamoiditis in the horse is usually difficult. This image demonstrates the pathological increase in bony activity of the sesamoid bone associated with established sesamoiditis

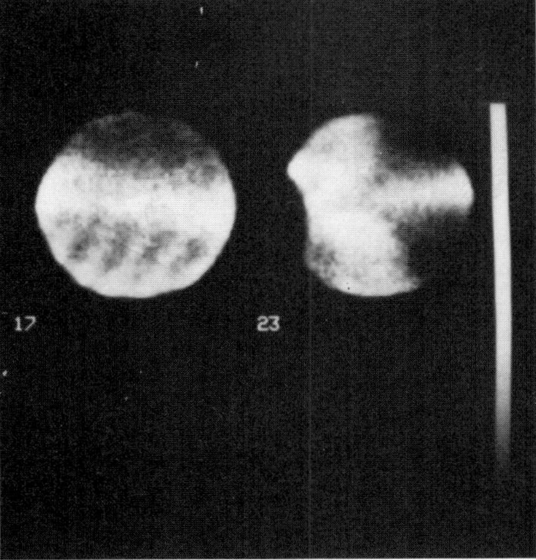

Fig. 12. An image of the lateral aspect of thoracic vertebrae of a hunter (left) and of the sacro-iliac joint (right)

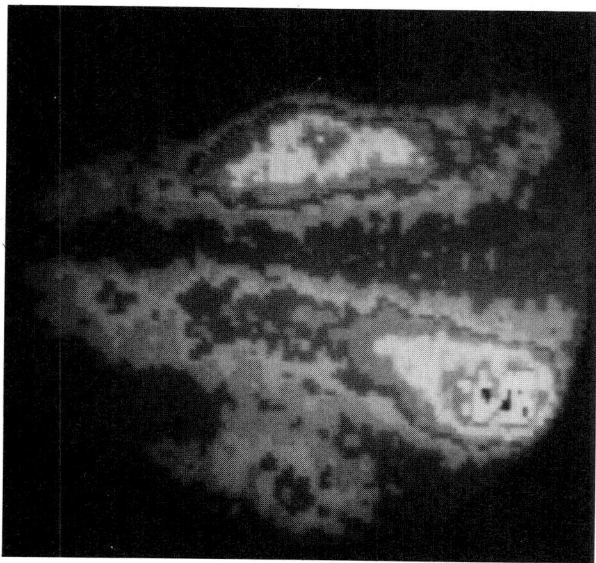

Fig. 13. Increased bony activity which can be associated with a bone infection. The diseased roots of two molar teeth are shown, one in the lower and the other in the upper jaw. This image is a lateral view of the two jaws.

The most useful application of the hand-held scanner is for bone scanning in both large and small animals. The whole of the skeleton of the small animal can be scanned and areas of localized increase in activity accurately detected and delineated.

It has been found by comparing the hand-held scanner results in the horse with those from the gamma camera (Attenburrow *et al.*, 1988), that very useful and accurate bone scanning of the bones of the lower limbs, cervical vertebrae and skull can be achieved with a hand-held detector. Imaging by gamma camera is preferable for all the vertebrae, pelvis and higher joints of both fore and hind limbs.

There can be difficulties in interpretation of scans from the bones of a limb contralateral to a limb with established bony pathology and severe lameness demonstrated over a prolonged period of time. In these cases increased uptake of radiopharmaceutical in the bones of the limb providing the major support to the horse can occur. This could be a result of remodelling of the bone under stress. Such physiological changes do not, however, impair the diagnostic value of skeletal scans.

REFERENCES

Attenburrow D. P., Bowring C. S. and Vennart W. (1984). Radioisotope bone scanning in horses. *Equine Vet. J.*, **16**, 121–124

Attenburrow D. P., Portergill M. J. and Vennart W. (1988) Development of an equine nuclear medicine facility for gamma camera imaging. *Equine Vet. J.* (in press)

Devous M. D. and Twardock A. R. (1984) Techniques and applications of nuclear medicine in the diagnosis of equine lameness. *J.Am.Vet.Med.Ass.* **184**, 318–325

Metcalf M. R. (1985) Preliminary clinical use of combined blood pool and bone phase radionuclide imaging in dogs. *Vet.Radiol.* **26**, 117–122

Tofe A. J., Lloyd G. G., Roenigk W. J., Francis M. D. (1974) The utilization of ^{99m}Tc-Sn-EHDP bone scanning agent for detection and clinical progress of abnormal bone metabolism: a case report. *J.Am.Vet.Radiol.Soc.* **15**, 87–92

Ueltschi G. (1977) Bone and join imaging with [99m]Tc- labelled phosphates as a new diagnostic aid in veterinary orthopaedics. *J.Am.Vet.Radiol.Soc.* **18**, 80-84

F. D. KIRBY

Some changes in infectious diseases of British farm livestock in the last two decades

INTRODUCTION

THE SURVEILLANCE of non-notifiable disease of farm animals is one of the functions of the Veterinary Investigation Service. The VIDA II system (Hall *et al.*, 1980) includes computerized records of all the diagnoses made by the laboratories since 1975. The records represent a sample of those diseases occurring in the farm animal population for which veterinary practitioners may seek laboratory diagnostic confirmation. Figure 1 gives an indication of how highly selected the disease records are. However, the selective bias is unlikely to vary greatly from year to year so that some

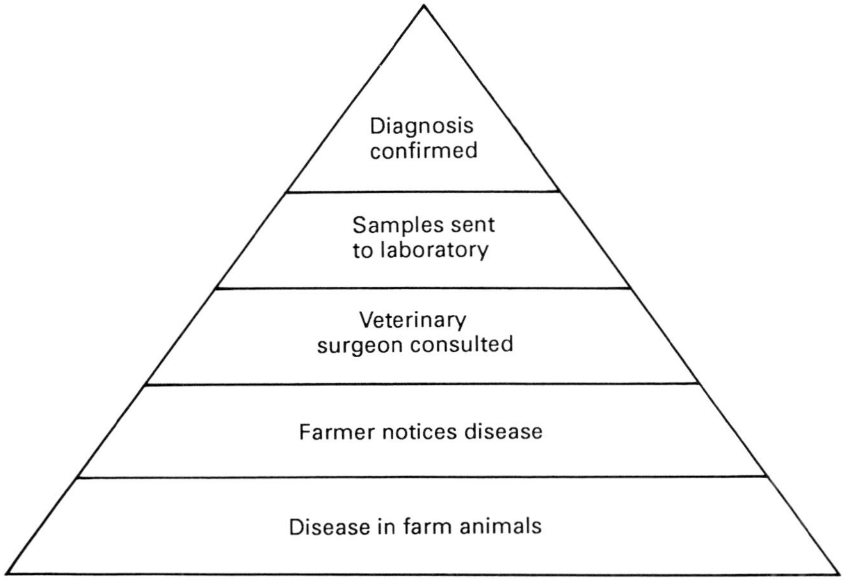

Fig. 1.

conclusions may be drawn about changes in the incidence of the diseases recorded by comparing the records over a period of some years.

Over the last 20 years some new laboratories have been added to the system and others have been closed. Changes in the charges made for diagnostic examinations and changes in the economics of animal farming, such as the imposition of milk quotas, could influence the number and type of samples received. The total number of submissions per year from cattle have remained fairly constant for the period of the record but annual submissions from pigs have increased by about 50% and annual submissions from sheep have increased approximately threefold.

To take this into account the records used as illustrations here have been reduced to a common base of 10 000 submissions for pigs and sheep and 100 000 annual submissions for cattle. This approximates the actual annual submission level for each species.

Comprehensive surveillance data is available for reportable and notifiable disease from the Animal Health Division of the State Veterinary Service. Other sources of information on particular diseases are special surveys, the Veterinary Laboratories of the Milk Marketing Board and the Veterinary Schools.

G. Davies (1982) described some farm animal disease trends in a previous edition of this publication. This paper considers some recent changes in the incidence of infectious diseases and why they may have occurred.

DISEASES PREVIOUSLY UNKNOWN IN THIS COUNTRY BUT WHICH HAD BEEN RECOGNIZED ABROAD FOR SOME TIME

Some previously unknown diseases may be associated with the importation of livestock or animal products. Some, such as maedi-visna (Dawson *el at.*, 1979) and enzootic bovine leucosis (Crowley, 1985), were first detected in flocks or herds containing recently imported stock. Other conditions that may have been imported during the last 20 years include diseases caused by *Haemophilus somnus* (Pritchard and MacLeod, 1977) and *Mycoplasma bovis* (Thomas *et al.*, 1975) as well as swine vesicular disease, which was first diagnosed in this country in 1972. It had been seen previously in Hong Kong in 1970 and Italy in 1966.

NEW DISEASES OF UNKNOWN ORIGIN

Some of these might arise from genetic mutation and others from infections spilling over into new species of host animal. Concurrent infection with different strains of influenza viruses may result in new strains arising from the recombination of genetic material from both parent strains.

Contagious equine metritis (Platt *et al.*, 1977) and bovine spongiform encephalopathy (BSE) (Wells *et al.*, 1987) are examples. BSE has some characteristics in common with scrapie but its distribution (Figure 2) does not reflect that of the sheep population. It has occurred principally in dairy cattle, which have less contact with sheep than beef breeds. Incorporation of rendered ovine material into cattle rations has been suggested as a route of transmission of infection (Morgan, 1988). VIDA figures show an increase in the number of scrapie diagnoses but this parallels the increased rate of submission of ovine material (Figure 3).

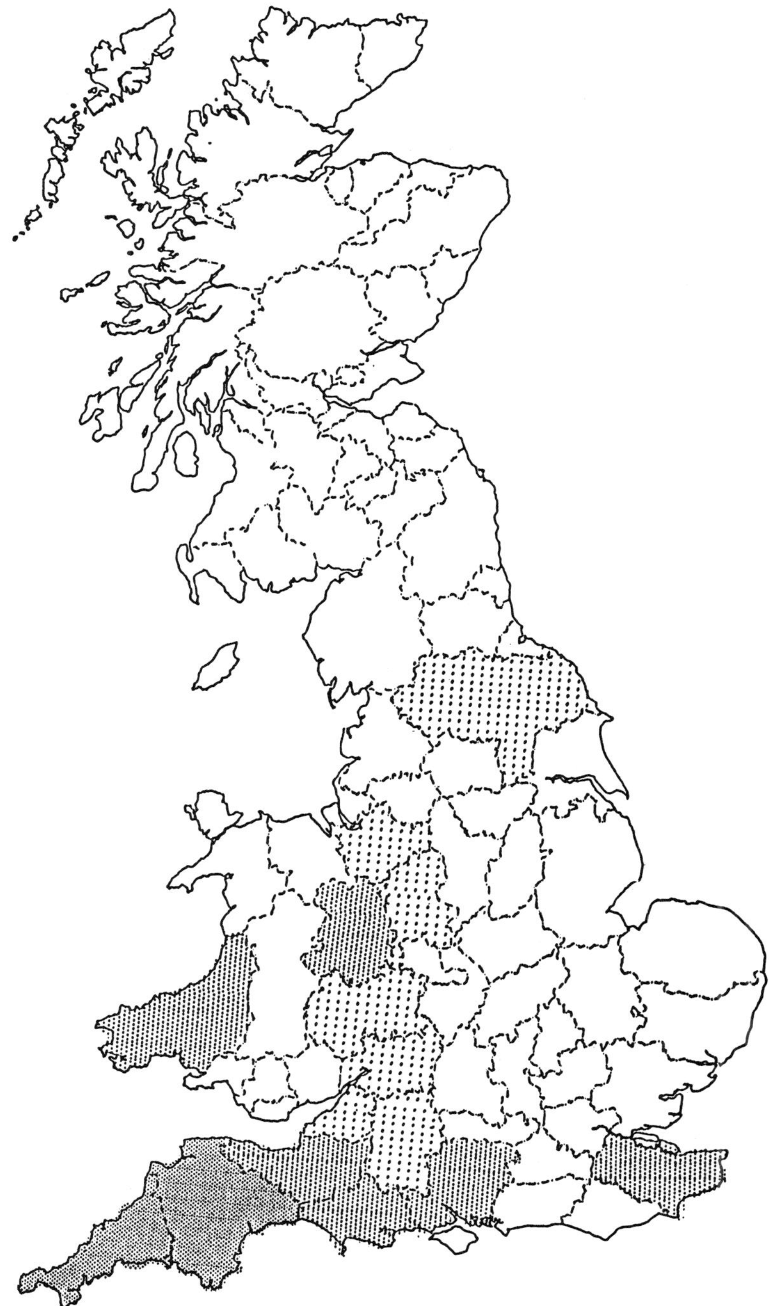

Fig. 2. Incidence of bovine spongiform encephalopathy. Infected farms per county in May 1988:□,0–9;⊡;10–19,⊞;20–49;▨,50+

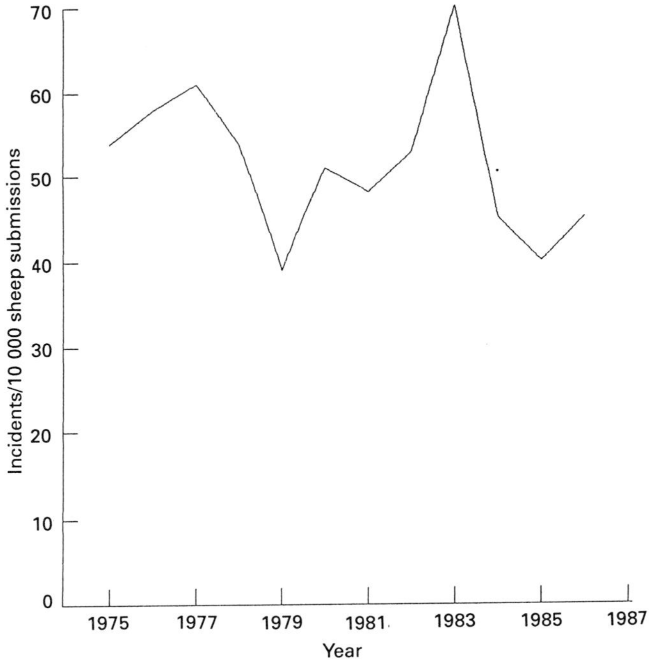

Fig. 3.

INFECTIONS FOR WHICH NEW DIAGNOSTIC TESTS HAVE BEEN DEVELOPED

Faecal electron microscopy led to the discovery of viruses that showed little pathogenicity to tissue cultures. White (1970) first reported a high incidence of rotavirus infection in diarrhoeic calves. Subsequently, other diagnostic methods that could be used in less well equipped laboratories were developed. The recent introduction of latex agglutination tests for rotavirus infection may be partly responsible for the apparent recent steep rise in the incidence of this infection in calves (Figure 4).

Some developments in human diagnostic medicine have had veterinary applications. Most human rotaviruses are antigenically similar to the strains found in calves and the infection may be zoonotic. The development of selective media for cultivation of campylobacters from faeces led to interest in the role of *C. jejuni* as a cause of diarrhoea. Though these organisms are thought to be a significant human pathogen, their frequent isolation from the intestines of healthy domestic livestock suggests that they are best considered as part of the normal intestinal flora (Garcia *et al.*, 1983).

INCREASED AWARENESS OF PATHOGENIC SIGNIFICANCE

In assessing the significance of a pathogen emphasis has shifted from experimental challenge with the pathogen to a comparison of its prevelance in diseased and healthy

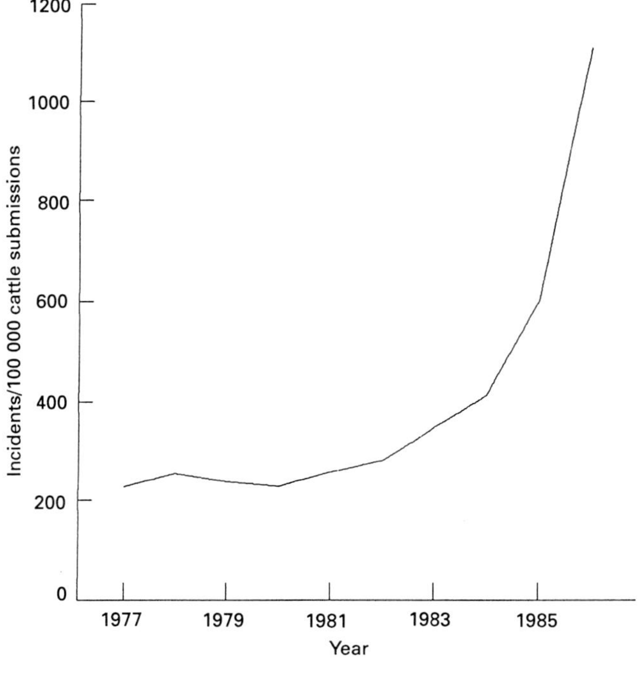

Fig. 4.

Table 1 PREVELANCE OF FIVE CALF ENTEROPATHOGENS IN TWO FIELD SURVEYS ON FIFTY-ONE FARMS

Pathogen	*Diarrhoeic calves*		*Healthy calves*	
	number/total	*%*	*number/total*	*%*
Rotavirus	252/567	44	60/434	14
Cryptosporidia	116/542	21	37/428	9
Coronavirus	77/567	14	2/434	0.5
Salmonella	53/550	10	10/434	2
Enterotoxigenic *E. coli*	17/419	4	10/434	2

animals in the field. Table 1 shows pooled results of two field surveys of calf enteropathogens (Snodgrass *et al.*, 1986, Reynolds *et al.*, 1986). Note the low significance of enterotoxigenic *E.coli* which were thought to be a major pathogen in calf diarrhoea 20 years ago. With experimental challenge it is difficult to be sure that the route, weight and frequency of the challenge equate to the field situation.

Cryptosporidia are protozoal parasites that were first described in 1907 but were not directly associated with diarrhoea in calves until 1975 (Shmitz and Smith, 1975). Interest in their pathogenicity followed the appreciation of their significance in immuno-compromised human patients, particularly those suffering from AIDS.

Zoonotic spread occurred from experimentally infected calves to their attendants at an American Veterinary School. New staining methods have improved diagnosis.

Following the control of *Brucella abortus* in cattle interest focused on other infectious causes of bovine abortion. Another zoonotic infection, caused by *Leptospira hardjo*, has been shown to be an important cause of bovine abortion. A fluorescent antibody test (FAT) has been developed using foetal kidney to supplement serological diagnosis. The marketing of a vaccine has encouraged practitioners to seek the diagnosis because effective control is now possible. Figure 5 illustrates the increased interest in this infection.

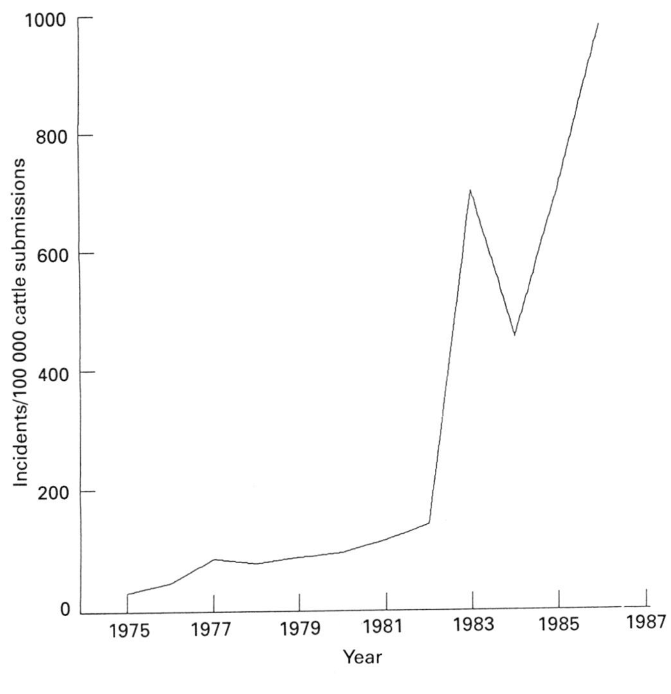

Fig. 5.

HUSBANDRY CHANGES

Pig husbandry has become more intensive and hysterectomy-derived nucleus breeding herds are kept with a high level of disease security. It has been suggested that the high levels of hygiene under which these animals are kept delays the establishment of a normal intestinal flora and permits pathogens that are uncommon under normal conditions, such as *Campylobacter sputorum*, to cause problems. Any infection established in nucleus herds could be widely disseminated through the multiplying herds to the commercial breeders and fatteners at the base of the pyramid. *Streptococcus suis II* may have been spread in this way (Figure 6).

High levels of hygiene in broiler units may mitigate against the early establishment of a normal flora and permit *salmonella* to establish themselves in the intestines.

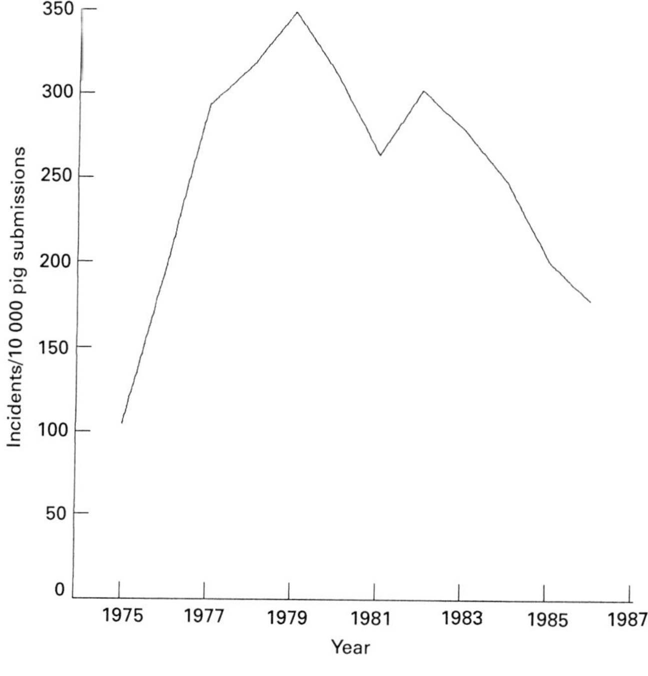

Fig. 6.

Nurmi and Rantalla (1973) proposed the oral administration of a bacterial cocktail to counteract this.

The introduction of cow cubicles in conjunction with a mastitis control scheme aimed principally at Gram-positive infections may have led to *E.coli* becoming more important as an udder pathogen.

Listeria monocytogenes can multiply in silage of a pH higher than 4.5. An increase in the amount of silage fed to sheep is thought to be the principle factor in the increasing incidence of ovine listeriosis (Wilesmith and Gitter, 1986). Figure 7 compares the incidence of listeriosis in cattle and sheep. *Listeria* can multiply at much lower temperatures than most bacterial pathogens. If the increasing incidence of ovine listeriosis is disregarded, the figure shows a very similar profile to bovine listeriosis. This might be due to the influence of weather conditions on the multiplication of *Listeria* within silage.

CONCLUSION

Infectious pathogens evolve at a much faster rate than their vertebrate hosts. A new and more serious disease may occur if a pathogen spreads to a new host species. Novel infections may be spread by the international trade in new animal breeds. The development of new and more sensitive tests are likely to reveal the presence of infections of which we are yet unaware. Who can say what the next 20 years will bring?

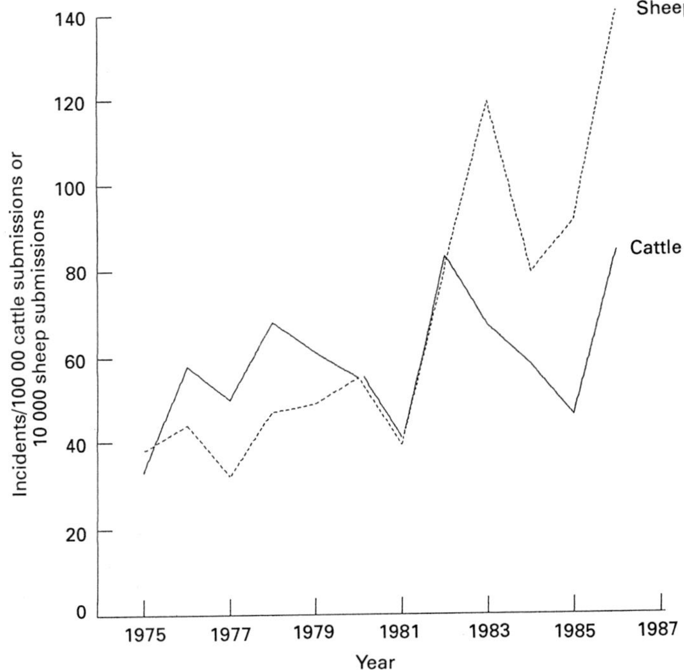

Fig. 7.

REFERENCES

Crowley, A. J. (1985) *Veterinary Annual*, 25th edn, Wright, Bristol.
Davies, G. (1982) *Veterinary Annual*, 22nd edn, Wright, Bristol
Dawson, M., Chasey, D., King A. *et al.*, (1979) *Vet. Rec.* **105,** 220
Garcia, M., Eaglesome, M. and Rigby, C. (1983) *Vet. Bull.* **53,** 800
Hall, S., Dawson, P. and Davies, G. (1980) *Vet. Rec.* **106,** 260
Morgan, K. (1988) *Vet. Rec.* **122,** 445
Nurmi, E. and Rantalla, M. (1973) *Nature* **241,** 210
Pritchard, D. and MacLeod N. (1977) *Vet. Rec.* **100,** 126
Platt, H. Atherton, J. and Simpson, D. (1977) *Vet. Rec.* **101,** 20
Reynolds, D., Morgan, J., and Chanter, N. *et al.* (1986) *Vet. Rec.* **119,** 34
Shmitz, J. and Smith, D. (1975) *J.Am.Vet.Med.Ass.* **167,** 731
Snodgrass, D., Terzolo, H., and Sherwood, I. *et al.* (1986) *Vet. Rec.* **119,** 31
Thomas, L., Howard, C. and Gourlay, R. (1975) *Vet. Rec.* **97,** 55
Wells, G., Scott, A., Johnson, C., *et al.* (1987) *Vet. Rec.* **121,** 419
White, R., Mebus, C. and Twiehaus, M. (1970) *Vet.Med.Small Anim.Clin.* **65,** 487
Wilesmith, J. and Gitter, M. (1986) Vet. Rec. **119,** 467

B. D. PERRY

The oral immunization of animals against rabies

INTRODUCTION

THE TREATMENT of the ancient and feared disease of rabies relied for centuries on practices such as local wound treatment of mad dog bites with caustic and corrosive substances, burning the site of a bite with a hot iron, and ingestion of a variety of remedies such as the liver of a mad dog, crayfish eyes, cock's brain and cock's comb (Wiktor, 1985). The first major turning point in the control of rabies came in 1885 with Pasteur's successful immunization of a 9 year old peasant boy who had been severely bitten by a rabid dog, into whom he injected a desiccated rabbit spinal cord rabies antigen preparation. This he repeated on 12 successive occasions with material of increasing virulence. Nervous tissue-derived injectable vaccines soon came into use for the post-exposure treatment of man, but it was not until over thirty years later that such vaccines, in the form of the phenol-inactivated Semple vaccine, were used on a large scale for the immunization of dogs. This vaccine is still used in many developing countries.

The second major turning point in the control of animal rabies was the introduction of effective potency tests for rabies vaccines (Habel, 1945) and the widespread use of the more immunogenic modified live virus (MLV) chick embryo vaccines, developed by Koprowski and Cox in 1948 (Koprowski and Cox, 1948). In combination with organized disease control programmes, rabies in domestic animals was then rapidly controlled in countries such as the United States (Winkler, 1983). The number of human cases in the US correspondingly fell dramatically from an average of 22 cases per year during the years 1946–1953 to an average of less than two cases per year during the years 1962–1985. Many of the cases during this latter period were acquired outside the US.

Two major goals of rabies control remain elusive. The first is the attainment of high levels of dog vaccination coverage in the developing world, where the overwhelming majority of rabies cases occur, as has been achieved in the US and elsewhere. The second is the control of rabies in wildlife in countries where successful dog rabies control has not eliminated the disease due to its persistence in wildlife populations. It is the latter situation which has provided the substrate for the third major turning point in the control of animal rabies, the development of oral rabies vaccines. This will undoubtedly have a considerable impact on both the remaining goals in rabies control.

ORIGIN OF ORAL RABIES VACCINES

During the 1960s, when the attention was, at least in Europe and North America, turning from dog rabies control to wildlife rabies control, the most important reservoir species in both continents at that time was the red fox *(Vulpes vulpes)*. Attempts to control fox rabies by reducing the fox population with trapping, poisoning and gassing of dens had not generally proved successful and were considered ecologically unacceptable by many.

The concept of immunizing wildlife populations was considered by a number of workers during the early 1960s (Ramsden and Johnston, 1975), and was taken more seriously following the work of Correa-Giron *et al.* (1970), who studied the pathogenesis of oral invasion of rabies virus in mice. Oral infection is not the normal route of infection of rabies, which is generally transmitted by the inoculation of virus-laden saliva from the bite of a rabid animal. They found that primary infection took place in the buccal and lingual mucosa. This prompted a series of studies on the oral immunization of the red fox, initiated by Black and Lawson, (1970) and Baer *et al.*, (1971). These studies demonstrated protection against challenge with street rabies virus following the oral administration of high titre attenuated vaccine. The vaccine used was the ERA vaccine (an acronym of the developers, Evelyn-Rokitnicki-Abelseth) derived from the SAD (Street-Alabama-Dufferin) strain of rabies virus (Abelseth, 1964) which had been grown on baby hamster kidney (BHK/21) cells to high titre.

Subsequent studies (Debbie *et al.*, 1972; Black and Lawson, 1973) confirmed that red foxes given commercial ERA vaccine orally by infusion or in a bait were protected, but that inactivated ERA vaccines and low egg passage (LEP) chick embryo vaccines did not provide protection by this route. Attempts were then made to develop systems for delivery of this vaccine to foxes under field conditions (Winkler *et al.*, 1975). Initial studies examined eggs (Debbie, 1974) and sausage baits (Winkler and Baer, 1976) for this purpose, and despite successful delivery of vaccine to lingual and buccal mucosa in experiments with foxes, further development of these baits was not pursued. This was due in part to the attractiveness of the baits to a wide variety of species other than foxes and the consequent potential for causing vaccine-induced rabies in rodents which consumed the baits (Winkler *et al.*, 1976). In addition, foxes tended to store eggs for later consumption, at which time the vaccine would probably have lost its viability.

Oral rabies vaccines can be targeted at the oropharyngeal mucosa or at the small intestine (Baer *et al.*, 1975; Johnston, 1975). Contact of food and liquid with the oropharyngeal mucosa in carnivores is generally brief so the choice of the small intestine as a target is attractive. However, the rabies virus is sensitive to an acid pH and to enzyme activity and does not readily pass the gastric barrier intact.

Inactivated vaccines, as killed products, would be much more acceptable for widespread use in wildlife populations than live attenuated vaccines. When surgically deposited into the lumen of the duodenum, inactivated vaccines have been shown to elicit serum neutralizing antibodies, albeit short-lived, in the red fox (Lawson *et al.*, 1982). However, inactivated vaccines do not appear to be immunogenic in the oropharynx of foxes (Black and Lawson, 1970). As no method has yet been determined of protecting inactivated vaccines during their passage through the stomach, most of the research into oral rabies vaccines has concentrated on live attenuated virus vaccines, targeted at the oropharyngeal mucosa.

DEVELOPMENT OF ORAL RABIES VACCINE SYSTEMS

AREAS OF RESEARCH

The subsequent research into the development of oral rabies vaccines has been concentrated on two component areas.
1. Development of safe and efficacious vaccines.
2. Development of effective bait delivery systems.

REQUIREMENTS OF ORAL RABIES VACCINE SYSTEMS

The requirements of vaccines and bait delivery systems have been outlined by Johnston (1975) and by Wandeler et al., (1988). They are summarized in Table 1.

In dog rabies control, it has been suggested that 70–80% of the dog population must be immunized to reduce the contact rate between rabid and susceptible dogs sufficiently to eradicate the disease. There is no target figure available for wildlife populations based on definitive field studies. However, mathematical models have suggested that an immunization cover of 60% in the European red fox population would be effective in eradicating the disease (Bacon and Macdonald, 1980). Given that not 100% of baits accepted by animals would immunize, bait acceptance rates in excess of 60% would be necessary to achieve this.

PROGRESS OF VACCINE DEVELOPMENT

After the flurry of activity by North American scientists in the early 1970s, research in the US on oral rabies vaccines declined during the subsequent decade. This was not, however, the case in Europe. Fox rabies, which had spread from Poland into East Germany in 1947 and from there to West Germany and much of central Europe (Steck and Wandeler, 1982) was moving progressively westwards at a rate of about 30 km per year (Bacon and Macdonald, 1980). Swiss scientists carried out a series of laboratory studies on the SAD strain of rabies virus grown in BHK/21 cells to determine the immunizing dose which could be delivered in a bait to the oropharyngeal mucosa of red foxes, and protect them against challenge with virulent fox rabies virus isolates (Hafliger et al., 1982; Steck et al., 1982). They chose a cloned SAD strain with a minimum of 10^7 TCID$_{50}$ (50% tissue culture infectious doses) dispensed in 1.8 ml aliquots into small plastic blister packages, which were fixed under the skin of slaughterhouse chicken heads, their selected bait.

Because of the concern about residual pathogenicity to rodents of the SAD strain vaccine (Winkler et al., 1976), the vaccine was tested in all the rodent species indigenous to Central Europe (Wandeler et al., 1982). In addition, an extensive field trial was carried out on an island in which vaccine was distributed in baits. Weanling mouse-inoculation studies for the presence of rabies virus were performed with tissues of the 760 small mammals subsequently trapped from the area. There was no indication that SAD virus became established in the small animal community (Wandeler et al., 1982).

In 1978, the Swiss scientists had an opportunity to test their system in the field, having obtained the necessary clearances to do so. They created an 'immune barrier' at the entrance to the Rhone valley, in the face of an advancing fox-rabies epidemic.

Table 1 REQUIREMENTS OF ORAL RABIES VACCINE SYSTEMS

Component	*Requirements*
Vaccine	1. Efficacy in target species. 2. Safety to target, non-target species and man. 3. Stability: a) At environmental temperatures for defined period. b) No reversion to greater pathogenicity. 4. No excretion. 5. Free of contamination. 6. Easily, produced in standard potent form 7. Inexpensive.
Bait	General: 1. Contain vaccine in sterile form. 2. Not interfere with efficacy of vaccine. 3. Immediately attractive to target species. 4. Non-attractive to non-target species and man. 5. Deliver vaccine into oral cavity. 6. Protect vaccine (temperature, rain, ultra-violet light). 7. Produceable in standard form under local conditions. 8. Capable of carrying a biomarker. 9. Inexpensive. 10. Withstand freezing without damage to integrity. Attractant: 1. Present optimal visual, olfactory, tactile and gustatory stimuli to target species. 2. Compatibility with bait and vaccine. 3. Remain palatable for a defined period. 4. Minimal attraction to non-target species and man. 5. Reproducible under local conditions in standard form. 6. Economical. 7. Tolerant of freezing. Biomarker: 1. Compatible with other bait components. 2. Safe for target and non-target species. 3. Adequate marking properties in target population over defined period. 4. Not present in subject population. 5. Economical.

This was done by distributing vaccine in chicken-head baits by hand at the rate of about 12 baits per km^2 (Steck *et al.*, 1982). Post-baiting evaluations estimated that about 60% of the fox population of the barrier had been immunized, and the advance of rabies along the Rhone valley was halted. Field trials were continued by the Swiss from 1978 to 1982. These freed the alpine zone of rabies. The trials progressed into a fully-fledged rabies eradication campaign, based on the hand placement of baits (although baited vaccine was dropped by helicopter in a few inaccesible areas). This resulted in the virtual eradication of the disease by the end of 1986 (Wandeler *et al.*,

1988). Rabies persists only in certain areas on the Swiss borders where it is endemic in the adjacent areas of neighbouring states.

In West Germany, using the SAD B19 vaccine at a virus titre of 10^7 TCID$_{50}$ per ml, similar success has followed initial field trials carried out in 1983 (Schneider *et al.*, 1983). However, the chicken head bait has been replaced by a machine-manufactured fat-based product (the Tubinger Fox Bait), which has allowed these studies to be carried out on a much larger scale in Germany (Schneider and Cox, 1988). Using this technology, rabies has subsequently been eradicated in Italy and the province of Vorarlberg in Austria. France, Belgium and Luxembourg, are now engaged in joint field trials (Wandeler, 1988), and it is to be expected that the eventual eradication of rabies will be attainable in Europe (Schneider and Cox, 1988).

In North America, the reluctance to deploy live attenuated vaccines in the field has continued, despite the successes gained in Europe. Nevertheless following recent safety studies in Canada with the ERA vaccine, (Lawson *et al.*, 1987) pilot field trials with this vaccine have begun. The safety studies showed that the 7 wild and domestic animal species fed up to 5 sponge baits each containing 14 ml of ERA vaccine at a titre of $10^{5.6}$ TCID$_{50}$ did not develop clinical signs of rabies. Vaccine-induced rabies did occur in wild mice (*Mus musculus*) but transmission to other animals was not reported (Lawson *et al.*, 1987). Pilot field studies used the commercial SAD-derived ERA strain of vaccine, initially with a titre of $10^{5.5} - 10^{6.5}$ median mouse intra-cerebral lethal dose (MICLD$_{50}$). Although bait acceptance rates were reasonably good (fox, 64%; skunk, 33%; raccoon, 43%), serological evidence suggested an immunization rate in foxes of only 12% (Johnston *et al.*, 1988). The poor response appeared to be due to a decline in vaccine potency following bait distribution. Subsequent studies have used higher titre virus grown on BHK/21 cells.

Oral rabies vaccines other than the attenuated SAD virus are also under development, and considerable success has been demonstrated in the laboratory with orally administered recombinant DNA vaccines. Kieny *et al.*, (1984) constructed a recombinant vaccinia virus containing the ERA strain rabies glycoprotein, the surface portion of the virus responsible for eliciting neutralizing antibody (Crick and Brown, 1969; Crick, 1981). This vaccinia recombinant rabies vaccine has been shown to be extremely effective in protecting against street virus infection by the intramuscular and oral routes in rabbits, raccoons, red foxes and skunks (Wiktor *et al.*, 1984; 1985; Blancou *et al.*, 1986; Rupprecht *et al.*, 1986; 1987; 1988; Tolson *et al.*, 1987). Indeed, the vaccine not only appears extremely immunogenic but also protects several different wildlife species when administered orally. It is unclear whether this latter desirable feature can be achieved with the SAD strain vaccines. Rupprecht *et al.*, (1986; 1988) confirmed a previous report (Baer, cited in Rupprecht *et al.*, 1988) that the ERA strain, effective by the oral route in red foxes (Lawson *et al.*, 1987) and by the intramuscular route in raccoons, did not protect by the oral route in raccoons. However, Schneider and Cox (1988) have demonstrated immuno-genicity of the SAD B19 strain in several species including the European martin, badger, wild boar, raccoon dog, domestic dog and pigs.

In summary, oral immunization against rabies can be successfully achieved in several species of wildlife with a live attenuated vaccine (SAD strain) and with a vaccinia recombinant virus vaccine. In spite of the risk of vaccine-induced rabies in non-target species with the SAD vaccines, Europe is well on the way to eradicating fox rabies without any evidence to date of this vaccine strain becoming established in nature. The apparently more broadly immunogenic vaccinia recombinant vaccines offer an alternative to live attenuated vaccines but they are not without their problems. There has been considerable international debate on the release of genetically engineered viruses and vaccines into the environment (Bishop, 1988). With the vaccinia recombinant rabies vaccine, concerns include safety and establishment in non-target species, long-term vaccine stability and public health issues (Rupprecht *et al.*, 1988). These concerns, although similar to those expressed about the widespread use of the attenuated SAD strain, deserve serious consideration given the extensive worldwide application such a vaccine could have. Nevertheless, genetic engineering offers the prospect of safe, broadly immunogenic and inexpensive oral rabies vaccines. A pragmatic, cautious but progressive approach is required whereby vaccinia recombinant virus vaccines, and indeed any other candidate vectors of the rabies glycoprotein, are evaluated as to their safety and efficacy in a wide range of target and non-target species, including humans.

Ironically, the oral rabies vaccine technology has, up to now, been directed towards controlling wildlife rabies in developed countries, whereas the vast majority of the world's rabies cases occur in dogs in developing countries. Both live attenuated SAD strain vaccines and recombinant DNA vaccines offer hopeful prospects for the control of dog rabies in the developing world (Perry, 1987), particularly for the dog populations whose unrestricted nature does not permit high levels of vaccination coverage by traditional injection techniques (Perry, Johnston *et al.*, 1988). Recent studies have indicated that the SAD B19 strain vaccine at high virus titre (10^8 TICD$_{50}$ per ml) will immunize dogs by the oral route (Schneider and Cox, 1988). In Tunisia, serological studies of dogs given this vaccine in the Tubinger Fox Bait have shown promising results (Schneider and Haddad, personal communication). In addition, a bait delivery system appropriate for dog populations has been tested in Zimbabwe (Perry, Brooks *et al.*, 1988). Chinese workers have also demonstrated that when a virus vaccine (designated CTN-1) attenuated by passage in adult mouse brain and human diploid cell cultures, was administered in dog food during house-to-house visits, 80–88% of over 19 000 dogs so immunized developed serum neutralizing antibodies (WHO, 1988).

PROGRESS IN BAIT DEVELOPMENT

BAIT

Following the initial studies of Debbie (1974), and Winkler and Baer (1976), using eggs and beef sausages, most of the bait systems tested have, like the vaccines, been directed at wildlife. The chicken-head bait developed in Switzerland has proved extremely effective as a bait for foxes. Even though the vaccine is contained within a separate 'blister pack' stapled under the skin of the head, it is readily presented to the oropharyngeal mucosa of the fox rather than being separated out and rejected.

Faced with vast areas over which foxes and skunks roamed, Canadian scientists turned to the concept of baits which were capable of being mass-produced, and distributed by aeroplanes rather than by hand. Initially, they studied 40 different bait types in captive animals (Johnston and Voigt, 1982) and selected a 30 g meatball in a plastic bag for more extensive field trials. This they distributed (without vaccine) by aeroplanes at varying target densities of baits per km^2 over an area of 50 000 hectares in five large scale field trials. Bait uptake rates of 63–74%, measured using the biomarker tetracycline, were achieved in target red fox populations. Rates of

25–57% were achieved in skunks and rates of 2–30% were achieved in raccoons (Johnston *et al.*, 1988).

Subsequent studies in Canada and the United States have examined the efficacy of man-made baits, particularly those based on a polyurethane sponge. A beef fat and wax coated polyurethane sponge bait of dimensions of $31 \times 31 \times 39$ mm has been shown to be an effective vehicle under laboratory conditions for delivering the live attenuated ERA vaccine to red foxes, (Lawson *et al.*, 1987) and the vaccinia recombinant rabies vaccine to raccoons (Rupprecht *et al.*, 1986). Initial field studies have given bait uptakes rates of 76% in raccoons following aerial dropping of these baits (again without vaccine) at densities of 120 per km^2 in Pennsylvania (Johnston, Voigt, MacInnes *et al.*, 1988). Hadidian *et al.*, (1988) distributed similar baits by hand in an urban national park in Washington DC at a density of 124 per km^2, and achieved a 63% bait uptake in the target raccoon population. Also in the eastern US, a non-coated polyurethane sponge, of dimensions $50 \times 35 \times 20$ mm enclosed in similar sized polyethylene sachets which were heat sealed, and contained in an outer polyethylene bag (15×15 cm) have been tested as a delivery system for raccoons (Perry, Garner *et al.*, 1988). These baits, containing a placebo and tetracycline as a biomarker, were distributed at bait densities of 120 and 450 per km^2 in two areas of Virginia. Bait uptake levels of 30.4–72.7% were recorded in the raccoon populations of these study sites.

This latter bait has also showed some promise as a delivery system for dogs in Africa (Perry *et al.*, 1988). In Zimbabwe, baits containing rhodamine B as a biomarker were distributed from bicycles in the vicinity of dwellings in two adjacent rural target areas; 79% of baits recovered 24 hours later had been significantly bitten and chewed, and 25% of dogs examined at the same time showed evidence of bait consumption.

In Germany, distribution of the SAD-B19 vaccine to foxes is now achieved using a manufactured fat-based bait (Tubinger Fox Bait) incorporating a fish meal attractant (Schneider and Cox, 1988). Vaccine is contained in a 'blister pack' within the bait, and uptake levels of around 78% have been achieved. This bait/vaccine combination has also been evaluated for use in dogs in Tunisia. Uptake rates of 32.4–51.7% have been reported there (Haddad, Matter and Schneider, personal communication).

ATTRACTANT

Suitable attractants, particularly important with manufactured baits such as the Tubinger Fox Bait and the polyurethane sponge baits, vary considerably from species to species. An attractant suitable for foxes will not necessarily be appropriate for raccoons or dogs. Generally, meat and fish based products have been found the most satisfactory for foxes and raccoons. Banana has also shown to be effective for raccoons (Rupprecht *et al.*, 1987). For dogs, an attractant originally developed for jackal traps (Foggin, 1988), prepared from a mixture of meat, offal, fish, blood, cheese and yeast and allowed to ferment and putrefy for several days at room temperature, proved extremely effective in field studies in Zimbabwe (Perry *et al.*, 1988). This attractant had the added quality of being repugnant to human beings, thus reducing the risk of baits and vaccine being inadvertently consumed by children.

Some attractants have been incorporated into the bait itself, such as the original Canadian polyurethane bait (with beef tallow) and the Tubinger Fox Bait (with fish meal). Others, such as the polyurethane sponge evaluated in raccoon and dog populations (Perry *et al.*, 1988; Perry, Brooks *et al.*, 1988; Perry, Johnston *et al.*, 1988) require the attractant to be contained in an outer plastic bag in close apposition to the bait but separated from it by its polypropylene sachet surround.

BIOMARKERS

In order to assess the uptake rate of a baiting system by a target population, it is necessary to incorporate a biomarker into the bait which can then be assayed in individual animals. Biomarkers which have been used in this context can generally be classified as surface markers, calciphilic markers and tissue markers. The surface marker commonly used has been rhodamine B, a potent stain which gives a vivid pink coloration to skin and mucous membranes for up to several days. It is useful as a preliminary indicator of bait attractiveness in cage trials and in field trials in dogs, where the acquisition of tooth or tissue samples is impractical. However, the duration of superficial staining is extremely variable.

Tetracycline is the calciphilic marker which has been widely used in the bait uptake studies in wildlife in Europe, Canada and the United States (Johnston *et al.*, 1987). Incorporation of approximately 150 mg oxytetracycline per bait will produce detectable deposits in tooth and bone within 48 hours, which will persist for years in adult animals. The disadvantage of the procedure is that a canine tooth and an adjacent portion of surrounding bone are required for the assay. This has meant that bait uptake studies have often been done in conjunction with the hunting season of the target wildlife species. Teeth and bone samples are then sectioned, and mounts of 60–150 microns examined under ultraviolet light on a microscope for the presence of fluorescing bands in the dentine and cementum layers of the teeth and adjacent bone (Johnston and Watt, 1981). Several bands may be seen in the growing teeth of juvenile animals, indicating multiple bait ingestion.

Tissue markers have been used very little in bait uptake studies but iophenoxic acid has recently been shown to be effective as a serum marker in carnivores (Baer *et al.*, 1985) and raccoons (Hadidian *et al.*, 1988). Iophenoxic acid is an organic iodine containing substance, previously used in human medicine as a diagnostic radiographic contrast agent. It can be detected by a serum iodine assay from 24 hours after oral ingestion, and persists for approximately eight weeks (Larson *et al.*, 1981). However, this method does not currently allow estimation of the number of baits ingested.

ACKNOWLEDGEMENTS

My colleagues David Johnston, Ministry of Natural Resources, Ontario, Canada; Suzanne Jenkins, Department of Health, Virginia, USA and Chris Foggin, Veterinary Research Laboratory, Harare, Zimbabwe have provided support, advice and collaboration in many ways, for which I am sincerely grateful.

REFERENCES

Abelseth, M. K. (1964) An attenuated rabies vaccine for domestic animals produced in tissue culture. *Can. Vet. J.,* **5,** 279–286

Bacon, P. J. and Macdonald, D. W. (1980) To control rabies: vaccinate foxes. *New Scientist,* **87,** 640–645

Baer, G. M., Abelseth, M. K. and Debbie, J. G. (1971) Oral vaccination of foxes against rabies. *Am. J. Epidemiol,* **93,** 487–490

Baer, G. M., Broderson, R. W. and Yager, P. A. (1975) Determination of the site of oral rabies vaccination. *Am. J. Epidemiol.,* **101,** 101–164

Baer, G. M., Shaddock, J. H., Hayes, D. J. and Savarie, P. (1985) Iophenoxic acid as a serum marker in carnivores. *J. Wildlife Management,* **49,** 49–51

Bishop, D. H. L. (1988) The release into the environment of genetically engineered viruses, vaccines and pesticides. *Trends in Ecology and Evolution,* **3,** 512–515

Black, J. G. and Lawson, K. F. (1970). Sylvatic rabies studies in the silver fox (*Vulpes vulpes*). Susceptibility and immune response. *Can. J. Comp. Med.,* **34,** 309–311

Black, J. G. and Lawson, K. F. (1973). Further studies of sylvatic rabies in the fox (*Vulpes vulpes*); vaccination by the oral route. *Can. Vet. J.* **14,** 206–211

Blancou, J., Kieny, M. P., Lathe, R., Lecocq, J. P., Pastoret, P. P., Soulebot, J. P. and Desmettre, P. (1986) Oral vaccination of the fox against rabies using a live recombinant vaccinia virus. *Nature,* **322,** 373–375

Correa-Giron, E. P., Allen, R., and Sulkin, S. E. (1970) The infectivity and pathogenesis of rabies virus administered orally. *Am. J. Epidemiol.,* **91,** 203–215

Crick, J. and Brown, F. (1969) Viral subunits for rabies vaccination. *Nature,* **222,** 92

Crick, J. (1981) Rabies. In *Virus Diseases of Food Animals,* Vol. 2 (Ed. E. P. J. Gibbs). Academic Press, London, pp. 469–516

Debbie, J. G. (1974). Use of inoculated eggs as a vehicle for the oral rabies vaccination of red foxes (*Vulpes fulva*). *Infection and Immunity,* **9,** 681–683

Debbie, J. G., Abelseth, M. K. and Baer, G. M. (1972) The use of commercially available vaccines for the oral vaccination of foxes against rabies. *Am. J. Epidemiol.* **96,** 231–235

Foggin, C. M. (1988) *Rabies and rabies-related viruses in Zimbabwe: historical, virological and ecological aspects.* Unpublished D. Phil thesis, University of Zimbabwe

Habel, K. (1945) Evaluation of a mouse test for the standardization of the immunising power of antirabies vaccines. *Public Health Reports,* **55,** 1473–1487

Hadidian, J., Jenkins, S. R., Johnston, D., Savarie, P. J., Nettles, V. F., Manski, D. and Baer, G. M. (1988) Oral bait acceptance in an urban raccoon population (Carnivora: Procyonidae). *J. Wildlife Diseases,* in press

Hafliger, U., Bichsel, P., Wandeler, A. and Steck, F. (1982) Zur oralen Immunisierung von Fuchsen gegen Tollwut: Stabilisiering und Koderapplikation des Impfvirus. *Zentralblatt fur Veterinaermedizin, Reihe B,* **29,** 604–618

Johnston, D. H. (1975) Principles of wild carnivore baiting with oral vaccines. WHO consultations in oral vaccination of foxes, Document No. 7, World Health Organisation, Geneva, 12 pp

Johnston, D. H. and Watt, I. D. (1981) A rapid method for sectioning undecalcified carnivore teeth for aging. In *Proceedings of Worldwide Furbearer Conference* (Annapolis, Maryland) (Eds J. A. Chapman and D Pursley) pp. 407–422

Johnston, D. H. and Voigt, D. R. (1982). A baiting system for the oral rabies vaccination of wild foxes and skunks. *Comp. Immunol. Microbiol. Infectious Diseases,* **5,** 185–186

Johnston, D. H., Joachim, D. G., Bachmann, P., Kardong, K. V., Stewart, R. E. A., Dix, L. M., Strickland, M. A. and Watt, I. D. (1987) Aging furbearers using tooth structure and biomarkers. In *Wild furbearer management and conservation in North America* (Eds M. Novak, J. A. Baker, M. E. Obbard and B. Malloch). Ontario Trappers Association, North Bay, Ontario, Canada, pp. 228–243

Johnston, D. H., Voigt, D. R., Matejka, F. O., Bachmann, P., Watt, I. D., MacInnes, C. D., Eare, B. D. and Rosatte, R. C. (1988) A baiting system to distribute rabies vaccine to wild carnivores by aircraft. *Wildlife Society Bulletin,* in press

Johnston, D., Voigt, D. R., MacInnes, C. D., Bachmann, P., Lawson, K. F. and Rupprecht, C. E. (1988) An aerial baiting system for attenuated recombinant rabies vaccines for foxes, raccoons and skunks. *Rev. Infectious Disease*, in press

Kieny, M. P., Lathe, R., Drillien, R., Spehner, D., Skory, S., Schmitt, D., Wiktor, T., Koprowski, H., and Lecocq, J. P. (1984) Expression of rabies virus glycoprotein from a recombinant vaccinia virus. *Nature*, **312**, 163–166

Koprowski, H. and Cox, H. R. (1948) Studies on chick embryo adapted rabies virus 1. Culture characteristics and pathogenicity. *J. Immunol.* **60**, 533–554

Larson, G. E., Savarie, P. J. and Okuno, I. (1981) Iophenoxic acid and Mirex for marking wild, bait-consuming animals. *J. Wildlife Management*, **45**, 1073–1077

Lawson, K. F., Johnston, D. H., Patterson, J. M., Black, J. G., Rhodes, A. J. and Zalan, E. (1982) Immunisation of foxes (*Vulpes vulpes*) by the oral and intramuscular routes with inactivated rabies vaccines. *Can. J. Comp. Med.*, **46**, 382–385

Lawson, K. F., Black, J. G., Charlton, K. M., Johnston, D. H. and Rhodes, A. J. (1987) Safety and immunogenicity of vaccine bait containing ERA strain of attenuated rabies virus. *Can. J. Vet. Res.*, **51**, 460–464

Perry, B. D. (1987) The control of rabies. *Trends in Ecology and Evolution*, **2**, 30–31

Perry, B. D., Brooks, R., Foggin, C. M., Bleakley, J., Johnston, D. H. and Hill, F. W. G. (1988) A baiting system suitable for the delivery of oral rabies vaccine to dog populations in Zimbabwe. *Vet. Rec.*, **123**, 76–79

Perry, B. D., Johnston, D. H., Jenkins, S. R., Foggin, C. M., Bleakley, J and Garner, N. (1988). Studies on the delivery of oral rabies vaccines to wildlife and dog populations. *Acta Veterinaria Scandinavia* (Suppl.), in press

Perry, B. D., Garner, N., Jenkins, S. R., McCloskey, K., and Johnston, D. H. (1988). A study of techniques for the distribution of oral rabies vaccine to wild raccoon populations. *J. Wildlife Diseases*, in press

Ramsden, R. O. and Johnston, D. H. (1975) Studies on the oral infectivity of rabies virus in Carnivora. *J. Wildlife Diseases*, **11**, 318–324

Rupprecht, C. E., Wiktor, T. J., Johnston, D. H., Hamir, A. N., Dietzschold, B., Wunner, W. H., Glickman, L. T. and Koprowski, H. (1986) Oral immunisation and protection of raccoons (*Procyon lotor*) with a vaccinia-rabies glycoprotein recombinant virus vaccine. *Proc. National Academy of Science, USA*, **83**, 7947–7950

Rupprecht, C. E., Dietzschold, B., Koprowski, H. and Johnston, D. H. (1987) Development of an oral wildlife rabies vaccine: immunisation of raccoons by a vaccinia-rabies glycoprotein recombinant virus and preliminary field baiting trials. In *Vaccines, 87: Modern Approaches to New Vaccines* (Eds R. M. Chanock, R. A. Lerner, F. Brown and H. Ginsberg). Cold Spring Harbor Laboratory, New York, pp. 389–92

Rupprect, C. E., Hamir, A. N., Johnston, D. H. and Koprowski, H. (1988). Efficacy of a vaccinia-rabies glycoprotein recombinant virus vaccine in raccoons (*Procyon lotor*). *Rev. Infectious Disease*, in press

Schneider, L. G., Wachendorfer, G., Schmittdiel, E. and Cox, J. H. (1983) Ein Feldversuch zur oralen Immunisierung von Fuchsen gegen Tollwut in der Bundesrepulik Deutschland. II. Plannung, Durchfuhrung und Auswertung des Feldversuch. *Tieraerztliche Umschau*, **38**, 476–480

Schneider, L. G. and Cox, J. H. (1988). Eradication of rabies through oral vaccination: the German field trial. *Rev. Infectious disease*, in press

Steck, F. and Wandeler, A. (1982) The epidemiology of fox rabies in Europe. *Epidemiologic Rev.*, **2**, 71–96

Steck, F., Wandeler, A., Bichsel, P., Capt, S., Hafliger, U. and Schneider, L. (1982) Oral immunisation of foxes against rabies: laboratory and field studies. *Comparative Immunology, Microbiol. and Infectious Disease*, **5**, 165–171

Tolson, N., Charlton, K. M., Stewart, R. M., Campbell, J. B. and Wiktor, T. J. (1987) Immune response in skunks to a vaccinia virus recombinant expressing the rabies virus glycoprotein. *Can. J. Vet. Res.*, **51**, 363–366

Wandeler, A. (1988). Control of Wildlife Rabies: Europe. In *Rabies* (Eds J. B. Campbell and K. M. Charlton) Kluwer Academic Publications, Boston, pp. 365–380

Wandeler, A., Bander, W., Prochaska, S., and Steck, F. (1982) Small mammal studies in a SAD baiting area. *Comp. Immunol., Microbiol. and Infectious Diseases,* **5,** 171–176

Wandeler, A., Capt, S., Kappeler, A. and Hanser, R. (1988). Oral immunisation of wildlife against rabies: concepts and first field experiments. *Rev. Infectious Diseases,* in press

WHO (1988). Report of WHO consultation on oral immunisation of dogs against rabies. *Document Rab. Res.* **88.26**, WHO, Geneva, 11 pp.

Wiktor, T. J. (1985) Historical aspects of rabies treatment. In *World's Debt to Pasteur* (Eds H. Koprowski and S. A. Plotkin). Alan R. Liss Inc., New York, pp. 141–151

Wiktor, T. J., Macfarlan, R. I., Reagan, K. J., Dietzschold, B., Curtis, P. J., Wunner, W. H. Kieny, M-P., Lathe, R., Lecocq, J-P., Mackett, M., Moss, B. and Koprowski, H. (1984) Protection from rabies by a vaccinie virus recombinant containing the rabies virus glycoprotein gene. *Proc. Nat. Acad. Sci.,* USA, **81,** 7194–7194

Wiktor, T. J., Macfarlan, R. I., Dietzschold, B., Rupprecht, C. E. and Wunner, W. H. (1985) Immunogenic properties of vaccinia recombinant virus expressing the rabies glycoprotein. *Annales de L'Institut Pasteur. Virologie.* **136E,** 405–511

Winkler, W. G. (1983). Rabies control for domestic animals. In *Report on Rabies.* Fromm Laboratories, New Jersey, pp. 17–22

Winkler, W. G., McLean, R. G. and Cowart, J. C. (1975) Vaccination of foxes against rabies using ingested baits. *J. Wildlife Diseases,* **11,** 382–388

Winkler, W. G. and Baer, G. M. (1976) Rabies immunisation in red foxes (*Vulpes vulpes*) with vaccine in sausage baits. *Am. J. Epidemiol.,* **103,** 408–415

Winkler, W. G., Shaddock, J. H. and Williams, L. W. (1976) Oral rabies vaccine: Evaluation of its infectivity in three species of rodents. *Am. J. Epidemiol.,* **104,** 294–298

A. R. MICHELL

Shock in companion animals

INTRODUCTION

SHOCK IS a form of circulatory failure characterized by inadequate capillary perfusion and its adverse systematic effects. Frequently, but not invariably, cardiac output is also reduced. Fundamentally, shock is a caricature of the physiological response to haemorrhage. It has all the recognizable features but they are exaggerated to an absurd and damaging degree. The underlying pathophysiology has been reviewed in some detail comparatively recently (Michell, 1985) and is only summarized here together with its therapeutic implications. Treatment of shock has also been reviewed recently (Michell *et al.*, 1988) and most of this chapter is therefore concerned with newer developments rather than an exhaustive reiteration of details.

Research on shock is profuse, sometimes savage and draws essentially on three pools:
1. Human clinical experience.
2. Veterinary clinical experience.
3. Animal experiments, frequently aimed at human medicine.

The caveats are obvious. The dominant features of shock are probably similar in all species but the details differ, for example, cats are more vulnerable to pulmonary oedema as a result of high infusion rates compared with dogs or humans (Mitchell *et al*, 1988). Dogs are peculiarly susceptible to gastrointestinal damage as a result of shock, to the extent that shock may cause intestinal haemorrhage as well as resulting from it (Hardie and Rawlings, 1983; Michell, 1985). The pattern of response to endotoxin shock, haemorrhagic shock and to anaphylactic shock is species-specific, particularly the vascular beds which are primarily affected (Collins, 1982; Bone *et al.*, 1987). Thus ponies happen to provide an excellent model for human septic shock (Sembrat *et al.*, 1979).

Mention of the different types of shock serves to emphasize that they are not the same, though they have sufficient in common for hypovolaemic shock to serve as a basic model for understanding shock in general. Hypovolaemic shock is often encountered as haemorrhagic or traumatic shock. Although they are overwhelmingly similar, even these three types of shock are not identical. For example, severe diarrhoea causes hypovolaemic shock but no loss of red cells (RBC). Traumatic shock usually, but not necessarily, involves haemorrhage. For example, there is often no haemorrhage associated with burns. Traumatic shock includes additional features due to tissue damage. Many of these increase the risk of pulmonary oedema (Pretorius *et al.*, 1987). Nevertheless, the pathophysiology of shock is best understood by considering hypovolaemic shock and perceiving that many of its

48

features originate as responses appropriate to the physiological defence against haemorrhage and its consequences.

PATHOPHYSIOLOGY

Established shock is characterized by vicious cycles (positive feedback loops) so that the longer it exists, the more it tends to progress. Most of these maladaptive and potentially lethal responses are based on appropriate responses to haemorrhage but they are too widespread and sustained for too long. They primarily involve the circulatory system including the vessels, the heart and the blood itself, which deteriorates in both composition and viscosity. There are also profound changes in cellular metabolism and organ function with particular impact on the heart, the liver, pancreas and intestine, and the lungs.

Most successful therapy is based on restoration of circulating volume, correction of cardiovascular function and, particularly, improvement of capillary perfusion. Nevertheless, these measures alone will still leave many individuals in a condition of irreversible shock. The emphasis in recent years has been on a better understanding, and therefore better treatment, of the cellular and metabolic changes (Michell, 1985). Whatever the therapeutic strategy, urgency remains the overriding priority.

The cellular changes include depression of both the metabolic and reticulo-endothelial functions of the liver, failure of cells to maintain their normal low sodium content and, as a result, cell swelling and leakage of potassium (Shires, 1984; Heath, 1985; Schumer, 1986; Kirby, 1987). The resulting hyperkalaemia is often exacerbated by acidosis, particularly lactic acidosis. Both adversely affect cardiac function (Horton, 1987a; Nagy, 1987). The presence of lactic acidosis can be conveniently assessed from the 'anion gap' and this may be a helpful contribution in prognosis (Gossett *et al.*, 1987). The cardiac changes include alterations in membrane permeability and cell volume within the myocardium and endocardium (Horton, 1987b). Even in septic shock, where cardiac output is often increased initially, cardiac efficiency is already reduced in the early stages (Rackow *et al.*, 1987). Among the contributory factors is the production of a potent myocardial depressant factor or factors (MDF) in most forms of shock, in most species studied (including dogs, cats and humans). This same factor depresses reticulo-endothelial function. It originates from the pancreas as a result of ischaemic damage caused by excessive vasoconstriction (Lefer, 1987).

Not surprisingly, acute pancreatitis is a potent cause of shock, which itself causes further pancreatic ischaemia. The result is a drastic reduction of cardiac output, circulating volume and renal function. The hypovolaemia results from changes in capillary permeability caused by circulating mediators and a specific benefit of the therapeutic use of plasma in the treatment of acute pancreatitis in that it contains factors which inhibit the formation of these mediators (Levy, 1986).

MEDIATORS

Among the other mediators involved in shock, attention has recently focused on tumour necrosis factor (TNF) which may underlie many of the features of endotoxin shock (Mannel, 1987) and the production of free radicals and activated forms of oxygen (H_2O_2, superoxides), especially from macrophages (Lee *et al.*, 1987; Till and

Ward, 1987; Floke, 1987). These may be particularly involved in pulmonary damage associated with shock (Trabe, 1985; Schumer, 1986). The possible beneficial effects of antioxidant drugs are already being tested (Ortolani *et al.*, 1987). Free radicals are, however, a very fashionable area of research and some consider that their importance in shock may have been exaggerated (Horton and Borman, 1987).

The possibility that histamine may be an important factor causing organ damage in various forms of shock, notably endotoxin shock in cats is increased by the suggestion that it may be locally generated in tissues, independent of mast cell activity (Parratt *et al.*, 1986). Nevertheless, anaphylactic shock remains the only form in which the role of histamine is well established (Neugebauer and Lorenz, 1987). The role of prostaglandins also remains uncertain because they have both beneficial and adverse effects in shock, though those of other eicosanoids, notably thromboxane A, are mainly detrimental. Not surprisingly, the usefulness of non-steroidal anti-inflammatory drugs for therapy remains ambiguous. Their main role seems to be in endotoxin shock and even this is not yet clear (Feuer-Stein and Hattenbeck, 1987).

VASOCONSTRICTION

Among these uncertainties, the fact that the central common feature in most forms of shock is excessive vasoconstriction remains essentially unchallenged (Hardaway, 1985; Shoemaker, 1987). It may not be present in the initial stages of endotoxin shock because this hyperdynamic phase involves wasteful overperfusion of areas affected by bacteria or toxins. Maintenance of arterial pressure imposes a need for vasoconstriction in other areas. Later, peripheral pooling so impedes venous return that this becomes the main factor underlying the reduced cardiac output of the hypodynamic phase. Restoration of *circulating* volume thus becomes an essential feature of treatment (Vincent *et al.*, 1987). Hypovolaemia also results from increased capillary permeability in endotoxin and septic shock. Hypoglycaemia is also a prominent feature (McAnulty, 1982; Heath, 1985). The distinction between endo-toxic or septic shock and haemorrhagic shock are blurred by the fact that intestinal ischaemia leads to invasion by enteric bacteria and bacteraemia is a common feature (Koziol *et al.*, 1988). Once again, the cause is excessive vasoconstriction and there is no role for vasoconstrictors in the treatment of shock except where all other measures fail to relieve hypotension or where they are used in low doses for their stimulating effect on the heart (Desjars *et al.*, 1987; Melchior *et al.*, 1987).

Vasopressin (ADH) is increased during shock. Its constrictor effects are initially beneficial by reducing splanchnic pooling but ultimately the effects become det-rimental and antagonists prolong survival in experimental shock models in dogs (Cronnenwett *et al.*, 1986).

BLOOD AND CIRCULATORY CHANGES

Not only the heart and vessels are adversely affected in shock but also blood itself. It is a thixotropic liquid, i.e. its viscosity increases when it ceases to flow. This is beneficial in a non-drip paint but disastrous in stagnant capillary beds! The viscosity of blood is greatly increased by a rising packed cell volume but plasma viscosity also rises in shock. Albumin and Dextran 40 are particularly *good* colloids for improving viscosity (Chien *et al.*, 1987). The other adverse change in blood is disseminated intravascular coagulation (DIC) which leads to further capillary damage and ultimately to a consumptive coagulopathy, i.e. inability to clot due to consumption of the necessary precursors. DIC is particularly associated with tissue damage, septic shock or the use of badly stored blood (Hardaway, 1985; Bennett and Towler, 1985; Heene *et al.*, 1986; Chien *et al.*, 1987).

Doubts have recently been raised about two commonly used clinical guides to the assessment of shock which are based on the cardiovascular changes. First, although the usual shock case has a rapid pulse, bradycardia is possible in acute severe haemorrhage (Barriot and Riou, 1987). Second, although vasoconstriction commonly leads to cold extremities and thus a widened gap between core temperature and peripheral temperature, even where core temperature falls, as it often does in shock, this core peripheral temperature gradient can no longer be regarded as a good guide to the severity of shock, at least in humans (Woods *et al.*, 1987). It correlates with neither cardiac output nor peripheral resistance, nor with their changes in individual cases.

The therapeutic implications of the pathophysiology are considered below.

RESTORATION OF CIRCULATING VOLUME

There are three questions which underlie most of the controversies in this area.
1. How important is blood in the treatment of haemorrhagic shock?
2. What are the relative merits of colloids and electrolyte solutions in treating hypovolaemia?
3. How should the acidosis be corrected?

The latter is a relatively simple matter and has recently been discussed in detail (Michell, 1988; Michell *et al.*, 1988). Suffice to say that although restoration of circulating volume, in itself, improves the acidosis by restoring renal hepatic perfusion, it is counter-productive to do this with a solution devoid of bicarbonate or its precursors. Among these, lactate is the most familiar (as in Hartmann's solution, *lactated* Ringer's). The merits of bicarbonate versus precursors are discussed in the reviews mentioned above.

The question of blood transfusion remains lively though the arguments have long been plain. The controversy, if there is one, is sustained by the human weakness for simple escapes from complicated problems. The fact that blood is lost does not make blood the ideal replacement fluid even in haemorrhagic shock (Michell, 1985), any more than the main priority for the victim of a cliff fall is climbing back to the top. The event changes the circumstances.

'Haemorrhage is much more than the temporary loss of circulating blood volume. It is properly and necessarily considered as a systemic disease...' (Collins, 1982). The problem in shock is not the loss of RBC but the fact that vasoconstriction and changes in viscosity make it almost impossible for them to circulate efficiently. There is, therefore, no advantage in a *PCV* above 30 units; there are possible adverse effects, notably on viscosity (Messmer, 1984; Hunt *el al.*, 1986; Fortune *et al.*, 1987). Thus a 30% loss of RBC is trivial in its effects whereas a 30% loss of plasma volume is disastrous (Muir, 1987). The exceptions are where pre-existing disease interferes with oxygenation so that the concentration of RBC becomes more important. Where transfusion is used, it should be aimed at restoring adequate haemoglobin, with other fluids used to restore circulating volume. Recently there has been a resurgence of interest in the re-use of the animal's own blood to deal with surgical haemorrhage (autotransfusion) (Patterson, 1987; Michell *et al.*, 1988).

The great debate on the relative merits of electrolyte or colloid solutions is similarly somewhat artificial. Colloids are clearly better than electrolytes at repairing *circulating* volume instead of ECF as a whole (Shoemaker, 1986; Michell *et al.*, 1988) and that is the primary concern in treating shock. Interstitial fluid, however, is also depleted and is the communication between the capillaries and the cells. It becomes a barrier if it is excessively depleted or expanded in volume (Demling, 1986; Kirby, 1987). Since colloids are more expensive, both the rationale and the economics support the use of both types of fluid (Smith and Norman, 1982), neither in excess.

Among the available artificial colloids, Dextran 40, Dextran 70 and Haemaccel (gelatin) are the most familiar (Michell *et al.*, 1988). They are less effective than albumin in boosting plasma volume, because they are uncharged (Michell, 1988) but they have other merits, including the beneficial effects of Dextran 40 on capillary bloodflow and the protective effects of Dextran 70 against pulmonary entrapment of potentially damaging agents including granulocytes (Modig, 1988). Dextran 70 can even give better correction of metabolic acidosis than acetated Ringer's solution, despite the latter's content of bicarbonate precursor.

The importance of Dextran 40 and 70 as allergens has been exaggerated (Michell, 1988). Their antigenicity has been reduced (Gammage, 1987) and the effect can be prevented by pre-injection of very low molecular weight dextran (Michell *et al.*, 1988). Hydroxyethyl starch is non-antigenic, and has no adverse effects on clotting or cross-matching (Gammage, 1987). However, any colloid will eventually impede clotting by causing haemodilution, hence the wisdom of keeping the dose below 20 ml/kg (20% of blood volume).

Gelatin, the most widely used colloid in veterinary practice, has neither the persistence of Dextran 70 nor the specific effects on capillary perfusion of Dextran 40. It may cause fewer side effects (which are few anyway) and it does not interfere with blood typing or cross-matching.

During intestinal obstruction, colloids have the particular advantage of not leaking into the gut lumen (Michell, 1988). The really contentious question in comparing colloids and crystalloids (electrolyte solutions), however, is which is more likely to cause/avoid pulmonary oedema?

PULMONARY OEDEMA

It used to be thought that the main cause of pulmonary oedema in shock (shock-lung, ARDS, etc.) was excessive use of electrolyte solutions. They certainly cause peripheral oedema but the factors leading to pulmonary oedema are rather different (Michell, 1985; Demling, 1986; Gammage, 1987). In particular, dilution of plasma albumin by crystalloids is not a potent factor. However, colloid leakage or excessive venous pressure are both potentially important, the latter because it impedes lymphatic drainage (Allen *et al.*, 1987) as well as raising capillary pressure.

The alveolar space is better protected against oedema than the pulmonary interstitial space but interstitial oedema has little effect on gas exchange and causes few clinical signs until it is advanced, when alveolar flooding occurs (Geiger, 1986). A more potent interference with pulmonary gas exchange in shock comes from loss of surfactant, collapse of alveoli and thus the shunting of 'venous' blood into the systemic arterial supply (Schumer, 1986; Seeger, 1987). Where pulmonary oedema does occur the main factor is not normally excessive infusion rates but the damaging effects on the lungs of tissue trauma, haemolysed blood or endotoxin (McAnulty, 1982; Seeger, 1987; Hardaway and Williams, 1987). Indeed, trauma causes damage which is detectable by conventional and electron microscopy before any change in X-rays or blood gases is apparent (Pretorius *et al.*, 1986). One fairly definite benefit of corticosteroids in the treatment of shock is that they help to prevent pulmonary oedema (Geiger, 1986).

Thus despite their greater ability to repair circulating volume (indeed because of it) colloids are not actually significantly safer than electrolytes with regard to pulmonary oedema. Electrolytes may be just as effective in improving pulmonary circulation (Pearl *et al.*, 1988). Ultimately, however, excessive infusion rates will cause pulmonary oedema with either type of solution, especially if there is pre-existing cardiac or respiratory dysfunction. Dogs are relatively resistant to the adverse effects of high infusion rates, perhaps because they tend to clear circulating bacteria via the liver rather than the lungs and thereby have some protection against one factor contributing to pulmonary oedema (Hardie and Rawlings, 1983). Cats, on the other hand, can only tolerate much lower infusion rates (Kitchell and Haskins, 1984; Boothe *et al.*, 1985).

CORTICOSTEROIDS IN SHOCK

There is no likelihood that corticosteroids have any useful effect on shock except at very high doses (pharmacological doses), repeated if necessary, and begun as early as possible. Even then, there is a conflict between a strong body of clinical opinion, both medical and veterinary, that they are useful, especially in endotoxin shock and there is an almost total lack of convincing evidence from adequately designed trials (Michell, 1985). Indeed, there is only one prospective randomized trial in humans with septic shock and a recent attempt to duplicate it failed (Kirby, 1987).

Yet the theoretical advantages based on the pharmacology of corticosteroids make them appear almost unbelievably appropriate to the treatment of shock, lacking only the ability to repair circulating volume (Bowen, 1980; Michell, 1985). They improve cardiac output, peripheral perfusion, prevent pulmonary oedema, reduce the release of MDF and protect cells and their membranes from some of the metabolic and permeability effects of shock. They are theoretically ideal but, after some 35 years, still practically unproven. The likely effectiveness of a particular steroid depends on the salt which is used, e.g. methylprednisolone is more effective as succinate than phosphate (Shafney *et al.*, 1982). The reason for the massive doses required in shock may be that, at least in experimental canine septic shock, there is a reduced population of glucocorticoid receptors. The same is true in human patients (Zonghai *et al.*, 1987). There was, until recently, little likelihood that corticosteroids did harm (Schumer, 1987), except possibly in some horses, e.g. by causing laminitis (Muir, 1987). Now, however, they are regarded as contraindicated in human patients with evidence of renal failure or endotoxin shock (Bone *et al*, 1987*b*). This is extremely worrying since it was the one condition in which anything other than clinical impressions or pharmacological theory stood in their favour.

The central problem in evaluating corticosteroids for the treatment of shock remains unchanged and applies to other drugs, notably non-steroidal anti-inflammatory drugs (NSAID). Studies still confuse the ability to prevent shock by pretreatment with the ability to remedy established shock (Michell, 1985; Hardaway and Williams, 1987). In experiments with endotoxic shock, animals frequently receive steroids within 15 minutes (White *et al.*, 1982). Few clinical cases will be so fortunate unless their veterinarian is a clairvoyant with a very fast car. Similarly, a recent study of the effect of ibuprofen on endotoxin shock in dogs used it either as pretreatment, or within 30 minutes of the introduction of endotoxin (Beck and Abel, 1987).

OTHER THERAPEUTIC MEASURES

NALOXONE

Following a strong growth in the belief that β-endorphins are important mediators in shock and that naloxone provides a useful component of its treatment, doubts have appeared. In dogs with haemorrhagic shock it appeared to confer no additional benefit to fluid therapy alone (Wagner-Mann and Gross, 1986; Gin *et al.*, 1987). In humans it appeared to have neither adverse nor beneficial effects. However, species differences may be important. Thus the main effect in cats is apparently to reduce MDF whereas in dogs there is a direct increase in cardiac output. Moreover, in the human study naloxone was used after a considerable delay (Allolio *et al.*, 1987). Another study of haemorrhagic shock in the dog saw improvements in arterial pressure through increased peripheral resistance, rather than cardiac output (Tooth, 1986). Because perfusion is the central problem in shock, improvement of arterial pressure is preferably achieved through increased cardiac output. The mode of action of naloxone apparently differs in haemorrhagic and endotoxin shock (Gurll *et al.*, 1987). A possible drawback of naloxone in some cases of shock would be to oppose the reduction in pain sensitivity which often occurs.

NSAID

In ponies, flunixin improved pulmonary circulation and prolonged survival compared with corticosteroids. However, this difference was not statistically significant and the steroids were not used at high doses (Templeton *et al.*, 1987). Other studies suggest that flunixin is beneficial in equine shock (Muir, 1987). In dogs, ibuprofen improved arterial pressure in experimental haemorrhagic shock but did so via peripheral resistance and failed to improve cardiac performance. Survival was not increased (Beamer *et al.*, 1987). Dogs may be susceptible to overdosage with ibuprofen, resulting in gastrointestinal haemorrhage (England, 1987).

HYPERTONIC SALINE

Substantial evidence has accumulated to suggest that small volumes of hypertonic saline provide a useful treatment for shock by acting via cardiovascular reflexes rather than replacement of circulating volume (Michell, 1985). This is, therefore, quite different from conventional fluid therapy. Despite a recent study of endotoxin shock in dogs in which the effects were short-lived and less satisfactory than

Hartmann's solution (Prough *et al.*, 1986), another study showed improved cardiac output and oxygen consumption in dogs with severe endotoxin shock (Luypaert *et al.*, 1986). In cats with experimental haemorrhagic shock, hypertonic saline reduced the production of MDF and, in combination with restoration of circulating volume, was a useful adjunct to treatment (Bitterman *et al.*, 1987). It remains to be seen whether hypertonic saline becomes established as part of the routine therapy for shock; if so, it will be relatively safe, simple and inexpensive.

ANTIBIOTICS

The importance of antibiotics arises from the fact that even in the absence of endotoxin shock or contaminated wounds, invasion by normal constituents of the gut flora is likely during shock. These invaders will not be subject to the normal defence offered by the liver and its reticulo-endothelial cells. Antibiotics are probably beneficial in hypovolaemic shock and essential in endotoxin or septic shock (Michell *et al.*, 1988). This is true despite the likelihood of increasing the release of endotoxin; the benefit arises from reducing the source (Shenep and Morgan, 1984; Jacobson and Young, 1985; Muir, 1987).

CONCLUSION

A variety of other measures have been suggested or tried in the treatment of shock, including positive inotropic agents, antihistamines, and adenosine triphosphate (ATP) (Michell, 1985). Real progress will occur when drugs become available to correct the cellular disturbance associated with shock and to restore the full protective function of the reticulo-endothelial system. In the foreseeable future the main and inescapable priority in treating shock will remain early, adequate and appropriate fluid therapy. Solutions to repair extracellular volume must contain plasma-like concentrations of sodium (Michell *et al.*, 1988). Further research is needed to clarify the importance of glucose in the treatment of shock, especially endotoxin shock with its tendency to progress rapidly towards hypoglycaemia.

Perhaps the real advance in the treatment of clinical cases of shock in animals will come when artificial blood becomes widely available at reasonable cost. There is a long way to go because current products require an oxygen-enriched atmosphere. The growing problems with using blood in humans, however, make it certain that the development of convenient, inexpensive substitutes will continue to be a high priority. When they appear they are likely to be usable in all species and to have better flow characteristics than blood itself.

REFERENCES

Allen, S. J., Drake, R. E., Williams, J. P., Laine, G. A. and Gabel, J. C. (1987) Recent advances in pulmonary edema. *Crit. Care Med.,* **15,** 923–929

Allolio, B., Fischer, H., Kaulen, D., Deuss, U. and Winkelmann, W. (1987) Naloxone in treatment of circulatory shock resistant to conventional therapy. *Klin. Wochenschr.,* **65,** 213–217

Barriot, P. and Riou, B. (1987) Hemorrhagic shock with paradoxical bradycardia. *Intensive Care Med.,* **13,** 203–207.

Beamer, K. C., Daly, T. and Vargish, T. (1987) Hemodynamic evaluation of ibuprofen in canine hypovolaemic shock. *Circ. Shock,* **23,** 51–57

Beck, R. R. and Abel, F. L. (1987) Effect of ibuprofen on the course of canine endotoxin shock. *Circ. Shock,* **23,** 59–70

Bennett, B. and Towler, H. M. (1985) Haemostatic response to trauma. *Br. Med. Bull.* **41,** 274–280

Bitterman, H. B., Triolo, J. and Lefer, A. M. (1987) Use of hypertonic saline in the treatment of hemorrhagic shock. *Circ. Shock,* **21,** 271–283

Bone, R. C., Jacobs, E. R. and Wilson, F. J. (1987) Increased hemodynamic and survival with endotoxin and septic shock with ibuprofen treatment. In *First Vienna Shock Forum (A)* (Ed. G. Schlag and H. Redl) Alan Liss, New York, pp. 327–332

Bone, R. C., Fisher, C. J., Clemmer, T. P., Slotman, G. J., Metz, C. A. and Balk, R. A. (1987*b*). A controlled clinical trial of high dose methyl prednisolone in the treatment of severe sepsis and septic shock. *New Eng. J. Med.* **317,** 653–665

Boothe, H. W., Clark, D. R. and Merton, D. A. (1985) Cardiovascular effects of rapid infusion of crystalloid in the hypovolaemic cat. *J. Sm. Anim. Pract.,* **26,** 477–489

Bowen, J. M. (1980) Are corticosteroids useful in shock therapy? *J. Am. Vet. Med. Assoc.,* **177,** 453–455

Chien, S., Dormondy, J., Ernst, E. and Matrai, A. (1987) *Clinical Hemorheology.* Martinus Nijhoff, pp. 311–338

Collins, J. A. (1982) Pathophysiology of haemorrhagic shock. *Prog. Clin. Biol. Res.,* **108,** 5–29

Cronnenwett, J. L., Bauer-Neff, B. S., Grekin, R. and Sheagren, J. N. (1986) The role of endorphins and vasopressin in canine endotoxic shock. *J. Surg. Res.,* **41,** 609–619

Demling, R. H. (1986) Effect of plasma and interstitial protein content on tissue oedema formation. *Current Studies in Haematology and Blood Transfusion,* **53,** 36–52

Desjars, P., Pinaud, M., Potel, G., Tasseau, F. and Touze, M. D. (1987) A reappraisal of norepinephrine therapy in human septic shock. *Crit. Care Med.,* **15,** 134–137

England, G. C. W. (1987) Suspected flurbiprofen toxicity and its treatment in a dog. *Vet. Rec.,* **120,** 599–560

Feuer-Stein, G. and Hallenbeck, J. M. (1987) Prostaglandine, leukotrienes and platelet activating factor in shock. *Ann. Rev. Pharm. Tox.,* **27,** 301–314

Floke, L. (1987) Oxygen-centred radicals in shock. *J. Clin. Chem. Clin. Biochem.,* **25,** 232–233

Fortune, J. B., Feustel, P. J., Sanfi, J., Stratton, H., Newell, J. and Shah, D. (1987) Influence of hematocrit on cardiopulmonary function after acute hemorrhage. *J. Trauma,* **27,** 243–249

Gammage, G. (1987) Crystalloid versus colloid: is colloid worth the cost? *Int. Anaesth. Clin.,* **25,** 19–36

Geiger, K. (1986) Clinical aspects of fluid transport and vascular permeability in the lung. *Klin. Wochenschr.,* **64** (Suppl. 7) 18–23

Gin, S. L., Dranen, S. C., Syverud, S. A., Barson, W. G. and Cunningham, C. A. (1987) Naloxone does not improve hemodynamics following graded hemorrhage in a canine model. *Am. J. Emerg. Med.,* **5,** 478–482

Gossett, K. A., Cleghorn, B. and Martin, G. S. (1987) Correlation between anion gap, blood L lactate concentrate and survival in horses. *Eq. Vet. J.,* **19,** 29–30

Gurll, N. S., Ganes, E., and Reynold, D. C. (1987) CNS is involved in the cardiovascular response to naloxone in canine endotoxin but not hemerrhagic shock. *Circ. Shock,* **22,** 115–125

Hardaway, R. M. (1985) Treatment of shock from a clinical viewpoint. In *Circulatory Shock: Basic and Clinical Implications* (eds. H. F. Jansen and C. D. Barnes) Academic Press, London, pp.197–235

Hardaway, R. M. and Williams, C. H. (1987) Influence of steroids on hemorrhagic and traumatic shock. *J. Trauma,* **27,** 667–670

Hardie, E. M. and Rawlings, C. A. (1983) Septic Shock. *Comp. Cont. Ed.,* **5,** 369–377

Heath, D. F. (1985) Subcellular aspects of the response to trauma. *Br. Med. Bull.*, **41**, 240–245

Heene, D. L., Kirchstein, W. and Dempfle, C. E. (1986) Shock induced alterations in haemostasis. *Klin. Wochenschr.*, **64**, (Suppl. 7), 14–17

Horton, J. W. (1987a) Cardiocirculatory function in the intoxicated shocked dog: acid–base derangements. *Circ. Shock*, **22**, 23–34

Horton, J. W. (1987b) Hemorrhagic shock impairs myocardial cell volume regulation and membrane integrity in dogs. *Am. J. Physiol.*, **252H**, 1203–1210

Horton, J. W. and Borman, K. R. (1987) Possible role of oxygen-derived free radicals in cardiocirculatory shock. *Surg. Gynec. Obstet.*, **165**, 293–300

Hunt, T. K., Rabkin, J. and van Smitten, K. (1986) Effects of edema and anemia on wound healing and infection. *Current Studies in Haemorrhage and Blood Transfusion*, **53**, 101–113

Jacobson, M. A. and Young, L. S. (1985) Gram-negative shock: approaches to treatment. *J. Roy. Coll. Phys.*, **19**, 214–217

Kirby, R. R. (1987) Shock: A systemic or cellular disease. *Int. Anaesth. Clin.*, **25**, 19–36

Kitchell, B. E. and Haskins, S. C. (1984) Feline trauma and critical care medicine. *Vet. Clin. N. Am. (Sm. Anim. Pract.)* **14**, 1331–1343

Koziol, J. M., Rush, B. F., Smith, S. M. and Machiedo (1988) Occurrence of bacteraemia during and after haemorrhagic shock. *J. Trauma*, **28**, 10–16

Lee, E. S., Greenburg, G., Maffinel, P. W., Meleker, E. D. and Velly, T. S. (1987) Superoxide radicals and hemorrhagic shock; are intravenous radicals associated with mortality? *J. Surg. Res.* **42**, 1–6

Lefer, A. M. (1987) Interaction between myocardial depressant factor and vasoactive mediators with ischaemia and shock. *Am. J. Physiol.*, **252R**, 193–205

Levy, M., Geller, R. and Hymovitch, S. (1986) Renal failure in dogs with experimental acute pancreatitis: role of hypovolaemia. *Am. J. Physiol.*, **251F**, 969–977

Luypaert, P., Vincent, J. L., Davies, M., Van den Linden, P., Blezic, S., Azimi, G. and Bernard, A. (1986) *Circ. Shock*, **20**, 311–320

Mannel, D. N. (1987) Tumour Necrosis Factor – a mediator of endotoxin shock. *J. Clin. Chem. Clin. Biochem.*, **25**, 209–211

McAnulty, J. F. (1982) Septic shock in the dog. *J. Am. An. Hosp. Assoc.*, **19**, 827–835

Melchior, J. C., Pinaud, M., Blanloeil, Y., Bourreti, B., Potel, G. and Souron, R. (1987) Haemodynamic effect of continuous norepinephrine infusion in dogs with and without hyperkinetic endotoxin shock. *Crit. Care Med.*, **15**, 687–691

Messmer, K. (1984) Blood substitutes in shock therapy. In *Shock and Related Problems* (ed. G. T. Shires), Churchill Livingstone, New York, pp. 191–205

Michell, A. R. (1985) What is shock? *J. Sm. Anim. Pract.*, **26**, 719–738

Michell, A. R. (1988) Drips, drinks and drenches; what matters in fluid therapy? *Irish Vet. J.*

Michell A. R., Bywater, R. J., Clarke, K. W., Hall, L. W. and Waterman, A. E. (1988) *Veterinary Fluid Therapy*, Blackwell, Oxford

Modig, J. (1988) Beneficial effects of Dextran 70 vs. Ringer's Acetate on pulmonary hemodynamics and survival in a porcine endotoxin shock model. *Resuscitation*, **16**, 1–12

Muir, W. W. (1987) Equine shock: the need for prospective studies. *Eq. Vet. J.*, **19**, 1–7

Nagy, S (1987) Cardiopressant and cardiostimulant factors in shock. In: *First Vienna Shock Forum (A)* (eds G. Schlag and H. Redl), Alan Liss, New York, pp. 599–610

Neugebauer, E. and Lorenz, W. (1987) Biogenic amines in circulatory shock: current status of histamine. *J. Clin. Chem. Clin. Biochem.*, **25**, 222–234

Ortolani, O., Biasiucci, A., Trebbi, A., Cianciulli, M. and Cuocolo, R. (1987) Antioxidant drugs and shock therapy. *Prog. Clin. Biol. Res.*, **263A**, 271–280

Parratt, J. R., Saleh, S. and Waton, N. G. (1986) Feline endotoxin shock: effect on tissue histamine. *Br. J. Pharm.*, **89**, 635–640

Patterson, A. (1987) Massive transfusion. *Int. Anaesth. Clin.*, **25**, 19–36

Pearl, R. G., Halperin, B. D., Mihan, F. G. and Rosenthal, M. H. (1988) Pulomonary effect of crystalloid and colloid resuscitation from hemorrhagic shock in the presence of oleic acid induced pulmonary capillary damage in the dog. *Anaesthesiology*, **68**, 12–20

Pretorius, J. P., Schlag, G., Redl, H., Botha, W. S., Coosen, D. J., Bosman, H. and van Geden, A. F. (1987) The 'lung in shock' as a result of hypovolaemia – traumatic shock in baboon. *J. Trauma*, **27**, 1344–1358

Prough, D. S., Carson Johnson, J., Stump, D. A., Stullkens, E. H., Poole, G. V. and Howard, G. (1986) Effects of hypertonic saline *versus* lactated Ringer's solution on cerebral oxygen transport during resuscitation from hemorrhagic shock. *J. Neurosurg.*, **64**, 627–632

Rackow, E. C., Kaufman, B. S., Falk, J. L., Astiz, M. E. and Weil, M. H. (1987) Haemodynamic response to fluid repletion in patients with septic shock. *Circ. Shock,* **22,** 11–22

Schumer, W. (1986) Cellular metabolism in shock. *Kiln. Wochenschr.,* **64,** (Suppl. 7), 7–13

Schumer, W. (1987) Corticosteroids in the treatment of septic shock. In *First Vienna Shock Forum (A)* (eds G. Schlag and H. Redl), Alan Liss, New York, pp. 249–260.

Seeger, W. (1987) Clinical features and pathophysiology of lung failure in shock. *J. Clin. Chem. Clin. Biochem.*, **25**, 209–211

Sembrat, R. F., DiStazio, J. and Stremple, J.F. (1979) The pony as a model for septic shock. *Adv. Shock Res.*, **2,** 137–151

Shafney, C. H., Lillehel, R. C., Dietzman, R. H., Romero, L. H. and Beckman, C. B. (1982) Influence of the salt moiety on the effectiveness of corticosteroid therapy in cardiogenic shock. *Circ. Shock,* **9,** 247–258

Shenep, J. L. and Mogan, K. A. (1984) Kinetics of endotoxin release during antibiotic therapy for experimental Gram-negative bacterial sepsis. *J. Inf. Dis.,* **150,** 380–388

Shires, G. T. (1984) *Shock and Related Problems.* Churchill Livingstone, New York, pp. 15–43

Shoemaker, W. C. (1986) Hemodynamic and oxygen transport effects of crystalloids and colloids on critically ill patients. *Current Studies in Haemorrhage and Blood Transfusion,* **53,** 101–113

Shoemaker, W. C. (1987) Circulatory mechanisms of shock and their mediators. *Crit. Care Med.,* **15,** 787–794

Smith, J. A. R. and Norman, J. N. (1982) The fluid of choice for resuscitation of severe shock. *Br. J. Surg.,* **69,** 702–705

Templeton, C. B., Bottoms, G. D., Fessler, J. E., Ewert, K. M., Roesel, O. F., Johnston, M. A. and Latshaw, H. S. (1987) *Circ. Shock,* **23,** 231–240

Till, G. O. and Ward, P. A. (1987) Oxygen radicals and lipid peroxidation in experimental shock. In *First Vienna Shock Forum (A)* (ed. G. Schlag and H. Redl), Alan Liss, New York, pp. 235–244

Tooth, P. D. (1986) Hemodynamic effect of naloxone on hemorrhagic shock in the beagle. *Circ. Shock,* **20,** 35–42

Trabe, D. L. (1985) Pulmonary dysfunction during shock. In *Circulatory Shock: Basic and Clinical Implications* (eds H. F. Janssen and C. D. Barnes), Academic Press, London, pp. 23–46

Vincent, J. L., Domb, M., Luypaert, P., De Boelpaepe, C., van der Linden, P. and Blecic, S. (1987) Endotoxin shock model in the dog: In: *First Vienna Shock Forum (A)* (eds G. Schlag and H. Redl), Alan Liss, New York, pp. 393–400

Wagner-Mann, C. C. and Gross, D. R. (1986) Effects of naloxone in treating hemorrhagic shock in dogs with maintained baroreceptor responsiveness. *Am. J. Vet. Res.,* **47,** 1763–1766

White et al (1982)

Woods, I., Wilkins, R. G., Edwards, J. D., Martin, P. D. and Faragher, B. (1987) Danger of using core-peripheral temperature gradient as a guide to therapy in shock. *Crit. Care Med.,* **15,** 850–852

Zonghai, H., Han, G. and Renbao, X. (1987) Studies on glucocorticoid receptors during intestinal ischaemic shock and septic shock. *Circ. Shock,* **23,** 27–36

G. A. H. WELLS

Bovine spongiform encephalopathy

INTRODUCTION

THE DEGENERATIVE brain changes characterized by neuronal vacuolation and grey matter spongiosis, called bovine spongiform encephalopathy (BSE) and the associated novel clinical syndrome were reported originally in six cows from four geographically separated dairy herds in England (Wells *et al.*, 1987). The new disease was considered similar to the transmissible spongiform encephalopathies caused by incompletely characterized or unconventional infectious agents (Table 1), the best understood representative of which is scrapie in sheep.

This article summarizes some of the rapidly evolving information on the disorder, with emphasis on the clinical signs.

Table 1 TRANSMISSIBLE SPONGIFORM ENCEPHALOPATHIES

Host	Disease	References
Sheep and goats	Scrapie	Kimberlin, 1981
Mule deer (*Odocoileus hemionus hemionus*)	Chronic wasting disease	Williams and Young, 1980
Mink (ranch reared)	Transmissible mink encephalopathy (TME)	Prusiner and Hadlow, 1979
Man	Kuru Creutzfeldt–Jakob disease	

EPIDEMIOLOGY

By the end of 1987 over one hundred cases of BSE had been confirmed with an average annual incidence in affected herds of 1% of milking cows. During 1988 the within herd incidence remained low with 75% of affected herds experiencing only single cases. The disease was reported initially only in Friesian/Holstein dairy cows but subsequently occurred in other breeds. There is no evidence of a breed predisposition. It was also identified in suckler herds but at a much lower incidence than in dairy herds. Affected cattle were 3–8 years old with the greatest incidence in

4-year old cows. A case described in a 3-year old bull (Gilmour *et al.*, 1988) was the first confirmed report of BSE in a male but the incidence in bulls is similar to that in dairy cows.

The original reports of BSE were from southern England. The earliest clinically suspected case presented in April 1985. Although the disease was later recorded from most other parts of Great Britain, the reporting rate remained highest in the south. No epidemiological associations were evident between disease occurrence and stage of breeding cycle or season of the year. No treatments, intoxicants or specific biological products were common to all outbreaks. The occurrence of the disease in multiple breeds argues against genetic determinance. The distribution and circumstances of occurrence were consistent with an extended common source epidemic without evidence of cattle-to-cattle contagion. Affected herds were scrutinized for associations with sheep but twenty per cent had had no sheep on the farm since 1980. Nevertheless, the data suggested an infectious aetiology and results of the epidemiological study (Wilesmith *et al.*, 1988) lead to the conclusion that cattle have acquired a scrapie-like agent via commercial feedstuffs containing meat and bone meal. Using computer modelling, the data is consistent only with exposure commencing 1981–1982, an incubation period of 2–8 years, and the majority of cattle becoming infected in calfhood.

CLINICAL SIGNS

The clinical signs of BSE are insidious in onset and progress over a period of weeks to months. Rarely, cases present more acutely and deteriorate rapidly. Variability of the disease course is reflected in accounts of the signs (Cranwell *et al.*, 1988; Gilmour *et al.*, 1988; Johnson *et al.*, 1988; Wells *et al.*, 1987; Wells, unpublished data; Whitaker and Johnson, 1988; Wilesmith *et al.*, 1988) but most cases show alterations in behaviour , posture, movement and sensorum, indicative of a diffuse central nervous system disorder. The signs most constant throughout the disease course are expressions of apprehension, hind limb gait ataxia, and loss of general bodily condition (Wilesmith *et al.*, 1988). The earliest signs are usually changes of behaviour suggestive of hypomagnesaemia or nervous ketosis. Kicking at milking, gait ataxia, reduced milk yield or liveweight loss are variably also presenting signs.

Apprehension or fear are often manifest in reluctance to enter the milking parlour or pass through a gateway and in escape activity when approached at pasture. There is hyperaesthesia, particularly to tactile and auditory stimuli. Kicking during milking is noted and attempts to handle the animal's head may be vigorously resisted. Ear twitching, constant changes in ear position or a stance with the ears held directed backwards (Figure 1) may be evoked by the slightest noise. In contrast to the normal ear movements in cattle, ear movements are exaggerated and persist even after familiarity with the stimulus.

Agonistic reactions (passive and active aggression) may be increased and include avoidance of other cows when loose or increased threats and butts toward others when bunched. Some affected cows indiscriminately charge among a yarded group. Interspecific aggression (to man) may be seen when in confined situations, cows may repeatedly butt and paw the ground. These changes may progress to frenzy but more usually locomotor signs complicate and dominate the later clinical picture.

Other behavioural signs include excessive or compulsive grooming, mainly licking

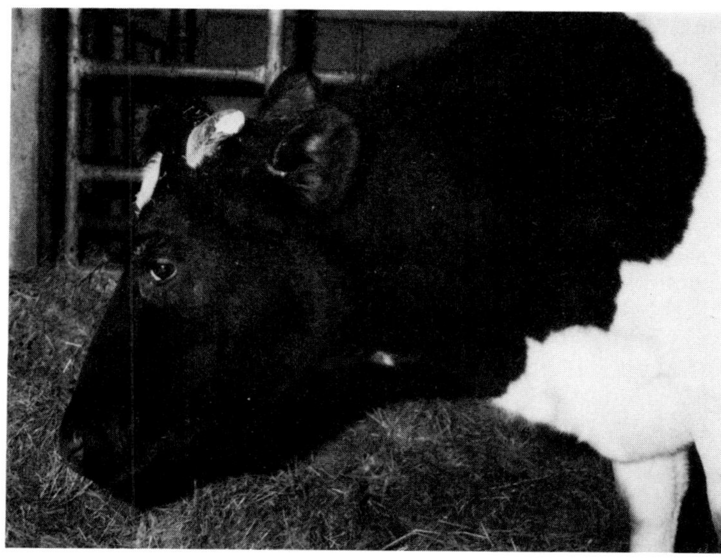

Fig. 1. Typical posture in a clinical case of BSE with low head carriage and ears held back.

the nose, shoulders or flank. Some affected cows habitually scratch their head, particularly the poll, with a hind foot or rub it against fixtures or learn to offer it to an attendant. In some cases palpation or stroking of the lumbo-sacral spine invariably induces extension of the neck and characteristic continuous lip movements similar to the nibbling reflex seen in sheep with scrapie. Evidence of severe pruritis is absent but small areas of hair loss and excoriation can result from rubbing. Teeth grinding episodes occur throughout the disease in some cases.

Concurrent with behavioural signs there are abnormalities of movement and posture. Early in the clinical course there is hind limb ataxia which worsens and is later accompanied and obscured by paresis. A shortened stride, a swaying gait and difficulty in negotiating turns are the first features. At pasture the ataxia is readily seen and includes hypermetria of the hind limb, and more rarely, the forelimb. The tail is sometimes raised when trotting. Asymmetry of gait may produce a 'crab-like' progression. A pacing type of gait at the trot, whereby both fore and hind limb of the same side are advanced simultaneously, has been noted (Cranwell *et al.*, 1988). Paraparesis contributes to later gait abnormalities especially in the negotiation of steps, slopes and slippery concrete floors.

Knuckling (involuntary flexion) of hind limb digital joints, stumbling and falling become evident. Recovery from falling is at first immediate but later there is prolonged or permanent recumbency. Instantaneous collapse into a sitting position with forelimbs rigidly extended sometimes results if cows are subjected to sudden loud noises. Recumbent animals, before advanced weakness, may make vigorous propulsive movements with partially flexed limbs resulting in progression with abortive or successful attempts to rise. In the late stages of the disease lateral recumbency may occur with extension of the neck and, rarely, brief seizures and nystagmus. Circling has been reported only rarely.

Adventitial involuntary movements include tremor, mainly localized to the head and neck, but sometimes diffuse, a myoclonic jerk repeated at regular intervals of a few seconds (resembling hiccups) and variably distributed muscle fasciculations.

Postural alterations may include a base wide stance, extension of the neck with low carriage (Figure 1) or lateral deviation of the head. A mild kyphosis, often called 'roach back', in the midthoracic region usually accompanies loss of weight and deteriorating general bodily condition.

Neurological signs fluctuate daily and external stimuli and stress seem to produce temporary exacerbations. Conversely, reduction of stress is associated with periods of clinical remission sometimes of several weeks.

Gradual loss of general bodily condition leading to generalized wasting may be a presenting sign but is also an indication of advanced disease. Appetite remains normal in most cases. Slaughter is necessitated on welfare considerations. Rarely, in the disease course, death occurs unexpectedly.

PATHOLOGY

There are no significant gross necropsy changes. Histological changes are character-istic and confined to the central nervous system with grey matter neuropil vacuolation and neuronal vacuolation distributed in a consistent, usually symmetrical, pattern involving mainly the brain stem. Scrapie associated fibrils (SAF) structures originally visualized by electron microscopy in detergent extracts of scrapie-infected mouse brain, are a feature of this group of transmissible spongiform encephalo-pathies in general and have been demonstrated in BSE (Wells *et al.*, 1987, Wells and Scott, 1988). SAF are composed of one major protein which is coded by the host but modified in the course of infection. It has been shown that the SAF protein in BSE is common with that in natural scrapie of sheep (Hope *et al.*, 1988). The possibility that the same protein also forms part of the infectious agent remains highly controversial. The first direct evidence that BSE is transmissible came with the production of a scrapie-like disease in mice inoculated with brain material from affected cows (Fraser *et al.*, 1988).

DIAGNOSIS

Clinical observations made on more than one occasion over a period of time, sufficient to appreciate progress of signs, provides a sound basis for clinical diagnosis. A good correlation exists between clinical diagnosis and histopathological diagnosis.

The early presenting signs must be differentiated from hypomagnesaemia and nervous ketosis. Clinical biochemistry has revealed no consistent abnormalities. The chronic nature of BSE contrasts with the more acute nature of most metabolic problems in dairy cows. Deviation of the head, the rarely observed circling and self isolation from the group could suggest encephalic listeriosis but other features of that disease are absent. Further differential diagnoses include, principally, lead poisoning, cerebro-spinal abscess or other space-occupying lesions and spinal trauma.

TREATMENT AND CONTROL

There is no effective treatment. Prospects for a control strategy are long term and must depend on the evolution of an understanding of BSE and on continuing progress in the field of spongiform encephalopathies of unconventional infectious agent origin. In the interim the statutory reporting, slaughter and destruction of affected cattle with suspension of the use of ruminant-derived protein in ruminant concentrate rations limits the likely common source of exposure and ensures continued monitoring (Order, 1988).

REFERENCES

Cranwell, M. P., Hancock, R. D., Hindson, J. C., Hall, J. S., Daniel, N. J., Hopkins, A. R., Wonnacott, B., Vivian, M. and Hunt, P. (1988) Bovine spongiform encephalopathy. *Vet. Rec.*, **122**, 190

Gilmour, J. S., Buxton, D., MacLeod, N. S. M., Brodie, T. A. and More, J. B. (1988) Bovine spongiform encephalopathy. *Vet. Rec.*, **122**, 142

Hope, J., Reekie, L. J. D., Hunter, N., Multhaup, G., Beyreuther, K., White, H., Scott, A. C., Stack, M. J., Dawson, M. and Wells, G. A. H. (1988) Brain fibrils of novel British cattle disease contain scrapie-associated protein. *Nature* (in press).

Johnson, C. T., Hancock, R. D., Gunning, R. F., Whitaker, C. J., Paul, N. J., Kupfer, J. A. M., and Morley, P. W. G. (1988) Bovine spongiform encephalopathy: clinical findings in four herds. *Vet. Rec.* Submitted for publication.

Kimberlin, R. H. (1981) Scrapie. *Br. Vet. J.* **137**, 105–112

Order (1988) The Bovine Spongiform Encephalopathy Order 1988, Statutory Instrument No; 1039. London, HMSO.

Prusiner, S. B. and Hadlow, W. J. (eds.) (1979) *Slow transmissible diseases of the nervous system. Vol.1 Clinical, Epidemiological, Genetic and Pathological Aspects of the Spongiform Encephalopathies.* Academic Press, New York

Wells, G. A. H. and Scott, A. C. (1988) Neuronal vacuolation and spongiosus; a novel encephalopathy of adult cattle. *Neuropathol. Appl. Neurobiol.*, **14**, 247 (abstract).

Wells, G. A. H., Scott, A. C., Johnson, C. T., Gunning, R. F., Hancock, R. D., Jeffrey, M., Dawson, M. and Bradley, R. (1987) A novel progressive spongiform encephalopathy in cattle. *Vet. Rec.* **121**, 419–420

Whitaker, C. J. and Johnson C. T. (1988) A neurological syndrome. *B.C.V.A. Proc.* (in press)

Wilesmith, J. W., Wells, G. A. H., Cranwell, M. P., and Ryan, J. B. M. (1988) BSE – Bovine spongiform encephalopathy epidemiological studies. *Vet. Rec.* (in press)

Williams, E. S. and Young, S. (1980) Chronic wasting disease of captive mule deer: a spongiform encephalopathy. *J. Wildl. Dis.* **16**, 89–98

J. ADRIAN LONGSTAFFE

Pruritus, pyrexia and haemorrhage syndrome in cattle

INTRODUCTION

SINCE 1976 there have been a number of reports describing a syndrome affecting adult dairy cattle that involves a combination of a pruritic papular dermatitis, an elevated body temperature and multiple haemorrhages (Hall, 1976; Thomas, 1979). These outbreaks have been described as Acute Fatal Haemorrhagic syndrome of dairy cattle and, more recently as the Pruritus, Pyrexia and Haemorrhage syndrome (PPH) (Matthews and Schreeve, 1978). This paper summarizes the findings to date, discusses aetiological theories and describes preliminary findings from an outbreak in 1985–1986 which is undergoing detailed study and follow-up.

EPIDEMIOLOGY

Almost without exception, the reported cases of PPH occur in adult dairy cattle. Morbidity varies from 1–22% but appears to be usually in the region of 4–8%. Mortality of affected animals is high, but difficult to estimate accurately. Although many animals die within a few days of showing signs, the remainder are slaughtered, either due to prolonged illness or, with recent outbreaks, in anticipation of this. This tendency for preemptive slaughter has made the disease difficult to investigate in depth. Dietary factors such as silage additives (Matthews and Shreeve, 1978; Turner *et al.*, 1978; Thomas, 1978;1979; Holden, 1980; Lawrie, 1983) moulds (Hall, 1976; Dyson and Reed, 1977; Petrie *et al.*, 1977) and di-ureido-isobutane (DUIB) (Breukink *et al.*, 1978) have been implicated in a number of cases. A high proportion of reported cases appears to have been associated with the first year of the introduction of treated silage (Matthews and Shreeve, 1978; Thomas, 1978;1979; Holden 1980; Lawrie, 1983).

CLINICAL SIGNS

When a clinical syndrome is not definitely categorized as a single disease, a spectrum of signs may be seen. Those described for PPH are as follows. Firstly, a pruritic papular dermatitis with patchy hair loss is seen which chiefly affects the head, neck, perineum and udder. Other affected sites can be the back, tail and limbs. Because of self trauma, further hair loss and excoriation with secondary infection can occur. Secondly, a variable pyrexia occurs which is usually resistant to treatment although spontaneous resolution can be seen. Finally, haemorrhage is observed which may consist of two types, frequently observed within the same animal. Capillary haemorrhage is seen as petechiation of visible mucosae, while gross haemorrhage is seen as a bloody diarrhoea, faecal blood clots, subcutaneous haematomata and epistaxis.

Some animals die within hours or days of showing the signs described above. Others show persistent dullness, inappetance and weight loss leading to death or emergency slaughter in 1 to 8 weeks.

A minority of animals show haemorrhagic signs only (Anderson, 1979; Cranwell, 1983). There is a mixture of capillary and gross haemorrhage but no skin lesions or elevated temperature.

LABORATORY FINDINGS

Several authors (Dyson and Reed, 1977; Turner *et al.*, 1978; Thomas, 1978;1979) have described a moderate anaemia with early leucopenia and later leucocytosis. Occasionally eosinophilia is observed (Hall, 1976; Thomas, 1979). Anderson (1979) reports a thrombocytopenia involving an entire herd. In many cases, however, haematological findings are within normal ranges. Serum biochemistry is usually unhelpful, and reflects only generalized signs of tissue damage (Turner *et al.*, 1978; Thomas, 1979).

Extensive serological and electron microscopic investigations for infectious agents have proved negative or not significant (Thomas, 1978;1979).

PATHOLOGICAL FINDINGS

Because of the frequency with which animals diagnosed clinically as PPH are sent for immediate slaughter, it is difficult to obtain the wide range of tissues necessary for a complete examination.

Reports of post-mortem findings (Hall, 1976; Dyson and Reed 1977; Turner *et al.*, 1978; Breukink *et al.*, 1978; Thomas, 1978;1979; Holden, 1980; Borthwick, 1983; Lawrie, 1983; Cranwell, 1983; Andrews *et al.*, 1983) include descriptions of either extensive haemorrhage (Hall, 1976; Breukink *et al.*, 1978; Cranwell, 1983) or little or none (Turner *et al.*, 1978; Thomas 1978;1979; Borthwick, 1983). Further post-mortem findings include enlarged kidneys with miliary pale lesions; softening of adrenals; pallor and flaccidity of the heart; enlargement and pallor of the liver; softening of lymph nodes and skin lesions.

Reports of histopathological changes relate only to outbreaks involving so-called 'classical' PPH (Thomas, 1979). In the skin, a non-specific crusting dermatitis is present. Within viscera, a granulomatous inflammatory infiltrate has been reported affecting a number of tissues including liver, myocardium, kidney, lymph nodes, pancreas, udder and salivary gland (Breukink *et al.*, 1978; Thomas, 1978;1979). Dyson and Reed (1977) describe degenerative changes in the liver and myocardium and Turner *et al.*, (1978) report a necrotizing cardiomyopathy with interstitial nephritis and non-suppurative encephalitis. There are no histopathological reports on the outbreaks which have apparently involved only haemorrhage.

INVESTIGATION OF A RECENT OUTBREAK (SW ENGLAND)

In the outbreak which is currently under investigation, 12 out of 600 cows on 3 associated farms using treated silage for the first time, showed signs of pruritus and pyrexia, haemorrhage of mucous membranes, dullness and loss of appetite. Two further animals presented with gross haemorrhage only (intestinal, nasal and retroperitoneal).

Gross post-mortem examination of 10 out of 12 animals showed multiple haemorrhages. These were present on the serosal surfaces of liver, kidney, heart, lung and mesentery. The only other change observed was the presence of miliary pale lesions in the kidney.

Histopathological examination shows non-specific inflammatory changes in skin. Infiltrates of eosinophils, histiocytes, macrophages and plasma cells were found throughout the kidney (10 out of 11), adrenal (9 out of 12), lymph node (9 out of 12), liver (7 out of 11), myocardium (6 out of 11), spleen (3 out of 10) and lung (3 out of 10). These were either focal or confluent. In five out of twelve cases giant cells were present, although not consistently within the same tissue. Identical changes were seen in the two animals showing haemorrhage only at post-mortem examination.

DISCUSSION

A number of questions regarding this poorly defined and understood clinical syndrome remain to be answered. Does the syndrome reflect more than one disease entity? What are the aetiological agents involved, and what is the pathogenesis of their action?

With regard to the number of disease entities involved, the syndrome appears to divide into two categories. The majority of reports describe the full spectrum of PPH with accompanying multisystemic granulomatous inflammation. A minority (Anderson, 1979; Cranwell, 1983; and one outbreak seen by the author), report multisystem haemorrhage only. Even in the case of classical PPH, some reports stress the haemorrhagic component whereas others hardly mention it. While it would seem that more than one pathogenetic mechanism is at work, some cases submitted to this laboratory and showing haemorrhage as the sole clinical sign, have been found to display the multisystemic chronic inflammatory lesions which we regard as histologically typical of PPH. Unfortunately, none of the apparent 'haemorrhage only' reports in the literature involved a histopathological evaluation.

With regard to aetiology, two main theories, those of mycotoxicosis and fungal hypersensitivity appear to be current. Many of the earlier reports suggest the involvement of mycotoxins in the aetiology of the disease (Hall, 1976; Petrie *et al.*, 1977; Dyson and Reed, 1977; Anderson, 1979), although this seems to be largely by comparison with other mycotoxic syndromes such as mouldy corn poisoning (Albright *et al.*, 1964). In the author's experience, there is much less of a degenerative and necrotic component in liver and kidney samples submitted from PPH outbreaks than is described for mouldy corn poisoning. Also, although Petrie *et al.*, (1977) identified a trichothecene metabolite T2, they were unable to quantify it, while Patterson *et al.*, (1979) have failed to cause haemorrhagic disease in calves and pigs with either trichothecene mycotoxins or whole cultures of *Fusarium tricinctum* and have concluded that mycotoxins have little or no part to play in the aetiology of feed associated haemorrhagic disease.

Andrews *et al.*, (1983) raise the possibility of a reaction to a fungal agent, *Sporothrix schenkeii* and, although subsequent investigations have failed to find further fungal material in lesions, the cellular reaction is suggestive of a hypersensitivity reaction (Thomas, 1978;1979; Holden, 1980). In addition to this, the history of the outbreak currently under investigation includes a report of facial/ocular swelling in many other cows at the time of the outbreak. Rapidly appearing and disappearing facial or ocular swellings of this nature are compatible with a Type 1 hypersensitivity. In addition, Dyson and Reed (1977) and Morris and McInnes (1978) report skin lesions which could be allergic in nature in 80% and 25% of affected herds respectively. Lesions of this type would suggest a mixture of inappropriate allergic reactions.

Although eight out of thirteen reports have associated PPH with the introduction of chemically treated silage, this association remains obscure. Direct toxic effects seem highly unlikely although it is possible that alteration to silage pH may allow altered growth or survival of allergenic fungi. This remains theoretical.

Two outbreaks have been linked with agents in the feed. Cranwell (1983) reports tissue levels of dicoumarol associated with the ingestion of sweet vernal grass and Breukink *et al.*, (1978) describe a syndrome apparently identical to PPH that they were able to reproduce experimentally by the administration of a feed additive di-ureido-isobutane (DUIB).

How are the clinical signs and pathological changes linked with the irreversible loss of condition and death of the majority of animals? Although the interstitial nephritis seen in some cases is sufficient to have caused renal failure, it is not so in others. It is possible that the very severe adrenal damage seen in five out of twelve recent cases may also contribute to the demise of the animal. Other possibilities are the impairment of cardiac or liver function by the lesions. None of these fully explains the almost inevitable death of clinically affected animals.

CONCLUSION

PPH is a syndrome affecting adult dairy cattle with a low (usually 4–8%) morbidity but high mortality. Although the incidence of this syndrome is low, this disease is of great importance to the affected farmer because it involves the deaths of adult dairy cows in full production. Further investigations are under way to further define the condition and clarify the aetiology.

ACKNOWLEDGEMENTS

The author wishes to thank Mr N. Todd, Mr C. Watson, Mr N. Gunning and other staff at the Langford Veterinary Investigation Centre for their help with the provision of material and the ongoing investigation of the syndrome at Langford. Thanks also to Dr G. R. Pearson for assistance in the preparation of this paper and Mrs B. Riddick and Mrs V. Godfrey for the typing of the manuscript.

REFERENCES

Anderson, M. A. (1979) Haemorrhagic syndrome in cattle. In: *Proceedings of the Third Meeting on Mycotoxins in Animal Disease.* (Eds G. A. Pepin, D. S. P. Patterson and B. J.

Shreeve) MAFF. Central Veterinary Laboratory, New Haw, Weybridge, pp. 51

Andrews, A. H., Longstaffe, J. A., Newton, A. C. and Musa, I. (1983) Acute fatal haemorrhagic syndrome in dairy cows. *Vet. Rec.*, **112**, 614

Albright, I. L., Aust, S. D., Byers, J. H., Fritz, T. E., Brodie, I. O., Olsen, R. E., Link, R. P., Simon, I., Rhoades, H. E. and Brewer, R. L. (1964) Moldy corn toxicosis in cattle. *J. Am. Vet. Med. Ass.*, **144**, 1013

Borthwick, B. R. (1983) Acute fatal haemorrhagic syndrome in dairy cows. *Vet. Rec.*, **112**, 394

Breukink, H. J., Gruys, E., Holzhauer, C. and Westenbroek, A. C. J. M. (1978) Pyrexia with dermatitis in dairy cows. *Vet. Rec.*, **103**, 221

Cranwell, M. P. (1983) Acute fatal haemorrhagic syndrome in dairy cows. *Vet. Rec.*, **112**, 486

Dyson, D. A. and Reed, J. B. H. (1977) Haemorrhagic syndrome of cattle of suspected mycotoxic origin. *Vet. Rec.*, **100**, 400

Hall, A. (1976) Haemorrhagic syndrome in dairy cows: a possible mycotoxicosis. In: *Proceedings of the Second Meeting of Mycotoxicosis in Animal Disease* (Aberdeen, 1976) MAFF. Central Veterinary Laboratory, New Haw, Weybridge. pp. 23

Holden, A. R. (1980) Two outbreaks of pyrexia with dermatitis in dairy cows. *Vet. Rec.*, **106**, 413

Lawrie, A. M. (1983) Acute fatal haemorrhagic syndrome in dairy cows. *Vet. Rec.*, **112**, 309

Matthews, J. G. and Shreeve, B. J. (1978) Pyrexia/pruritus/haemorrhagic syndrome in dairy cows. *Vet. Rec.*, **103**, 408

Morris, J. and McInnes, I. J. (1978) Pyrexia with dermatitis in dairy cows. *Vet. Rec.*, **102**, 368

Patterson, D. S. P., Matthews, J. G., Shreeve, B. J., Roberts, B. A., McDonald, S. M. and Haye, A. W. (1979) The failure of tricho-thecene mycotoxins and whole cultures of *Fusarium tricinctum* to cause experimental haemorrhagic syndromes in calves and pigs. *Vet. Rec.*, **105**, 252

Petrie, L., Robb, J. and Stewart, A. F. (1977) The identification of T-2 toxin and its association with a haemorrhagic syndrome in cattle. *Vet. Rec.*, **101**, 326

Thomas, G. W. (1978) Pyrexia with dermatitis in dairy cows. *Vet. Rec.*, **102**, 368

Thomas, G. W. (1979) Pyrexia with dermatitis in dairy cows. *In Practice*, **1**, 16

Turner, S. J., Kelly, D. F. and Spackman, D. (1978) Pyrexia with dermatitis in dairy cows. *Vet. Rec.*, **102**, 488

M. EYSKER

The epidemiology of lungworm infections in cattle

INTRODUCTION

IN MOST countries in Northwestern Europe dictyocaulosis (husk) is still an important disease in cattle despite the availability of a vaccine. The disease usually is seen at the end of the first grazing season, particularly when the summer has been wetter than usual.

Husk occurs predominantly in young animals. Older cattle have an acquired immunity. This immunity can only be developed when the incidence of infections is high. In the Netherlands, sero-epidemiological studies showed an incidence of husk of close to 100% on dairy cattle farms (Boon *et al.*, 1982; 1984). These results also indicate that on many farms first season grazing animals acquire infections without showing clinical signs. Apparently there is a 'race' between the acquisition of infections and the development of immunity in susceptible animals. The outcome controls whether clinical disease will occur.

Occasionally, outbreaks of husk also are seen in older cattle in the Netherlands. The reasons for these outbreaks are not known but it seems likely that they result from a lack of immunity. This is supported by the situation in Denmark where there is a low incidence of husk. As a result, the occasional outbreaks tend to occur in all age groups (Jørgensen, 1981). Obviously, there can be a considerable variation between farms and regions in the build up of population and the build up of immunity to lungworm infections.

SOME CHARACTERISTICS OF THE LIFE CYCLE

The adult parasites live in the bronchi where the eggs containing the first stage larvae (L1) are deposited. The eggs are coughed up and ingested. The larvae hatch during passage in the gut. The larvae develop in the faeces to the infective third stage (L3). They use their intestinal granules as nutrition.

A very crucial characteristic in the epidemiology of lungworm infections is that development and subsequent translation to pasture can occur within a week (Michel and Rose, 1954; Jørgensen, 1981; Eysker and van Miltenburg, 1988) during the grazing season. Translation of the rather sluggish larvae occurs mainly in the sporangia of the corprophagous fungus *Pilobolus* (Jørgensen *et al.*, 1982; Somers *et al.*, 1985). Recent results indicate that most translation by this fungus will occur within eight days (Eysker and de Coo, 1988). Other factors involved in translation are diarrhoea (Michel and Rose, 1954), rain, earthworms (Oakley, 1981) and insects.

The infection is also spread by mechanical means on boots, hooves and machines. In the summer the larvae will generally not survive for more than several weeks (Jørgensen, 1981; Jacobs *et al.*, 1985; Eysker and van Miltenburg, 1988). In autumn and winter, development, translation and survival takes longer and over-wintering has been demonstrated (Jarrett *et al.*, 1955; Enigk and Düwel, 1961; Gupta and Gibbs, 1970; Oakley, 1977; Duncan *et al.*, 1979; Jørgensen, 1981). However, it is an inconsistent phenomenon (Jørgensen, 1981).

After ingestion by the host, the larvae penetrate the intestinal mucosa, moult in the mesenteric lymph nodes, migrate via the lymph and the blood to the lungs and break out from the capillaries to the alveoles after approximately one week. In the bronchioles the final moult occurs some days later. The young adults move to the bronchi and mature. The pre-patent period is three weeks. Patent infections will not last much longer than a few months in most animals. However, patency may persist much longer in some animals (Jarrett *et al.*, 1955; Gupta and Gibbs, 1970; Supperer and Pfeiffer, 1971). These carriers are very important epidemiologically. The presence of carriers in the spring is mainly associated with resumption of development of larvae which survived in an inhibited early L5 stage in the host (Supperer and Pfeiffer, 1971, Eisenegger and Eckert, 1975; Inderbitzin, 1976).

SOURCES OF INITIAL INFECTIONS

In the epidemiology of lungworm the acquisition of the initial infections is of vital importance. The following possibilities will be discussed below: over-wintered infection on pasture; carriers; prolonged survival in soil or on pasture until summer and infections indoors.

There are regional differences in the over-wintering on pasture of lungworms. In Switzerland and Austria (Eisenegger and Eckert, 1975; Supperer and Pfeiffer, 1971) the epidemiological role of over-wintering on pasture is thought to be insignificant. In the British Isles it is more important, particularly in the mild and damp western areas (Jarrett *et al.*, 1955; Allen and Baxter, 1957; Downey, 1973; Oakley, 1977; Baxter and Allen, 1977). According to Jørgensen (1981) the size of the herd and the time of turnout is important because pasture infectivity declines rapidly to very low levels in spring. Consequently, the chance of some animals acquiring initial patent infections in the spring will be higher when large herds are turned out early.

In Switzerland (Eisenegger and Eckert, 1975), Austria (Supperer and Pfeiffer, 1971) and lower Saxony (Bürger, 1979) over-wintering in carriers is thought to be the main source of initial infections in susceptible animals. The significance of carriers in the epidemiology of lungworms has also been demonstrated in Britain (Jarrett *et al.*, 1955; Michel, 1955; Michel and Shand, 1955). Generally carriers will be second-year grazing animals but adult animals cannot be excluded.

Roe, fallow and red deer are a different category of carriers. Their importance is not clear because their lungworm may be *Dictyocaulus eckerti*. Nevertheless, patent infections have been obtained in calves infected with material originating from roe deer (Hildebrandt, 1962).

Duncan *et al.*, (1979) and Oakley (1979) observed outbreaks of lungworm infection in calves turned out on pastures which contained lungworms in previous years. Their explanation was that lungworm larvae over-wintered in the soil and emerged onto the grass in summer. However, Jørgensen (1981) cast some doubts on their interpretation. As alternative explanation for the results of Duncan *et al.* (1979) he suggests pasture to pasture contamination by *Pilobolus*. He believes Oakley's (1979) results are due to indoor infection of one of the 120 calves used.

Although lungworm infections are mainly transmitted in pasture, indoor infections have been observed (Michel and Parfitt, 1956; Enigk and Düwel, 1962). These can occasionally result in outbreaks (Simionescu *et al.*, 1972, Jørgensen *et al.*, 1985). Generally infections in housed stock are caused by ingestion of infected drinking water or food which has been contaminated by housed carriers. Recently, the role of *Pilobolus* in the transmission of these infections has been demonstrated experimentally (Grønvold and Jørgensen, 1987). Technically, lungworm vaccination is also a housed infection. Some of the irradiated larvae may reach maturity and vaccinated animals may excrete lungworm larvae at turn out.

BUILD UP OF INFECTIONS TO POSSIBLE DISEASE LEVELS

Michel (1969) indicated that outbreaks of husk would occur in the first, second or third generation after initial infection depending on infection levels and suitable conditions for translation of larvae to pasture.

Considering the pre-patent period of three weeks and the translation time of approximately one week, this implies that outbreaks occur approximately one, two or three months after initial infection. This would mean that most outbreaks will not result from the acquisition of over-wintered larvae because the outbreaks occur later than July. Thus, disease will probably result mainly from initial infections obtained from carriers or possibly from over-wintered larvae which emerged from the soil in summer.

According to Michel and Parfitt (1956), the environmental conditions in summer generally are too dry for optimal translation of lungworm larvae. The consequence of this may be a poor development of infections in summer leading either to development of immunity or, possibly, to outbreaks later on.

In any case, the factors which control the outcome of the race between lungworm population build-up and build-up of immunity in susceptible animals are far from clear.

CONCLUSION

To some extent the epidemiology of lungworm infection is predictable. It is obvious that throughout most of the grazing season a pasture will be infective one week after contamination as a result of the very efficient translation of the infection. However, the quantitative effect of moisture on this translation is not yet well known, though it is obvious that translation is more efficient under moist conditions. It is clear that this rapid translation makes control by grazing management very difficult because this control should theoretically, imply a weekly move to clean pasture.

The reason why the epidemiology of lungworm infections is not predictable is because it is not certain when initial infections will be acquired and what the extent of these infections will be. This is because it is not certain whether silent carriers are present or whether larvae can over-winter on pasture. Therefore, the pattern of pasture infectivity will be extremely variable in time and place. Nevertheless, there must be a seasonal trend in pasture infectivity because the higher incidence of husk at the end of the grazing season must reflect higher overall pasture infectivity levels at that time.

Further research on different aspects of the epidemiology of lungworm infections is necessary.

REFERENCES

Allen, D. and Baxter, J. T. (1957) *Vet. Rec.*, **69**, 717
Baxter, J. T. and Allen, D. (1977) *Vet. Rec.*, **110**, 394
Boon, J. H., Kloosterman, A. and van den Brink, R. (1982) *Vet. Quart.*, **4**, 155
Boon, J. H., Kloosterman, A. and van der Lende, T. (1984) *Vet. Quart.* **6**, 13
Bürger, H. J. (1979) *Facts and Reflections*, **3**, 137
Downey, N. E. (1973) *Vet. Rec.*, **93**, 505
Duncan, J. L., Armour, J., Bairden, K. *et al.*, (1979) *Vet. Rec.*, **104**, 274
Eisenegger, H. and Eckert, J. (1975) *Schweiz. Arch. Tierheilkd.*, **117**, 255
Enigk, K. and Düwel, D. (1961) *Tierärztl. Umsch.*, **16**, 415
Enigk, K. and Düwel, D. (1962) *Dtsch. Tierärztl. Wochenschr.*, **78**, 102
Eysker, M. and de Coo, F. A. M. (1988) *Res. Vet. Sci.*, **44**, 178
Eysker, M. and van Miltenburg (1988) *Vet. Parasitol* (in press)
Gupta, R. P. and Gibbs, H. C. (1970) *Can. Vet. J.*, **11**, 149
Grønvold, J. and Jørgensen, R. J. (1987) *Prev. Vet. Med.*, **5**, 43
Hildebrandt, J. (1962) *Thesis*, University of Hannover, Hannover, Germany
Inderbitzin, F. (1976) *Thesis*, University of Zurich, Zurich, Switzerland
Jacobs, D. E. and Fox, M. T. (1985) *Vet. Rec.*, **116**, 75
Jacobs, D. E., Fox, M. T. and Koyo (1985) *Vet. Rec.*, **116**, 492
Jarrett, W. F. H., McIntyre, W. J., Urquhart, G. M. *et al.*, (1955) *Vet. Rec.*, **67**, 820
Jørgensen, R. J. (1981) *Acta Vet. Scand. Suppl.*, **76**, 1
Jørgensen, R. J., Rønne, H., Helsted, C. *et al.*, (1982) *Vet. Parasitol.*, **10**, 331
Jørgensen, R. J., Bisgaard Madsen, E., Grønvold, J., *et al.*, (1985) *Dansk Vet. Tidesskr.*, **68**, 358
Michel, J. F. (1955) *J. Comp. Pathol. Ther.*, **65**, 149
Michel, J. F. (1969) *Vet. Rec.*, **85**, 326
Michel, J. F. and Parfitt, J. W. (1956) *Vet. Rec.*, **68**, 229
Michel, J. F. and Rose, J. H. (1954) *J. Comp. Pathol.*, **64**, 195
Michel, J. F. and Shand, A. (1955) *Vet. Rec.*, **67**, 249
Oakley, G. A. (1977) *Vet. Rec.*, **101**, 187
Oakley, G. A. (1979) *Vet. Rec.*, **104**, 460
Oakley, G. A. (1981) *Res. Vet. Sci.*, **30**, 255
Simionescu, E. D., Orbelescu, D., Boloanta, T. *et al.*, (1972) *Seria Med. Vet.*, **13**, 181
omers, C. J., Downey, N. E. and Grainger, J. N. R. (1985) *Vet. Rec.*, **116**, 657
Supperer, R. and Pfeiffer, H. (1971) *Berl. Münch. Tierärztl. Wochenchr.*, **84**, 386

P MSOLLA

Bovine parasitic otitis : An up-to-date review

INTRODUCTION

BOVINE PARASITIC otitis which was first reported by Malloy in 1959 (Jibbo, 1966) and later described in detail by Jibbo (1966) is now well established in the predominantly hot and humid coastal regions of Tanzania, as well as up-country regions. Although initially observed in ranch and traditional herds, the disease is now gaining a foothold in a number of dairy farms and causing serious economic losses as a result of chronic wasting. This necessitates culling of beef animals before slaughter weight, a sharp drop in milk production, infertility and deaths (Msolla *et al.*, 1987).

EPIDEMIOLOGY

Bovine parasitic otitis is caused by a small (1–2 mm long) free living viviparous nematode *Rhabditis bovis* (Kreiss, 1964; Jibbo, 1966). However, recently another unnamed oviparous species of *Rhabditis* has been found in mixed clinical infections with *Rhabiditis bovis* (Lweno *et al.*, 1983; Walter, 1985 and Msolla, Matandala *et al.*, 1986). The exact role of this new isolate in the pathogenesis of the disease is yet to be determined. The nematodes can be cultured in bovine and equine serum agar. A number of coliforms, most commonly *Staphylococcus* spp., *Corynebacterium bovis*, *Pseudomonas* spp. and *Streptococcus* spp. have been isolated from clinical cases along with the nematodes but they seem to play a secondary role in the pathogenesis of the disease (Msolla, Matandala *et al.*, 1986).

Although the exact pathogenesis of bovine parasitic otitis is not known, it seems that once in the ear the nematode causes loss of the integrity of the ear epithelium resulting in ulcerations. These are then invaded by the pyogenic coliforms causing severe aural inflammation (Lweno *et al.*, 1983). However, warmth and humidity of the ear canal are important in the stimulation of excessive glandular secretion which, together with the adherent organic particles, provides a favourable media for bacterial and saprophytic activity. The fairly long external acoustic meatus of boss indicus may play a predisposing role in this respect although boss taurus are also equally affected.

So far, cattle are the only known hosts but rabbits have been infected under experimental conditions (Msolla, Matandala *et al.*, 1986). Although cattle of all ages are susceptible, immature animals seem to suffer a more severe clinical disease possibly because they have less immunological tolerance. The âetiological agent, *Rhabditis bovis* multiplies freely and lives in manure as a saprophyte (Jibbo, 1966;

Msolla, Matandala *et al.*, 1986) Their multiplication and survival is enhanced by warm, humid weather.

The incidence of the disease is highest along the coastal belt and during the rainy season. The incidence is also higher amongst dipped (70%) than in sprayed (5%) animals. Viable nematodes have been recovered from 0.25% toxaphene dip wash tanks where clinically infected animals were being routinely dipped. These worms are introduced by the infective aural discharges and manure or soil carried in between hooves of the animals being dipped. The nematodes have been shown to multiply and survive in 0.25% toxaphene (Msolla, Matafu *et al.*, 1986). Chronically infected animals are responsible for the introduction of the disease in virgin areas.

Flies (*Muscae* spp.) have also been incriminated in the transmission of the disease because they are attracted to the infected offensive smelling aural discharges and carry the minute nematodes in their feathery legs to other susceptible animals (Jibbo, 1966; Msolla, Matafu *et al.*, 1986). It is also possible that the minute larvae may be carried in the intersegmental abdominal furrows of the flies (Bovien, 1987). The highest incidence of the disease also coincides with the high fly activity.

Bovine parasitic otitis is also known to occur in Botswana, Kenya, Uganda, Zimbabwe, and Sudan (Msolla, Matandala *et al.*, 1986) and Brazil (Walter, 1985).

CLINICAL SIGNS

The initial symptoms may pass unnoticed. In severe cases, the affected animals are dull and inappetant with a bloody aural discharge. In long standing acute cases, there is usually a dirty dark brown (mixture of blood and pus) aural discharge which soils the hair below and in front of the affected ear. This discharge has an offensive smell which can be perceived from a distance.

With time the discharge dries on the skin below and in front of the ear. When it peels off substantial amounts of hair are removed leaving an alopecic area. There is swelling on the external auditory meatus which may distort or occlude the lumen of the meatus completely. Both the root of the ear, the eyelids and the local lymph nodes may be swollen. The majority of the cases have a bilateral ear infection. In a few cases the base of the ear may be completely undermined by severe ulceration resulting in dropping of the ear flap. Involvement of the middle ear may cause severe pharyngitis by extension of the infection through the pharyngotympanic tube. This is a painful condition. The animal does little, if any, grazing and swallowing is impaired. This results in lodging of the cud between the gums and the cheek of the affected ear.

Ultimately, the infection passes through the inner ear and into the brain. This results in typical central nervous system abberations whereby the affected animal manifests a stiff neck with the head held low. The animal tends to circle towards the affected ear and occasionally exhibits head shaking in an attempt to expel the debris from the ear canal. Such severely affected animals become recumbent with paddling limb movements prior to death (Jibbo, 1966; Msolla *et al.*, 1985).

In the chronic and neglected cases, secondary myiasis resulting from larvae emerging from eggs deposited in the ear by *Chrysomyia bezziana* is a common feature. This makes the clinical picture even more severe. The overall morbidity is over 70%; the mortality is roughly 10%. In view of this, bovine parasitic otitis should be considered as a herd infection requiring herd, rather than individual, treatment.

PATHOLOGY

General emaciation is the main feature in long standing neglected cases. The lesions are restricted to the head region. In the very early stages there is usually hyperaemia of the mucous membranes of the auditory meatus with few visible motile nematodes. Later there are ulcerations which may involve much of the external ear.

In such cases, the conchal cartilage may be perforated. This may ultimately lead to dropping of the ear flap. On removal of the aural debris from the external ear, red raw areas of ulcerations are evident (Jibbo, 1966; Lweno *et al.*, 1983). There is also a marked swelling of the external auditory meatus which may distort or occlude the lumen of the meatus completely. Pharyngitis and lymphadenitis of regional lymph nodes occurs when the infection has extended through the eustachian tube from the middle ear. The brain changes are limited to the lateral aspects of the medulla oblongata and cerebellum and are gangrenous in nature (Jibbo, 1966). In other cases haemorrhagic foci and micro-abscesses are evident (Msolla, Matandala *et al.*, 1986).

Microscopically, there is epithelial cell desquamation in the external ear. In some cases there is severe loss of epithelium down to the subepithelium. The exudate overlying the epithelium consists of necrotic epithelial cells, lymphocytes, plasma cells, macrophages and neutrophils in variable degrees of disintegration. There is also a mononuclear and polymophonuclear cell infiltration with plasma cell lymphocytes and macrophages being predominant (Lweno *et al.*, 1983).

DIAGNOSIS

Advanced cases of bovine parasitic otitis are diagnosed on clinical grounds. Early cases may be missed unless ears are examined individually. Detailed examination of the infected ear reveals putrid material in which numerous, very tiny, actively moving organisms can be seen. A swab taken from such aural debris and washed in physiological saline solution and examined under a stereo microscope reveals the nematodes.

TREATMENT

Topical drugs and acaricide mixtures have been used for the treatment of bovine parasitic otitis with varying degrees of success. Re-infection is common and frequent treatment is vital (Jibbo, 1966).

Ivermectin, when given subcutenously at 10 mg/50 kg body weight, has been found to be over 95% effective. (Msolla *et al.*, 1985). The drug has a wide margin of safety but it is expensive considering that herd treatment and reinfection occurs within 60–90 days in a small proportion of treated cases. This is because the animals go back into the nematode-infested dip tanks (Msolla, Matafu *et al.*, 1986).

CONTROL

Treatment of 0.25% toxaphene dip wash tanks with approximately 2 p.p.m. nicotine has been found to be 95% effective in the treatment and control of bovine parasite otitis (Msolla *et al.*, 1987). Nicotine has been used as an insecticide since 1960 when tobacco waste was used to control pear lace bug on pear trees in France. Nicotine sulphate (black leaf) has been used to control infestation of cattle by *Hypoderma* larvae (Jones and John, 1943; McGrath and Campbell, 1944). In southern Africa, 0.04% nicotine was used to check tick resistence in arsenic dip tanks (Falmer-Hansen, 1984 personal communication). When used alone, nicotine is unstable and does not have a long residual effect. The tobacco dust used for the extraction of nicotine is cheap, as is the extraction process. There are a number of advantages in using dip-wash treated with nicotine. These include:

1. Animals are treated for two conditions at the same time, thus reducing labour costs
2. The combination of acaricide and nicotine might reduce any tendency towards tick resistence against acaricide

However, it is important to monitor the rate of nicotine replenishment in the dipwash because of the residual effect on animal tissue and the need to counter the development of resistance in the animal. The animal product may also be toxic to the consumer.

ECONOMIC IMPORTANCE

The disease is much more widespread in Tanzania than was the case 25 years ago when the country had less than two hundred dip tanks. Today Tanzania has more than 2000 dip tanks. The disease causes severe economic losses due to chronic wasting, heavy culling and emergency slaughter of stock which would not benefit from any form of treatment before attaining slaughter weight. This upsets the breeding, sales and management programmes of many farms. In lactating animals, there is a severe drop in milk production and overall infertility in breeding stock due to silent heat.

REFERENCES

Bovien, P. (1937) Some types of association between nematode and insects. *Vidensk. Medd. Naturh. Foren. Kbh,* **10,** 1–114

Jibbo, J. M. (1966) Bovine parasitic otitis. *Bull. Epizoot. Dis. Africa* **14,** 59–63

Jones, T. H. and John, F. V. (1943) *Vet. Rec.* **55,** 243

Kreiss, H. A. (1964). Ein Never Nematodes ah dem aiiserven Gehorgang Von Zeburidern in Ostafrika, *Rhabditis bovis* n.sp. *Schweizenarch Tieheik,* **106,** 372-378

Lweno, M., Semuguruka, W. D. and Mhoma, J. R. (1983) Nematode otitis. Etiological and pathological aspects. *Tanzania Vet. Bull.* **5,** 8–17

McGrath, R. E. and Campbell, D. (1944) *Vet. Rec.* **56,** 64–65

Msolla, P., Falmer-Hansen, J. Musemakweli, J. and Monrad, J. (1985) Treatment of bovine parasitic otitis using ivermectin. *J. Tropical Animal Health and Production* **17,** 166–168

Msolla, P., Matafu, E. P. M. and Monrad, J. (1986) Epidemiology of bovine parasitic otitis. *J. Tropical Animal Health and Production,* **18,** 51–52

Msolla, P., Matandala, M. T., Kassuku, A. A. and Semuguruka, W. D. (1986). Bovine parasitic otitis: a constraint to livestock productivity: Further epidemiological studies. *Proc. Tanzania Vet. Assoc. Scientific Conference* **4**

Msolla, P., Mmbuji W. E. O. and Kassuku A. A. (1987). Field control of bovine parasitic otitis. *Tropical Animal Health and Production* **19**, 179–183

Walter, M. Jr. (1985) Isolation of new *Rhabditis* spp. from clinical cases of otitis. *Mem. Inst. Oswaldo Grux, Rio de Janeiro* **80**, 11–16

G. O. ODIAWO

Mucormycosis infection in cattle

INTRODUCTION

MUCORMYCOSIS (ZYGOMYCOSIS) is an infection caused by fungi of the Mucoraceae family, class, Zygomycetes and genera *Absidia, Mucor* and *Rhizopus*. They are characterized morphologically by the presence of aseptate, broad, ribbon-like hyphae. They are ubiquitous; on suitable media, they grow rapidly with loose, grey and cottony colonies in 2–5 days. The mycellia consist of slender stalks. The sporangiophores contain sporangiopores, the asexual spores in the sporangia. Members of the *Absidia* and *Rhizopus* genera produce rhizoids but those of the genera *Mucor*, do not.

INCIDENCE

The incidence of mucormycosis in animals is low. However, it is increasing because mucorales hitherto rarely encountered even as contaminants, are now being reported as causative agents of the disease in humans (Dean *et al.*, 1977; Kien *et al.*, 1979).

Members of the Mucoraceae family have little ability to produce disease on their own in the absence of other stress factors within the animals. They are, therefore, regarded as opportunistic agents. They require some predisposing factors such as prolonged antibiotic and/or steroid therapy (Gleiser, 1953), a compromised immune system (Martin *et al.*, 1954); chronically debilitated individuals, and metabolically unbalanced animals, together with the presence of concurrent diseases (Baker *et al.*, 1957; Sidransky and Pearl, 1961; Seeling, 1965; Mills and Hirth, 1967; Spratling *et al.*, 1968 and Chick *et al.*, 1975). Butterworth *et al.*, (1982) reported that *Schistozomes* cause immuno-suppression by cleaving a peptide from the immuno-globulin G (IgG) and thus inhibit many cellular immune responses. In my study (Odiawo *et al.*, 1986, unpublished report) intestinal bovine mucormycosis was diagnosed on three occasions on a single farm where infections by *Schistozoma mattheei* is known to be enzootic. Ruminal acidosis in cattle with grain engorgement has also been suggested as one of the other predisposing factors (Schwartz *et al.*, 1977).

TRANSMISSION

Mucorales are saprophytes found mostly in organic matter. Therefore, infections are always derived from sources in the environment where the growth rate of the fungus is determined by the soil moisture content, temperature and humidity. Inhalation of dust containing fungal elements is the principal mode of transmission. The primary focus of infection is in the lungs. Ingestion of feed (hay and silage) contaminated with fungal agents is another route of infection. It is suggested (Cordes, *et al.*, 1967) that when infection is via the alimentary canal, there is a possibility that the infection will spread and localize in pregnant uteri. Haematogenous spread to other organs is also possible (Gitter and Austwick, 1959; Kharole *et al.*, 1988).

PATHOGENESIS

The sporangiospores germinate and the hyphae invade the small blood vessels causing thrombosis, infarction and necrosis (Davis *et al.*, 1955). The pathobiosis is characterized by massive infiltration of neutrophils, lymphocytes, plasma cells, macrophages and the presence of giant cells forming a true pyogranulomatous reaction in the affected organs (Figure 1). The cellular and tissue necrosis is followed by calcification. Ulceration and perforation of part of the gastrointestinal tract may result in severe peritonitis with ultimate spread to the uterus in the case of mature and pregnant animals. Occasional haematogenous spread from the primary focus to other organs including the brain, pregnant uteri and orbital tissue have been described (Cordes *et al.*, 1967; Kharole *et al.*, 1988; Knudtson *et al.*, 1975).

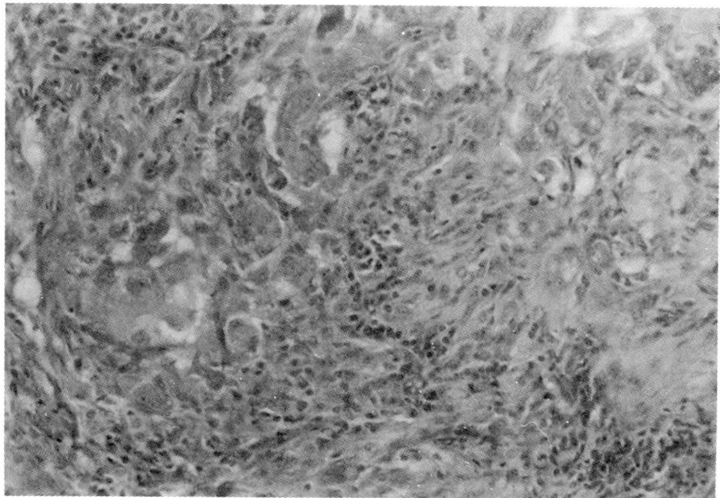

Fig. 1. Section of the intestinal wall of a one-year old steer showing a granulomatous reaction with neutrophils, mononuclear leukocytes and giant cells. H & E Magnification × 260.

CLINICAL SIGNS

The clinical signs are non-specific because of the variation in the organs in which the infection localizes. Calcified granulomas that involve the mesenteric lymph nodes can easily be confused with those of bovine tuberculosis affecting the same organs (Davis *et al.*, 1955). Yearling animals with the infection are likely to appear depressed, thin and hide-bound with a rough coat and poor growth rate; even though they maintain a normal appetite. The temperature and heart rates are usually unaffected. Respiratory dyspnoea, however, may be seen if the infection involves the lungs. If the gastrointestinal tract is involved, and depending on the portion of the gut, the condition may be characterized by rumenal stasis due to rumenitis, diarrhoea or passage of scanty, mucoid and sometimes blood-tinged faeces, especially if the intestinal walls are involved. In my experience, if the animal has markedly lost condition, and the mesenteric lymph nodes are affected, it is possible to palpate the granulomas through the intact external abdominal wall as readily as per rectum. However, this is by no means confirmatory.

Diarrhoea due to gastroenteritis has been described in young calves (Gitter and Austwick, 1959; Mills and Hirth, 1967). Severe peritonitis may result from a perforated abomasal or rumenal ulcers. Mycotic abortions due to necrotizing placentitis have been reported in cattle 3–7 months pregnant. The aborted fetuses have ringworm-like lesions on the skin (Austwick and Venn, 1962; Munday, 1967).

DIAGNOSIS

Clinical diagnosis is not always easy. This is because the condition resembles many other afebrile conditions. The mere isolation of the fungi from faeces may not constitute infection because of their ubiquitous nature. There are no serological tests available for disease confirmation. Biopsy specimens taken from the affected organs and tissues for both mycological and histopathological diagnosis are usually the best. The presence of aseptate fungal elements in a biopsy specimen stained with haematoxylin and eosin among necrotic and typical pyogranulomatous reaction (Figure 2) is confirmatory. Cases of osseous metaplasia have been reported (Odiawo *et al.*, 1986, unpublished report). (Figure 3).

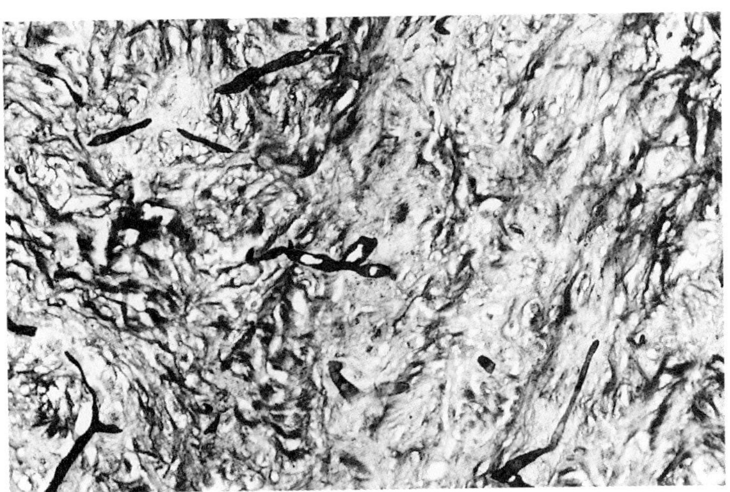

Fig. 2. Non-septate fungal elements in mesenteric lymph node granuloma of an 18-month old Sussex steer. Hexamine silver stain; magnification × 450

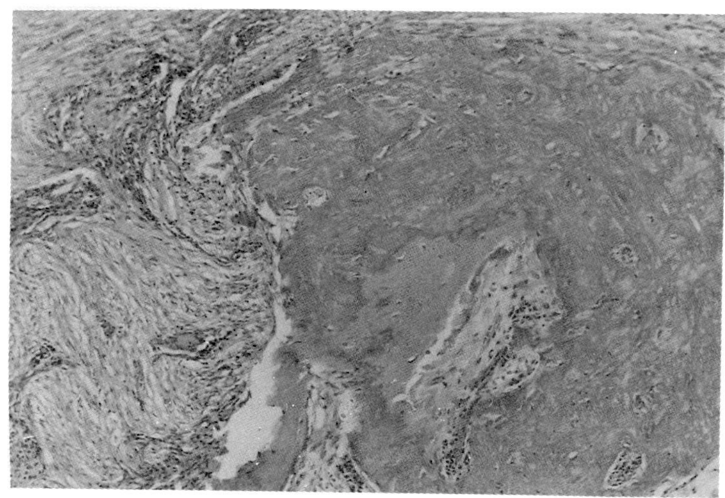

Fig. 3. Metastatic pulmonary granuloma showing osseous metaplasia. Magnification × 260.

TREATMENT

Treatment is rarely attempted because the disease is almost always diagnosed at post-mortem examinations. However, copper sulphate solution administered in drinking water has been shown to be an effective agent in controlling the gastrointestinal form of the disease in calves (Blood *et al.*, 1985).

REFERENCES

Austwick, P. K. C. and Venn, J. A. J. (1962) In: *Proceedings Fourth International Congress of Animal Reproduction* (The Hague) **3**, 562

Baker, R. D., Bassert, D. E. and Ferrington, E. (1957) *Am. Med. Assoc. Arch. Pathol.* **631**, 176–182

Blood, D. C., Radostits, O. M. and Henderson, J. A. (1985) Mucormycosis. In: *Veterinary Medicine*, 6th ed, Pitman, Bath, pp. 858–859

Butterworth, A. E., Taylor, D. W. and Veith, M. C. (1982) *Immunol. Rev.*, **61**, 5

Cordes, D. O., Royal, W. A. and Shortridge, E. H. (1967) *NZ Vet. J.*, **15**, 143

Chick, E. W., Balows, A. and Furcolow, M. L. (1975) Opportunistic fungal infections. In: *Proceedings of the Second International Conference* Charles C. Thomas, Springfield, Illinois

Davis, C. L., Anderson, W. A. and McCrory, B. R. (1955) *J. Am. Vet. Med. Assoc.*, **126**, 261–267

Dean, D. F., Ajello, L., Irwin, R. S., Woelk, W. K. and Sharulis, G. J. (1977) Cranial Zygomycosis caused by *Saksenaea vasiformis*. *J. Neurosurg*, **46**, 97–103

Gitter, M. and Austwick, P. K. C. (1959) *Vet. Rec.*, **71**, 6

Gleiser, A. (1953) *J. Am. Vet. Med. Assoc.*, **123**, 441–445

Kharole, M. U., Chand, P., Monga, D. P. and Sadana, J. R. (1988) *Vet. Rec.*, **122**, 236

Kien, T. E., Edwards, F., Armstrong, D., Rosen, P. P. and Weitzman, I. (1979) Pneumonia caused by *Cunninghamella bertholletiae* complicating chronic lymphatic leukemina. *J. Clin. Microbiol.*, **10**, 140

Knudtson, W. K., Bergeland, M. E. and Kivkbride, C. A. (1975) *Sabouraudia,* **13,** 299

Martin, F. P., Lukeman, J. M., Ranson, R. F. and Geppert, L. J. (1954) *J. Paediatrics,* **44,** 437

Mills, J. H. L. and Hirth, R. S. (1967) *J. Am. Vet. Med. Assoc.,* **158,** 862

Munday, B. L. (1967) *NZ Vet. J.,* **15,** 149

Seeling, M. S. (1965) *Bact. Rev.,* **30,** 442–459

Sidransky, H. and Pearl, M. A. (1961) *Chest Diseases,* **39,** 630–642

Spratling, F. R., Sparrow, D. S. H. and Nielson, S. W. (1968) *Vet. Rec.,* **82,** 282–284

Schwartz, J. N., Donnelly, E. H. and Klintworth, G. K. (1977) Ocular and orbital phycomycosis. *Surv. Orphthalmol,* **22,** 3–38

SUSAN P. YEO

Bovine neonatology

INTRODUCTION

IN HUMAN medicine the study of the physiology and immunology of the young and of childhood diseases has long been recognized as a separate field of expertise. In the veterinary field neonatology is not widely recognized as a separate topic for study or specialization. To attempt to treat the neonate as a miniature adult of the species may be unwise because the neonate differs in respect of physiology and immunology.

Minute but detectable amounts of immunoglobulin M (IgM) and immunoglobulin G (IgG) are present in the bovine foetus by day 145 of gestation (Schultz, Dunne and Heist, 1973). However, calves, like other ruminants, are essentially agammaglobulin-aemic at birth and acquire immunoglobulins by ingestion of the immunoglobulin-rich first milk or colostrum. IgG_1 is the predominant immunoglobulin in bovine colostrum, but appreciable amounts of IgA and smaller quantities of IgM and IgG_2 are also present (Brandon, Watson and Lascelles, 1971). During the first 8–24 hours of life the small intestine is permeable to such macromolecules as immunoglobulins, and circulating levels of IgA, IgM and IgG rise during the first 24–48 hours of life. After this time immunoglobulin levels fall. For the rapidly redistributed IgA and IgM this occurs over the first 2–3 weeks of life, but IgG_1 is catabolized more slowly ($T_{1/2} = 18$ days) (Logan and Penhale, 1971) and appreciable quantities of passively transferred IgG, may be detected at 2–3 months of age.

The protection conferred to the newborn calf by passively transferred antibodies thus depends on this immunological experience of the dam and on the biological properties of the class(es) of antibody transferred. Thus the protection against coliform septicaemia afforded by passive transfer of IgM (Logan and Penhale, 1971) may be due to the ability of IgM to fix, complement and promote phagocytosis. IgA and IgG_1 are relatively ineffective at complement-mediated phagocytosis when compared with IgG_2 and IgM.

Inadequate intake of colostrum, i.e. low circulating levels of IgA, IgG_1 and IgG_2, at 2 weeks of age, has been correlated with the occurence of clinical respiratory disease at 2 months of age (Williams, Spooner and Thomas, 1975) and with increased morbidity and mortality rates from coliform septicaemia (Logan, McBeath and Lowman, 1974). The high immunoglobulin content of the milk during early lactation may give further local protection from enteric infection (Evans, 1981; Logan and Penhale, 1971).

Humoral immunity (antibody) is only a part of the body's defence system against invading pathogens and many defence mechanisms require antibody and cellular cooperation, e.g. opsonization of particles prior to phagocytosis. Antibody production itself is a function of cells (B lymphocytes) and other cells of the immune system include T lymphocytes (cytotoxic cells, killer cells, helper and suppressor cells), macrophages and neutrophils.

Cellular and humoral (antibody) aspects of the immune system begin to develop sequentially in the foetus. Cell-mediated responses as indicated by delayed type hypersensitivity response and lymphocyte transformation have been demonstrated at birth in calves inoculated *in utero* with a variety of antigens (Rossi, *et al.*, 1978). However, *in utero* infections with Blue Tongue virus and Bovine Virus Diarrhoea–Mucosal Disease virus may result in foetal death, the development of immunological tolerance, i.e. the birth of a viraemic, antibody negative animal, or the birth of a virus negative antibody positive individual, depending on the maturity of the foetal immune system at the time of infection (McClurkin *et al.*, 1984).

CELLULAR IMMUNOLOGY

In the newborn the peripheral blood lymphocyte to neutrophil ratio is 0.6:0.7 and the calf is lymphopaenic, eosinopaenic and neutrophilic when compared to the adult (Lamotte and Eberhart, 1976). The differences in leucocyte parameters in the newborn have been attributed to the rise in foetal cortisol which occurs 10–15 days before birth and is thought to trigger parturition. By 8 weeks of age an adult type leucocyte population is present.

Antibody (B cell) responses are present at birth, but are poorer than in older calves (Husband and Lascelles, 1975). When passively-derived (maternal) specific antibody is present in the circulation, a marked unresponsiveness to antigen has been reported by several workers (Husband and Lascelles, 1975; Stott and Taylor, 1985). Endogenous production of IgG_1 and IgA have also been reported to occur earlier and to reach higher concentrations at 128 days of life in colostrum-deprived calves than in colostrum-fed calves (Husband and Lascelles, 1975). Cell-mediated responses have been less well studied. At birth, calves reject skin grafts as vigorously as adults, which indicates the presence of an active cell-mediated immune system (Billingham and Lampkin, 1957).

In children defects in neutrophil and monocyte function, when compared with those of cells taken from adults, are well recorded (Miller, 1979). Neutrophils from calves have been shown to be deficient in their ability to phagocytose opsonized particles and in their ability to kill bacteria intracellularly (Hauser, Koob and Roth, 1986), to have a reduced capacity to kill cells by antibody-dependent cell cytotoxicity (Mossman *et al.*, 1984), and to have deficient *in vitro* locomotion (Yeo, 1987). Bacterial killing (Hauser, Koob and Roth, 1986) and neutrophil locomotion (Yeo, 1987) have been demonstrated to reach adult levels only after the first year of life. Most of these deficiencies have been demonstrated in *in vitro* assays but it would seem likely that *in vivo* a similar state of affairs exists.

MUCOSAL IMMUNE SYSTEM

In utero, the gastrointestinal and respiratory tracts are bathed in fluid. The lung is involved in the secretion of fluid which the gut absorbs. Thus at birth there is a major change of function.

At birth the local immune system is poorly developed in the gut (Husband, 1984) and in the lung (Anderson *et al.*, 1986). Plasma cells are present in both systems by the end of the first week of life, and plasma cells producing IgA predominate at mucosal surfaces by 4 months of age. IgG is the predominant immunoglobulin in respiratory tract secretions until 9–14 weeks of age, when the relative concentration of IgA exceeds that of IgG, a situation which persists in the adult (Morgan and Bourne, 1978). There is considerable evidence that the IgG_1 in respiratory tract secretions during the first week of life is derived passively from colostrum via the serum (Sullivan *et al.*, 1969; Pederson, 1973).

At 24 hours of age the predominant cell type recovered from the lung is the neutrophil (Fogarty, Quinn and Hannan, 1984), but by the end of the second week of life the alveolar macrophage predominates. Initially alveolar macrophages and neutrophils from young calves actually support the intracellular growth of bacteria, but by 12 weeks of age there is evidence of bacterial killing (Fogarty, Quinn and Hannan, 1984; Yeo, 1987).

IMPLICATIONS FOR THERAPY OF THE BOVINE NEONATE

Whilst much evidence has been cited to demonstrate the function, reduced or otherwise, of the neonatal immune system, it remains unclear as to when in the life of a calf its immune system is capable of affording protection against invading pathogens.

The neonate's body weight is 70–75% water, compared to 50–60% of the adult's body weight. The neonate is very susceptible to dehydration. Care should therefore be taken to maintain hydration at all times by the use of oral electrolytes or parentral infusions.

Phagocytes (neutrophils and macrophages) from young calves of less than 12 weeks of age are likely to support the intracellular growth of bacteria. Antibiotics must be given at doses and frequencies which will achieve minimum inhibitory concentrations in blood and tissue fluids to kill bacteria. Fortunately during the first month of life many natural barriers to the transport of antibiotics, e.g. the blood – brain barrier, are not fully developed and it may be easier to obtain therapeutic levels of drugs in the central nervous system than at any other time (Short and Clarke, 1984).

However, some excretory pathways are not fully developed in the young calf. Renal excretion of tetracyclines is likely to be reduced during the first month of life and, except in the treatment of septicaemias, the dosing interval should be increased by up to one-third. Metabolism of macrolide antibacterial drugs is unlikely to be a problem in calves as it is in foals. Oral administration of antibiotics is unlikely to be effective beyond the first month of life when rumen function becomes established (Short and Clarke, 1984).

Such cellular immune functions as bacterial killing, cell cytotoxicity and leucocyte movement are energy-dependent processes. Young animals have poor reserves of glycogen and glucose precursors. Therefore, care should be taken to provide sick calves with an adequate energy and protein supply. Many biological processes, including bacterial killing and protein synthesis for repair of damaged tissues, are enzyme-controlled reactions, and as such they may proceed more rapidly at temperatures one or two degrees above 37°C. However, pyrexia is not beneficial if the body temperature rises to a level where feed intake is depressed or convulsions intervene. Conversely metabolic processes are slowed in hypothermia and efforts should be made to maintain body heat in sick calves by the provision of an external heat source such as an infra red lamp or the use of thick layers of straw, a rug, sack or old woolly jumper.

CONCLUSIONS

The young calf differs from the adult bovine in many aspects of its immunology and physiology. Therapy of the young calf should therefore consist of the provision of an adequate dosage regime of a suitable chemotherapeutic agent and the provision of adequate supportive care.

REFERENCES

Anderson, M. L., Moore, P. F., Hyde, D. M. and Dungworth, D. L. (1986) Immunoglobulin containing cells in the tracheobronchial tree of cattle: relationship to age. *Res. Vet. Sci.*, **41**, 221–227

Billingham, R. E. and Lampkin, G. H. (1957) Further studies in tissue transplantation in cattle. *J. Embryol. Exp. Morphol.*, 351–356

Brandon, M. R., Watson, D. L. and Lascelles, A. K. (1971) The mechanism of transfer of immunoglobulins into mammary secretions of cows. *Aust. J. Biol. Med. Sci.* **49**, 613–623

Evans, P. A. (1981) Immunological studies of the porcine gut and mammary gland. *PhD. Thesis*, University of Bristol, Bristol UK

Fogarty, U., Quinn, P. J. and Hannan, J. (1984) Pulmonary alveolar macrophages: a study of their activity in young calves. In: *CES Seminar on Cell-Mediated Immunity* (ed. P. J. Quinn) CEC, Luxemburg. pp. 64–80

Hauser, M. A., Koob, M. D. and Roth, J. A. (1986) Variation of neutrophil function with age in calves. *Am. J. Vet. Res.*, **47**, 152–153

Husband, A. J. (1984) Ontogeny of the gut associated lymphoid system. In *The Ruminant Immune System*. (ed. J. E. Butler) *Adv. Exp. Med. Biol.*, **137**, 633–647

Husband, A. J. and Lascelles, A. K. (1975) Antibody responses to neonatal immunisation in calves. *Res. Vet. Sci.*, **18**, 201–207

Lamotte, G. B. and Eberhart, R. J. (1976) Blood leucocytes and plasma corticosteroids in colostrum-fed and colostrum-deprived calves. *Am. J. Vet. Res.*, **37**, 1189–1193

Logan, E. F. and Penhale, W. J. (1971) Studies on the immunity of the calf to colibacillosis. 1. The influence of colostral when and immunoglobulins on experimental colisepticaemaia. *Vet. Rec.*, **88**, 222–228

Logan, E. F., McBeath, D. G and Lowman, B. (1974) Quantitative studies on serum immunoglobulin levels in suckled calves from birth to 5 weeks. *Vet. Rec.*, **94**, 367–370

McClurkin, A. W., Littledike, E. T., Cutlip, R. C., Frank, G. H., Coria, M. F. and Bolin, S. R. (1984) Production of cattle immunotolerant to Bovine Virus Diarrhoea virus. *Can J. Comp. Med.*, **48**, 156–161

Miller, M. E. (1979) Phagocytic function of the neonate : selected aspects. *Paediatrics*, **64**, 709–712

Morgan, K. L. and Bourne, F. J. (1978) The respiratory tract immune system. In *Respiratory diseases in cattle,* (ed. W. B. Martin) Martinus Nijhoff, The Hague

Mossman, H., Schmitz, B., Bamberger, U., Gerhung, M. and Hammer, D. K. (1984) Antibody-dependent cell cytotoxicity in cattle with special reference to the newborn calf. In *Cell-Mediated Immunity* (ed. P. J. Quinn) CEC, Luxemburg

Pederson, K. B. (1973) The origin of immunoglobulin G in bovine tears. *Acta. Path. Microbiol. Scan. Sect B.*, **81**, 245–252

Rossi, C. R., Keisel, G. K., Kramer, T. T. and Hudson, R. S. (1978) Cell-mediated and humoral responses of cattle to *B.abortus*, *M.bovis and Tetanus toxoid*. Immunisation of the foetus. *Am. J. Vet. Res.*, **39**, 1742–1747

Schultz, R. D., Dunne, H. W. and Heist, C. W. (1973) Ontogeny of the bovine immune response. *Infection and Immunity*, **7**, 981–291

Short, C. R. and Clarke, C. R. (1984) Calculation of dosage regimens of antimicrobial drugs for the neonatal patient. *J. Am. Vet. Med. Assoc.*, **185**, 1089–1093

Stott, E. J. and Taylor, G. (1985) Respiratory Syncitial virus. *Arch. Virol.*, **84**, 1–52

Sullivan, A. L., Prendergast, R. A., Antunes, L. J., Silverstein, A. M. and Tomasi, T. B. (1969) Characterisation of the serum and secretory immune system of the cow and sheep. *J. Immunol.*, **103**, 334–344

Williams, M. R., Spooner, R. L. and Thomas, L. H. (1975) Quantitative studies on bovine immunoglobulins. *Vet. Rec.*, **96**, 81–84

Yeo, S. P. (1987) *PhD Thesis*, University of Bristol, Bristol, UK

K. A. LINKLATER

Watery mouth in lambs

INTRODUCTION

WATERY MOUTH in lambs is a condition which has been well recognized in the Scottish/English Border counties for many years. More recently it has been reported throughout the UK and is now considered to be one of the most important causes of mortality in young lambs. It is also known by the terms slavers, slavery mouth and rattle belly. Sporadic cases occur in many flocks but the condition can reach epidemic proportions under certain types of management.

CLINICAL SIGNS

Lambs from 12 to 72 hours old are affected. They are usually normal at birth before showing increasing signs of dullness, inappetence and lethargy. As the name suggests there is a characteristic profuse drooling of saliva from the mouth (Figure 1) and the lamb ceases to suck. Distension of the abdomen is a frequent sign and a splashing sound may result if the lamb is gently shaken. Bowel movements cease and meconium is frequently, but not always, retained. In the early stages of the condition rectal temperature is normal but as the condition progresses the affected animal becomes hypoglycaemic and hypothermic and will die unless remedial therapy is quickly instigated. Due to the abdominal distension, affected lambs may appear to be well nourished. Scouring is a rare sign unless the bowels stasis is successfully reversed.

DIAGNOSIS

In the early stages diagnosis presents no problems. However, lambs which are sick from other conditions such as scours and joint ill/navel ill may also salivate excessively though not as profusely as in watery mouth. As the condition progresses differentiation from starvation, hypothermia and colisepticaemia becomes progressively more difficult. At post-mortem examination, the findings are not pathognomonic though the signs of gut stasis, distension of the abomasum and possible retention of meconium along with the history are usually enough to confirm the diagnosis. Quantities of clear mucin are usually found in the abomasum and any milk present is unclotted. The distension of the abomasum is exacerbated by gas, which may also be found in the small intestine. There is usually a mild enteritis. In animals untreated with antibiotics prior to death, *Escherichia coli* can readily be isolated from gut and all other organs.

88

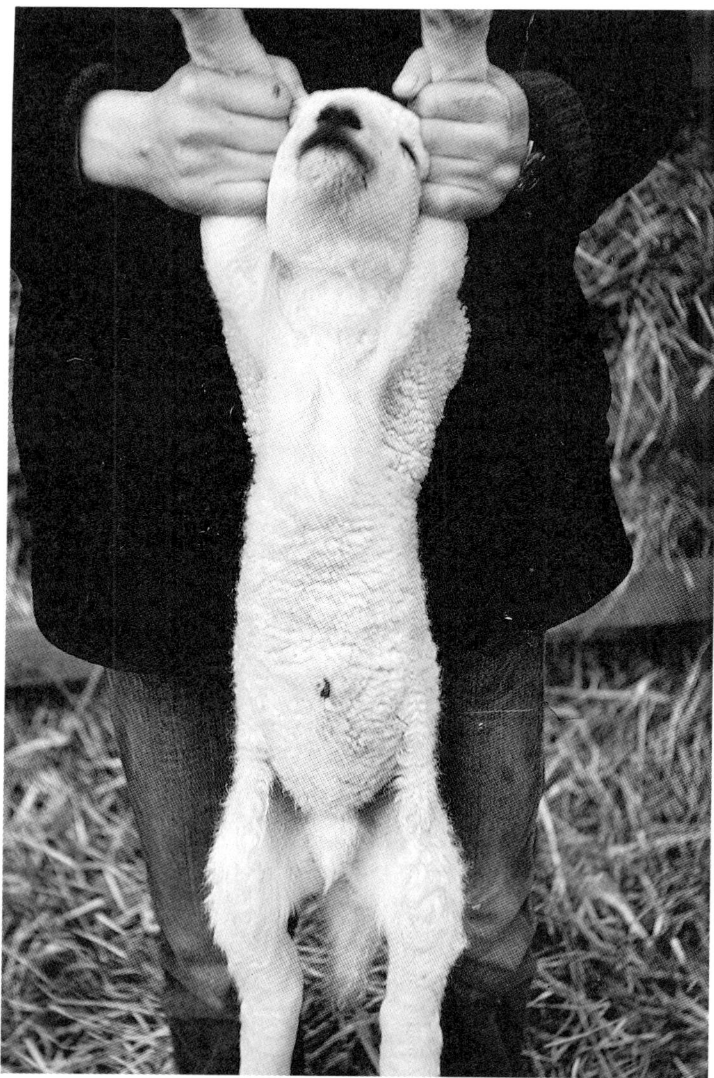

Fig. 1. Lamb affected with watery mouth showing profuse salivation and distension of the abdomen.

EPIDEMIOLOGY

Watery mouth is most common in intensive systems of management. It is rarely seen on the hills or in other systems where the ewes lamb out in the open fields. Unhygienic dirty surroundings in lambing areas or buildings predispose to the development of the condition. In flocks where watery mouth is a problem other conditions such as naval ill, joint ill, scour and hypothermia are often concurrently seen. Many of the more intensive low ground flocks claim to have an annually recurring problem with the condition.

Eales *et al.*, (1986) studied eleven flocks in which watery mouth was confirmed and reported flock incidences of from 1 to 24% and mortalities of from 7 to 83%. They also showed that watery mouth is more common in twins and triplets than in singles. The weight of the lamb did not appear to be significant. Twins born to lean ewes are more likely to be affected than those born to ewes in better bodily condition. With triplets no such distinction could be shown, presumably because the dams of these are generally all in relatively poor condition.

In another study of six flocks in the Scottish Borders, Collins *et al.*, (1985) reported a mean rate of morbidity in 6224 lambs of 1.6% and a mortality rate of those affected of 41%. They suggested that anything which interferes with sucking in the first twelve hours of life (e.g. castration or docking with rubber rings) is likely to increase the incidence of watery mouth.

CLINICAL CHEMISTRY AND HAEMATOLOGY

Collins *et al.*, (1985) were unable to demonstrate any relationship between susceptibility to watery mouth and plasma levels of either glucose or IgG. However, low plasma glucose levels were found in lambs which died. This is not surprising because these lambs would normally have been anorectic for some time. More extensive studies by Eales *et al.*, (1986) confirmed these earlier findings and also showed that a wide range of other biochemical parameters were not significantly different from those of normal lambs. The parameters looked at were total protein, albumin, calcium, magnesium, inorganic phosphate, copper and zinc.

More recently Hodgson *et al.*, (1988) have shown that lambs in which watery mouth has been experimentally reproduced have higher plasma lactate, creatinine and urea concentrations and lower plasma glucose levels than controls maintained under the same system of management. These same workers described a leucopenia in experimentally affected lambs. In contrast, Eales *et al.*, (1986) showed normal white cell counts in field cases.

AETIOLOGY

Field studies have suggested that *E.coli* plays a major role in the aetiology of the condition (Gilmour *et al.*, 1985). That organism was cultured from the gut contents of 25 lambs on which they carried out autopsies. Bacteraemia was also frequently detected. However, the strains isolated did not carry the K99 antigen which is commonly associated with the enterotoxigenic activity of *E.coli*.

Recent work by Hodgson and others (1988) has shown that signs of watery mouth can be reproduced experimentally using field strains of *E. coli*. Two strains isolated from the blood of lambs naturally affected with the condition and another strain not associated with watery mouth induced watery mouth disease in all of eight gnotobiotic colostrum-deprived lambs dosed orally at two hours of age with these strains. Typical signs of watery mouth were noted 12–18 hours after infection in seven of the lambs and at 40 hours post infection in the eighth. The clinical outcome appeared independent of the strain of *E.coli* used. Biochemical and haematological findings (*vide supra*) were consistent with those seen in endotoxic shock.

These findings give further credence to the hypothesis put forward by Eales (1987) for the pathogenesis of watery mouth. He suggests that newborn lambs pick up *E.coli* from their dams and the environment soon after birth. The bacteria can pass unhindered through the abomasum which has a pH of 7 at that time. The *E.coli* can then multiply, unless suppressed by colostrum or agents such as antibiotics. The bacterial products may reduce gut tone and motility which is already depressed in lambs of this age (Eales *et al.*, 1985). Partial or complete gut stasis encourages further bacterial multiplication. This results in invasion of the blood stream (bacteraemia) and the production of gas in the abomasum which leads to tympany and abdominal distension. Affected lambs stop eating and die of starvation, bacteraemia and respiratory embarrassment.

TREATMENT

For treatment to be successful it must be initiated as soon as possible after the signs have been identified. Basically, the aim is to promote gut motility, reverse the hypoglycaemia and control the coliform infection.

Eales (1987) suggests the following regime which he claims to be effective in 85% of cases where treatment is commenced early in the course of the condition:
1. Inject the lamb daily with broad spectrum antibiotics.
2. Feed the lamb by stomach tube three times daily. Each feed should consist of 100 to 200 ml of glucose/electrolyte solution containing the recommended dose of an appropriate antibiotic. One of the proprietary calf scour mixtures is suitable but the glucose content should be increased to 10% by the addition of powdered glucose.
3. Reverse the gut stasis either by use of oral purgatives or an enema (20 ml of soapy water injected about 5 cm into the rectum).
4. Leave the lamb with its dam unless it is too sick to look after itself.
5. Continue treatment until all signs have gone and the lamb is sucking normally from the ewe.

PREVENTION

Prevention is based on the hypothesis for the pathogenesis which has already been described. The first essential is to ensure that newborn lambs ingest adequate amounts of colostrum within one to two hours of birth. Any not sucking properly should be fed colostrum by stomach tube at the rate of 50 ml per kg body weight. This is especially important for any lambs which are weak at birth, e.g. small triplets. Ewes should be well fed in the latter third of pregnancy to ensure a good supply of colostrum. Any other factors which interfere with sucking, such as the application of rubber rings for docking and castration, should be postponed until the lambs are at least 24 hours of age.

Lambing quarters should be kept as clean as possible to cut down on environmental contamination. This applies to the pre-lambing areas as well as the individual pens. Ideally the latter should be cleaned out and disinfected between occupants. If problems with watery mouth arise, depopulation and thorough disinfection may be the only solution.

Oral antibiotics have been shown to be effective in preventing watery mouth. They should be administered as soon as possible after birth, preferably within 15 minutes. It is not a good idea to use antibiotics prophylactically until they are truly indicated, because strains of *E. coli* in many flocks tend to become resistant to a wide range of antibiotics very quickly. The longer the use of antibiotics can be postponed, the greater the chance they will be effective when really required.

Purgatives are widely used in some areas to prevent watery mouth. All lambs are given preparations such as Beechams Pills soon after birth to promote gut motility. If the hypothesis for the pathogenesis is correct, these preparations may have a part to play in the prevention of this still puzzling condition.

REFERENCES

Collins, R. O., Eales, F. A. and Small, J. (1985) Observations on watery mouth in newborn lambs. *Br. Vet. J.*, **141**, 135–140

Eales, F. A., Small, J., Murray, L. and McBean, A. (1985) Abomasal size and emptying time in healthy lambs and in lambs affected by watery mouth. *Vet. Rec.*, **117**, 332–335

Eales, F. A., Small, J., Gilmour, J. S., Donachie, W., Fitzsimons, J. and Dingwall, W. S. (1986) A field study of watery mouth : clinical, epidemiological, biochemical, haematological and bacteriological observations. *Vet. Rec.*, **119**, 543–547

Eales, F. A. (1987) Update: watery mouth. In *Practice,* supplement to *Vet. Rec.*, **9**, 12–17

Gilmour, J. S., Donachie, W. and Eales, F. A. (1985) Pathological and microbiological findings in 38 lambs with watery mouth. *Vet. Rec.*, **117**, 335–337

Hodgson, J. C., King, T. J., Hay, L. A. and Elston, D. A. (1988) Biochemical and haematological evidence for the involvement of endotoxin in the pathogenesis of watery mouth disease in lambs. *Res. Vet. Sci.*, in press

B. O. HOSIE

Infectious keratoconjunctivitis in sheep and goats

INTRODUCTION

INFECTIOUS KERATOCONJUNCTIVITIS (IKC) is a contagious disease of sheep and goats characterized by conjunctivitis and keratitis.

The synonyms include contagious conjunctivo-keratitis (CCK), contagious ophthalmia, inclusion keratoconjunctivitis, pink eye, heather blindness and snow blindness.

INCIDENCE

Infectious keratoconjunctivitis occurs throughout the world wherever sheep are kept. Cases are seen in lambs, hoggs, and adults. In the United Kingdom most outbreaks are dealt with by flock masters with or without veterinary assistance and very few are recorded by the veterinary investigation service (Anon, 1987). The disease appears to be painful but of little economic consequence unless it occurs among highly productive sheep at critical periods of the year. Axelsen (1961) reported that Merino ewes affected with keratoconjunctivitis between 4 and 2 weeks before mating and Border Leicester cross ewes affected during mating produced significantly fewer twins. Pregnancy toxaemia and agalactia may occur if heavily pregnant ewes cannot feed properly due to blindness.

AETIOLOGY

Although numerous infectious agents have been associated with keratoconjunctivitis in sheep, only two, *Chlamydia psittaci ovis* and *Mycoplasma conjunctivae*, are considered to be primary pathogens. Both agents have been isolated from the eyes of affected sheep in many parts of the world. In the United Kingdom *M. conjunctivae* is frequently isolated in outbreaks of ovine keratoconjunctivitis but there is only one report of *Chlamydia*-associated keratoconjunctivitis (Andrews *et al.*, 1987). All but one of the 300 ewes in the flock were severely affected.

CHLAMYDIA PSITTACI OVIS

Cooper (1974) reproduced keratoconjunctivitis in sheep by the intraocular inoculation of *Chlamydia*. Jones (1983) commented that the techniques employed could not exclude the possible concommittent presence of mycoplasmas. However, in a study of keratoconjunctivitis in feed lot lambs in the United States, Hopkins *et al.*, (1973) isolated *Chlamydia* from 42% of affected lambs. Complement fixing antibodies were detected in 43% of the lambs. In the United Kingdom, Andrews *et al.*, (1987) isolated *Chlamydia* from all five affected ewes sampled.

MYCOPLASMA CONJUNCTIVAE

This organism has been isolated from cases of infectious keratoconjunctivitis in Australasia, Europe and North America. The disease was reproduced in sheep by Jones *et al.*, (1976) and in goats by Trotter *et al.*, (1977). Following intraocular instillation of *M. conjunctivae* in sheep or subconjunctival inoculation of *M. conjunctivae* in goats the course of the disease lasted for about 18 days. However, *M. conjunctivae* was recovered for up to three months after an apparent recovery. This persistance of the infection is important in the spread of the disease both between and within flocks.

OTHER INFECTIOUS AGENTS

Acholeplasma oculi was isolated from the eyes of goats with keratoconjunctivitis and conjunctivitis was reproduced in experimental goats by Al-Aubaidi *et al.*, (1973). Arbuckle and Bonson (1980) isolated *A. oculi* together with *M.conjunctivae* from a flock of ewes in England but the relative significance of the concurrent isolations was not investigated.

Branhamella ovis (previously *Neisseria ovis*) is frequently isolated from both normal and affected eyes. *Moraxella bovis* and *Listeria monocytogenes* are rarely isolated. Several authors have suggested that these bacteria may monopolize on the primary lesion caused by *Chlamydia* or *Mycoplasma* and cause a more severe form of the disease. Experimental evidence for this proposition is lacking.

CLINICAL SIGNS

The descriptions of the clinical appearance of ovine keratoconjunctivitis are all essentially the same regardless of the causal agent identified. One or both eyes may be affected and animals frequently stand with the affected eye closed. Initially, there is a conjunctivitis with a great excess of clear lachrymal fluid, blepharospasm and cloudiness of the cornea. As the disease progresses vascularization extends inwards from the periphery of the cornea until the whole cornea becomes involved and the animal has difficulty in seeing. In severe cases corneal ulceration may ensue and the lachrymal discharge becomes muco-purulent.

The disease is frequently less severe in lambs than in adults. In lambs many cases do not progress through all the stages described and ulceration is rare in lambs. Uveitis associated with interstitial keratitis was reported by Andrews *et al.*, (1987) in ewes severely affected by *Chlamydia*-associated keratoconjunctivitis. In the USA polyarthritis may affect up to 85% of feed lot lambs with *Chlamydia*-associated keratoconjunctivitis (Hopkins *et al.*, 1973). This feature was not observed in outbreaks in the UK (Andrews *et al.*, 1987) or New Zealand (Cooper, 1974).

PATHOLOGY

In acute cases of keratoconjunctivitis numerous neutrophils, some lymphocytes and plasma cells and groups of two or three epithelial cells are found in smears of tears and in conjunctival scrapings stained by Giemsa. In *Chlamydia*-associated keratoconjunctivitis intracytoplasmic inclusion bodies may be found in 50% of affected animals. They stain purple with Giemsa stain and will fluoresce when stained with fluorescent antibody against the common group antigen (Bogaard, 1984; Moore and Whitley, 1984).

In *Mycoplasma*-associated keratoconjunctivitis Jones (1983) found large number of uni-, bi-, or tri-polar bodies associated with the epithelial cells in tears or corneal or conjunctival scrapings stained with May–Grunwald–Giemsa stain. These bodies were specifically stained in the fluorescent antibody test using antiserum to *M. conjunctivae*. Histopathology at the acute stages of infection with *M. conjunctivae* revealed the cornea infiltrated by polymophonuclear and mononuclear cells.

DIAGNOSIS

IKC is the most common cause of keratoconjunctivitis in sheep and goats and clinical diagnosis is relatively easy once foreign bodies and entropion are eliminated. Other conditions to consider include pine or cobalt deficiency, bluetongue and pasteurellosis.

Confirmation of the diagnosis is based on the following:

1. Isolation of one of the casual organisms from swabs taken from early clinical cases. The swabs should be placed immediately into Stuarts transport medium, *Mycoplasma* transport medium and *Chlamydia* transport medium. The bacteria associated with ovine keratoconjunctivitis are readily cultured aerobically on 5% sheep blood agar. With appropriate high quality artificial media *M. conjunctivae* should be cultured from a high proportion of the swabs. Embryonated eggs or specially treated tissue cultures are required to isolate *Chlamydia*.

2. Demonstration of organisms in tears or conjunctival scrapings. Both *Chlamydia* and *Mycoplasma* may be detected in smears stained by Giemsa, but fluorescent antibody tests, using specific antiserum are preferable because interpretation of stain preparations may be confused by the presence of melanin granules.

3. Examination of sera for antibodies to *Chlamydia*. Paired serum samples taken 14 days apart can be examined by the complement fixation test for evidence of a rising titre.

EPIDEMIOLOGY AND TRANSMISSION

Immunity to both *Chlamydia*-associated and *Mycoplasma*-associated keratoconjunctivitis is poor and relapses in individual animals and recurrence of outbreaks in flocks is common. *M. conjunctivae* may persist in the eyes and the nares for months after clinical recovery from the disease. Therefore, apparently unaffected animals may introduce the disease to previously unaffected flocks. Purchased rams are probably important in the spread of keratoconjunctivitis to closed flocks (Hosie, 1988; Konig, 1983).

Outbreaks may occur at any time of the year but most are seen in the autumn. Typically, a high proportion of a flock is affected and transmission is probably by contact. Weaning, gathering of lambs for marketing, gathering of ewes for mating together with the introduction of rams facilitate the rapid spread of the disease in the autumn. Outbreaks in the spring in pregnant or recently lambed ewes and their lambs can be particularly troublesome. The close contact in lambing pens and around feeding troughs is probably responsible for the spread.

The disease in the adults is often more severe and less responsive to treatment than the disease in lambs or hoggs (Hosie, 1988). The reason is not known but some immunological phenomenon may be responsible. Cheviot ewes were thought by Wall (1982) to be more susceptible to keratoconjunctivitis than Scottish Blackface ewes and Eales (personal communication) made a similar observation with Cheviot and Blackface lambs. However, Hosie (1988) found no difference in the susceptibility of the two breeds.

TREATMENT AND CONTROL

Although success is claimed for a wide variety of topical and parenteral antibiotic treatments, Hosie (1988) and Konig (1983) found that on critical evaluation oxytetracycline was the most effective antibiotic for the treatment of keratoconjunctivitis in sheep. A single intramuscular injection of a long acting formulation of oxytetracycline is an effective treatment for adult sheep. In serious cases an application of aureomycin topical powder in addition to the parental treatment may be worthwhile.

Parenteral oxytetracycline is also effective in suckling and weaned lambs with *Mycoplasma*-associated keratoconjunctivitis. Because the disease is seldom severe in this age group, treatment with aureomycin topical powder is generally sufficient. Although a single application was found satisfactory in a hill flock (Hosie, 1988), several daily applications may be required for more intensively managed lambs. Parenteral antibiotic is probably appropriate for lambs affected by *Chlamydia*-associated keratoconjunctivitis, particularly where polyarthritis is a sequelae.

Despite the use of effective antibiotic therapy, relapses are common and treatment may prolong the duration of outbreaks of keratoconjunctivitis. Initially, affected sheep should be isolated to prevent the spread of infection. In the face of a severe and widespread outbreak of keratoconjunctivitis parenteral treatment of all animals in the flock with a long acting formulation of oxytetracycline may have to be considered in an effort to eliminate the infection. Purchased rams should be treated prophylactically with oxytetracycline to prevent the introduction of keratoconjunctivitis to closed, previously unaffected flocks.

REFERENCES

Al-Aubaidi, J. M., Dardiri, A. H., Muscoplatt, C. C. and McCauley, E. H. (1973) Identification and characterization of *Acholeplasma oculusi* sp. Nov. from the eyes of goats with keratoconjunctivitis. *Cornell Vet.*, **63**, 117–129

Andrews, A. H., Goddard, P. C., Wilsmore, A. J. and Dagnell, G. J. R. (1987) A chlamydial keratoconjunctivitis in a British sheep flock. *Vet. Rec.*, **120**, 238–239

Anon (1987) Veterinary Investigation Diagnosis Analysis II 1986. Epidermiology Unit, Central Veterinary Laboratory, Weybridge, UK

Arbuckle, J. B. R. and Bonson, M. D. (1980) The isolation of *Acholeplasma oculi* from an outbreak of ovine keratoconjunctivitis. *Vet. Rec.,* **106,** 15

Axelsen, A. (1961) Effect of contagious ophthalmia on multiple lambing and sheep liveweight. *Aust. Vet. J.,* **37,** 60–62

Bogaard, A. E. J. M. (1984) Inclusion keratoconjunctivitis ('pink eye') in sheep. *Vet. Quart.,* **6,** 229–235

Cooper, B. S. (1974) Transmission of a *Chlamydia*-like agent isolated from contagious conjunctivokeratitis of sheep. NZ Vet. J., **22,** 181–184

Hopkins, J. B., Stephenson, E. H., Storz, J. and Pierson, R. E. (1973) Conjunctivitis associated with chlamydial polyarthritis in lambs. *J. Am. Vet. Med. Assoc.,* **163,** 1157–1160

Hosie, B. D. (1988) Keratoconjunctivitis in a hill sheep flock. *Vet. Rec.,* **122,** 40-43

Jones, G. E. (1983) Ovine keratoconjunctivitis. In *Diseases of Sheep.* (ed. W. B. Martin) Blackwell, Oxford, pp. 214–217

Jones, G. E., Foggie, A., Sutherland, A. and Harker, D. B. (1976) Mycoplasmas and ovine keratoconjunctivitis. *Vet. Rec.,* **99,** 137–141

Konig, C. D. W. (1983) 'Pink eye' or 'zere oogjes' or keratoconjunctivitis infectiosa ovis (KIO). Vet. Quart., **5,** 122–127

Moore, C. P. and Whitley, R. D. (1984) Ophthalmic diseases of small domestic ruminants – in large animal ophthalmology. In *Veterinary Clinics of North America, Large Animal Practice* (ed. C. P. Moore) Wisconsin, pp. 433–676

Trotter, S. L., Franklin, R. M., Baas, E. J. and Barile, M. F. (1977) Epidemic caprine keratoconjunctivitis: experimentally induced disease with a pure culture of *Mycoplasma conjunctivae. Infection and Immunity,* **18,** 816–822

Wall, A. E. (1982) Breed susceptibility to infectious keratoconjunctivitis. *Vet. Rec.,* **110,** 457

M. DAWSON

The caprine arthritis encephalitis syndrome

INTRODUCTION

THE SIGNIFICANCE of lentiviruses, which are non-oncogenic retroviruses, as pathogens for a variety of mammalian hosts is becoming increasingly apparent. Two lentivirus diseases, equine infectious anaemia (EIA) and maedi-visna (MV)/ovine progressive pneumonia are historically well known. Early reports of disease which ultimately proved to be associated with the caprine arthritis encephalitis (CAE) syndrome appeared twenty or so years ago. More recently, the human acquired immune deficiency syndrome (AIDS) has emerged together with what appear to be closely related diseases in domestic cats and cattle. No doubt others will emerge in the future.

To date, three basic immunopathological processes have been identified in lentivirus pathogenesis:

1. Immune complex-mediated haemolytic anaemia in EIA.
2. Immune deficiency associated with lymphocytopenia in AIDS and probably in the related feline and bovine diseases.
3. Lymphoproliferation and degenerative mononuclear cell inflammatory disease, which is found to a greater or lesser extent in all lentivirus diseases.

The latter predominates in the pathogenesis of MV and CAE. There is no evidence that the other components contribute significantly to the pathological process. This article reviews the main features of CAE and the properties of its causative virus.

AETIOLOGY

The CAE lentivirus establishes a persistent infection, and, like its ovine counterpart, MV virus, replicates in monocytes and macrophages via proviral DNA copies of its RNA genome. CAE and MV viruses share significant antigenic cross-reactivity on all structural and non-structural proteins. There is minimal expression of the proviral genome in monocytes, but replication is more permissive in macrophages.

DISTRIBUTION

Infection has been identified in many parts of the world, and in particular has been associated with the distribution of dairy-type goats of European origin. The

98

prevalence of seropositive, and thus infected, goats is high in North America, parts of Europe and Australia and the disease is a major problem. Indigenous feral breeds in countries into which dairy goats have been imported appear to have been previously free of infection.

THE SITUATION IN THE UK

Caprine lentivirus infection was first identified in 1982, and a serological survey two years later revealed a seroprevalence of 4%. Infection was present in 1 in 10 herds sampled. Although these figures presented a favourable situation compared to that elsewhere, there was substantial evidence that infection had been introduced recently in several herds.

PATHOGENESIS

The majority of infected animals show little clinical evidence of infection, a fact that can be attributed to the low level of expression of virus genome in the host. However, virus expression increases on macrophage maturation. In some individuals this change can induce degenerative lympho proliferative inflammation in one or more organs or tissues, for example, synovitis and bursitis, leucoencephalomyelitis, interstitial pneumonitis, interstitial indurative mastitis and glomerulonephritis.

The fate of infection in individuals is probably influenced by host factors, such as the density of expression of virus receptors on target cells and the immunogenetic regulation of the lymphoproliferative response. Environmental factors may dictate the degree of initial, and possibly continuing, exposure to CAE virus infection. Concurrent infections with a variety of pathogens may contribute to the pathogenesis by inducing macrophage recruitment and activation.

CLINICAL SIGNS

Although lesions of indurative mastitis are widespread, its clinical perception is not. Arthritis is the most commonly reported clinical component of the CAE syndrome.

Arthritis is a disease of sexually mature goats. Its onset is sudden or progressive. Any peripheral joint can be affected, though carpal arthritis, often bilateral, is the most commonly encountered. Evidence of lameness is variable. Some individuals appear to be suffering considerable discomfort, while others are able to walk soundly despite the obvious enlargement of joints. The latter tend to be those in which the disease has progressed insidiously over months or years. Acutely affected goats with painful arthritis should be destroyed. Treatment with anti-inflammatory drugs will afford temporary respite at best. A deterioration in general bodily condition is reflected in the poor quality of the coat; the hair tends to be dry and brittle.

Encephalitis, unlike arthritis, is mainly a disease of young kids. Most cases occur in animals under 4 months of age. Early signs of an awkward hind limb gait progress rapidly to hind limb paralysis and then quadriplegia. An alert disposition and appetite are usually maintained but spontaneous recoveries are rare and virtually all cases require euthanasia.

Indurative mastitis, though a widespread lesion in CAE virus-infected goats, is clinically less obvious than arthritis or encephalitis and is probably under-reported. Indurative changes, granular or diffuse, progress gradually and the milk quality is unaltered. The owner of an affected goat is presented with an individual that is not milking to potential. There are none of the signs commonly associated with mastitis such as an inflamed udder which produces milk with clots and/or blood. This may direct attention away from the udder as the source of the problem. The adverse economic consequences of widespread CAE virus infection in a large dairy herd are self evident.

Interstitial pneumonitis rarely advances to the stage of producing clinical pulmonary insufficiency, though cases of progressive pneumonia affecting adult goats, similar in character to ovine maedi, have been recorded.

VIRUS TRANSMISSION

Because virus replication increases when monocytes mature into macrophages, milk is much more infectious than blood. The feeding of pooled milk and colostrum to kids has been a major factor in the spread of infection and has contributed significantly to the emergence of CAE in several countries where such husbandry practices have been commonly adopted as part of modern progressive dairy goat practice. At mating, infected females are more likely to transmit to males than vice versa. This is possibly because of the greater macrophage content of vaginal secretions compared to that of semen. Infectivity of semen has not been demonstrated. A significant minority of kids born to infected dams are themselves infected before, or during, parturition. Lateral transmission can occur between individuals kept under conditions of intensive management, presumably by oro-nasal exposure to infected nasal secretions. Milk aerosols generated in dairy parlours may be significant sources of infection, and carry-over of infection on milking clusters cannot be discounted.

Although blood is potentially infective, in practice, the likelihood of transmission occurring during common husbandry practices, such as the ear marking of groups of kids, or vaccination, is remote. This is because virus is present in only a small proportion of circulating monocytes, and then in a relatively non-infectious form.

DIAGNOSIS

DIAGNOSIS OF INFECTION

CAE virus infections are persistent. Therefore, the detection of actively acquired antibody indentifies an individual as a virus carrier. Unfortunately, the period required for sero-conversion is variable and may be several months or longer. It is possible that a small proportion of infected goats remain antibody negative. In these individuals virus replication may be insufficient to induce an antibody response. Having sero-converted, a positive antibody status is maintained in most, but not all, cases. In a minority of 'previously tested positive' cases a negative result can be obtained subsequently. In such an event, owners must be cautioned against mistakenly interpreting the result as evidence that the goat is no longer infected. The detection of colostral antibody in kids is evidence that, unless the colostrum had been heat treated, they have almost certainly been exposed to virus.

DIAGNOSIS OF DISEASE

Serology is of limited value in diagnosing the disease. In addition to the problem of 'false negatives', it is apparent that the signs associated with the various components of the CAE complex could be attributed to causes other than CAE virus, i.e. the presence of CAE virus infection may be incidental. Confirmation of disease, as opposed to infection, requires a necropsy and the histological examination of the appropriate tissues, including the brain, spinal cord, joint capsules, tendon sheaths, bursae, udder, lungs and possibly kidneys, for evidence of the characteristic mononuclear cell inflammatory response and associated degenerative changes.

CONTROL

As with all currently known lentivirus diseases, options for control are limited. In the absence of effective treatments or vaccines, control strategies are based on identifying sources of infection and limiting further spread.

Blood testing can be used to identify infected goats. However, serology has its limitations and a single negative result on an individual cannot be interpreted as evidence of freedom from infection. In the Ministry of Agriculture, Fisheries and Food's (MAFF) Sheep and Goat Health Scheme, accredited status is conferred on a herd when all adults in the herd have tested negative on two successive herd tests with an interval of six months. The accredited status is protected by requiring adequate physical isolation for the scheme herd and by imposing movement and purchasing restrictions. The maintenance of accredited status is monitored by periodic surveillance tests.

The British Goat Society (BGS) administer a less restrictive scheme, the CAE Monitored Herd Scheme, which operates by regularly monitoring the antibody status of member herds. However, the onus is on the owner to protect that status. Movement restrictions are not imposed but members are educated as to the possible risks associated with potential sources of infection.

The MAFF CAE scheme, and to a lesser extent the BGS scheme, offer relatively safe sources of stock for prospective purchasers. Embryo transfer technology and artificial insemination will be used increasingly as options for improving the genetic status of herds without exposing them to risk of buying-in infected stock.

For the eradication of existing infection from herds, serological reactors and their progeny should be culled, together with any kids which are known or thought to have received suspect colostrum and/or milk. Any existing stocks of suspect colostrum or milk should be discarded. Future policy should be to ensure that kids receive colostrum and milk only from their dam, so that the further spread of infection from any reactors disclosed in the future can be more accurately predicted.

The artificial rearing of kids 'snatched' from infected dams and subsequently reared on heat treated (56° for 60 min) goat colostrum and milk, or bovine colostrum and milk substitute, has been only partially successful in breaking the chain of transmission.

RELATIONSHIP TO MV

The potential for cross-species transmission, sheep to goat and vice versa, has been clearly demonstrated in experimental studies, which include the feeding of infected goats' milk to lambs. The possibility that cross-species transmission could occur as a result of natural exposure should not be discounted.

FURTHER READING

Adams, D. S., Klevjer-Anderson, P., Carlson, J. L., McGuire, T. C. and Gorham, J. R. (1983) Transmission and control of caprine arthritis-encephalitis virus. *Am. J. Vet. Res.*, **44**, 1670–1675

Adams, D. S., Oliver, R. E., Ameghino, E., De Martini, J. C., Verwoerd, D. W., Houwers, D. J., Waghela, S., Gorham, J. R., Hyllseth, B., Dawson, M., Trigo, F. J. and McGuire, T. C. (1984) Global survey of serological evidence of caprine arthritis-encephalitis virus infection. *Vet. Rec.*, **115**, 493–495

Cork, L. C., Hadlow, W. J., Crawford, T. B., Gorham, J. R. and Piper, R. C. (1974) Infectious leukoencephalomyelitis of goats. *J. Infectious Diseases*, **129**, 134–141

Crawford, T. B., Adams, D. S., Sande, R. D., Gorham, J. R. and Henson, J. B. (1980) The connective tissue component of the caprine arthritis-encephalitis syndrome. *Am. J. Path.*, **100**, 443–454

Dawson, M. and Wilesmith, J. W. (1985) Serological survey of lentivirus (maedi-visna/caprine arthritis-encephalitis) infection in British goat herds. *Vet. Rec.*, **117**, 86–89

Gonzalez, L., Gelabert, J. L., Marco, J. C. and Saez-de-Okariz, C. (1987) Caprine arthritis-encephalitis in the Basque country, Spain. *Vet. Rec.*, **120**, 102–109

Norman, S. and Smith, M. C. (1983) Caprine arthritis-encephalitis: Review of the neurologic form in 30 cases. *J. Am. Vet. Med. Assoc.*, **182**, 1342–1345

Robinson, W. F. and Ellis, T. M. (1986) Caprine arthritis-encephalitis virus infection: from recognition to eradication. *Aust. Vet. J.*, **63**, 237–241

M. R. MUIRHEAD

Factors affecting efficient growth rate in the feeding pig

INTRODUCTION

OVER THE years a great deal of information and effort has been provided to increase efficiency in the breeding side of the pig farm. Little, however, has been written about the methods by which poor growth can be determined and corrective actions taken in the feeder pig. Indeed, on many feeding farms, performance is poorly documented, if at all.

Efficient growth rates in the pig are dependent upon the rate of deposition of lean meat. This deposition is determined by the genetic programming of the pig and the rate at which it grows. Growth rates are further influenced by the type of pig, the quality of nutrition and the methods by which it is fed. The influence of the environment on the utilization of feed by the pig is probably the most important single factor that influences growth. However, the presence of disease, particularly in its acute form, could impair the efficiency by which feed is converted into meat by as much as 0.4. The factors influencing growth rate are shown in Table 1. The work of the veterinarian on the farm to both diagnose poor growth rate and direct corrective actions is an important one.

THE PIG

The modern pig, through a process of continual selection, has the capacity to convert its food into lean meat at a much greater age than the pig of 15 years ago. In some breeds this deposition of lean meat will continue up to 60 kg liveweight before the deposition of fat increases. The amount of energy required to produce fat is approximately four times as much as that necessary to produce lean meat. Thus a rapid growth rate, particularly in the early stages of the pig's life, is an important area to be monitored on the farm.

The rate of deposition of lean meat is also dependent upon the sex of the pig. The continual move towards the production of more boar meat illustrates this. It is now possible to feed the boar *ad libitum* through to 90 kg at a probe measurement (P2) of less than 12 mm. Gilt performance is more efficient than the castrate.

NUTRITION

Feed can account for up to 85% of the cost of output of a feeding unit. The greatest impact on economic efficiency on the pig farm is determined by the choice of feed.

103

Table 1 FACTORS INFLUENCING GROWTH RATE IN THE PIG

The pig	Age/weight Breed/sex Group size Genetics
Nutrition	Protein levels/quality Amino acid/lysine levels Energy levels
Feed	Growth promotors Intake Palatability Water *Ad libitum*/restricted Trough/floor fed Wet feeding
The environment	Air speed Ventilation rate Temperature Airbourne dust. Micro-organisms Noxious gases
Housing	Insulation Floor type/bedding Floor space Humidity Method of dung disposal
Disease	Specific diseases Management of disease Therapy
Management	Correct decisions Constant monitoring Attention to detail

The correct type of feed is one which provides the nutrition requirements for maintenance and growth for that pig in that environment and yields maximum kilogrammes of meat. The two major components are the energy content of the diet and the quality of the protein levels. The energy content of pig feed is measured by its digestable energy (DE), expressed as megajoules per kilogramme (MJ/kg) of feed. The actual concentration of the energy in the feed and the daily requirements for that particular weight of pig determine the weight of the feed that is necessary.

The ratio between the concentration of energy and protein to maximize growth should be a constant one. Diets for the pig at weaning contain energy levels of up to 14.5–15 MJ/kg. During the weaning period these levels would be 13.6–14 MJ/kg and in the latter stages would vary from 13.4 MJ/kg upwards. However, such energy levels must also take into account the pig's appetite and the total energy necessary to satisfy environmental needs, maintenance and growth.

Protein is required for both the maintenance and production of lean tissue. Because lean tissue contains approximately 75% water, it is much more efficient to convert feed in to lean meat than into fat, which contains only 12% water. The quality of the protein in any diet is determined by the levels of essential amino acids. The most important and limiting amino acid is lysine. Methionine, cystine and tryptophan are also important. The quality of the protein used is therefore a vital factor.

Maximizing growth rate requires restricting energy intake to reduce fat deposition. However, this can increase the maintenance requirements due to longer finishing periods and conversion efficiency. It is important to determine the point at which lean meat deposition remains constant and fat deposition continues to increase. Approximately 35% of dietary energy is used by the pig for maintenance and 25% for growth. In total approximately 60% is lost from the body as heat. *Ad libitum* feeding in the early growing period is essential to maximize daily liveweight gain and lean meat deposition.

The lysine content of the diet is particularly important, not only in its contribution to the deposition of lean meat but also to growth rates. With the modern lean pig the requirements for this essential amino acid have gradually increased. Diets containing as much as 1.4% lysine are now commonplace in the early growing phase.

FEEDING THE PIG

The methods by which pigs are fed can have an effect on feed intake but once daily feeding is as effective as twice daily feeding. Wet feeding gives better results than dry feeding. Where floor feeding takes place, pellets are more efficient than meal. The greatest improvement in efficiency of feeding has been the change from floor feeding to hopper feeding. Floor feeding results is an enormous wasteage and soiling of feed with reduced palatability and intake. Feed conversions have improved by up to 0.3% following such changes with economic returns of an extra £5 per pig.

The availability of highly palatable, dry feed, not contaminated by dung or urine, is essential to achieve high levels of feed intake during the first 14 days post weaning. If this is maximized in the first week after weaning, improvements of up to 15% in daily gain and food conversion may be seen in the pig from weaning to 30 kg.

THE ENVIRONMENT

The pig has poor thermoregulatory mechanisms. Genetic selection has markedly reduced levels of back fat. Because heat is lost through radiation, convection, conduction and evaporation, the influence of the environment is very marked on this lean animal.

AIR TEMPERATURE

The range of air temperature within which heat production is independent of air temperature is described as the thermo-neutral zone with its upper (UTC) and lower critical temperatures (LCT). Factors determining the LCT are shown in Table 2.

Table 2 FACTORS AFFECTING THE LOWER (LTC) AND UPPER (UTC) CRITICAL TEMPERATURES OF THE PIG

Factors are dependent on:

Weight of the pig
Level of feed intake, e.g:

wt pig (kg)	Feed intake per day	LCT
40	1.5 kg	14°C
40	2.0 kg	8°C

Energy level of the ration
Fat depths of the pig
Group size
Stocking density
Air speed over the pigs
Quality of insulation of housing
Type of floor surface
Type and amount of bedding
Wet floors
Every 1°C below LCT equals 12 g/day loss in daily gain

When pigs are kept below their lower critical temperature a proportion of the feed is used to maintain body heat. Thus, growth rate will be retarded. Bruce and Clark (1979) have developed mathematical models for determining this zone.

The type of flooring, whether of slats, perforated metal or insulated concrete, has a very marked effect on the LTC. There is also a very marked increase in the LCT at the point of weaning due to the inability of the pig to increase its energy intake. This factor is particularly important in the predisposition to post-weaning diarrhoea.

In practice it is usual to hold the environmental temperature towards the lower part of the thermo-neutral zone in the growing phase because this will help increase feed intake and therefore growth rates. At the other end of the scale, as the temperature approaches the upper limit, pigs tend to wallow and there is a marked reduced feed intake. The level of feed intake and energy are major factors in determining the LTC. In addition, air temperature, body size and body insulation will also affect the level of heat production. The rate of heat loss is affected by the size of the pig and the numbers within the group, the type of floor and the presence of absence of bedding, the air speed at pig level and the air temperature and humidity. Generally, small pigs loose more heat than larger pigs. In particular there is a marked cooling effect when the air speed is increased over the pig. Heat loss is also dependent on the wetness of the floor and the type of floor. Such environmental changes can have a marked influence on growth rate. As a guide, the temperature requirement of a 15 kg pig on straw would be 18–23°C. On a totally slatted floor, this would rise to 22–27°C. If a pig is grown at one degree below its lower critical temperature, this will add a cost of approximately 94p on a £165 per tonne ration cost. However, five degrees below the LCT, the extra feed cost will be £5.11. Heat loss through radiation and convection is dependent on the insulation of the pig building. The control of the temperature is dependent on the ventilation rate, cubic capacity and critical temperatures. Therefore, measurement of temperature within the house over 24-hour periods is an important tool for assessment.

MANAGEMENT

For the veterinarian to assist in the differential diagnosis of poor growth rate on the farm the availability of record information is vital. A method of approach has been described by Muirhead (1987). It is important to be able to look at the weight of the pig at various ages and compare this to a standard, considered efficient (Table 3). When assessing the information in this table, be aware of the many variables that

Table 3 SUGGESTED REFERENCE DATA FOR EFFICIENT GROWTH USING SPECIFIC DIETARY PROTEIN AND ENERGY LEVELS. PIGS FED *AD LIBITUM* TO 74 KG LIVE WEIGHT

Age of pig	Weight (kg) at age	DLWG* at age (g/day)	From 21 days to age	FCE[†] at age	From 21 days to age	Content of diet — Protein %	Energy (MJ/kg)
Birth	1.20						
Weaning:							
21 days	5.75	250				22.5	15.0
24 days	6.50	250					
28 days	8.00	375					
35 days	10.25	320	321				
Week 6	12.75	360			1.20		
7	15.25	460	339	1.7	1.25	22.0	14.55
8	20.00	600			1.3		
9	25.50	770	464	1.9	1.35		
10	31.00	790			1.4		
11	36.50	780	544	2.0	1.5		
						18.5	13.50
12	42.00	780			1.6		
13	46.50	780	578	2.1	1.75		
14	52.00	800			1.85		
15	57.50	800	613	2.2	2.0		
16	63.50	860			2.1		
17	69.50	860	647	2.4	2.2		
18	74.50	800			2.3		
						17.5	13.20
19	80.00	780	660	2.6	2.4 ⎫		
20	85.00	740			2.5 ⎬ Feed restricted		
21	90.00	740	660	2.7	2.5 ⎭		

* Daily live weight gain.
[†] Feed conversion efficiency.

contribute towards its information. The information in the table can be used to plot a growth curve and the actual figures produced on the farm can be related to this. This immediately identifies the points at which growth is disadvantaged. It is important, however, to include in the overall farm assessment, detailed, clinical observations by an experienced observer.

DISEASE

The identification of poor growth rate associated with disease is dependent upon three factors: observation, pathological examinations and information. By critically examining the groups of pigs at points of variable growth, assessments can be made of all the interelated factors described in Table 1.

These factors include the appearance of the pigs and the environment in the house together with ventilation and humidity. Levels of active disease should also be noted together with and their effects on growth rate. These observations can then be

Table 4. FACTORS AFFECTING FEED CONVERSION EFFICIENCY AND THE METHODS OF IMPROVEMENT IN THE FEEDING PIG

Factors	*Methods of improvement*
Breed of pig. Genotype	Selection
Sex: males/females/castrate	Split sex pens

Age: worse with age
    1.1 to 1 at   4 weeks
    1.5 to 1 at   8 weeks
    4   to 1 at 24 weeks
	Grow faster
	Better feeds

Feed routine: *Ad libitum*/wasteful with food trough
    Wet better than dry
    Pellets better than meal
	Reduce waste

Amount fed: Waste/maximize lean tissue growth	Manage. Increase intake
Trough feeding: Better feed conversion efficiency	
Feed composition: Protein Energy Quality Lysine Growth promotors	 Type Quality Levels
Environment: Temperature, ventilation, humidity	Management
Health	Control
Management	Your efficiency

supported by information from the records which should include the daily gain, cost per kg of liveweight gain, the feed intake and food conversion efficiency. The factors that effect food conversion and the methods of improvement are shown in Table 4.

The effects of specific diseases will vary from one farm to another and are dependent on the actual severity. When disease is first introduced into a herd, the effects of a poorer conversion and daily gain are much greater during the acute phase than when the condition has settled and moved into chronic phase. Of the major infectious diseases present in the UK the pneumonia complex (including enzootic and haemophilus pneumonias) together with swine dysentery are the most important from an economic view. The ranges of effects noted on farms for the important specific diseases are shown in Table 5. The diagnosis and significance of these on the farm is vital. This is a job for the veterinarian.

Table 5 THE EFFECTS OF THE MAJOR INFECTIOUS DISEASES ON FOOD CONVERSION EFFICIENCY AND GROWTH RATES ON A HERD BASIS. PIGS SLAUGHTERED AT 90 KG LIVE WEIGHT

Disease	Acute disease increases in FCE*	Days increase to 90 kg	Endemic disease increases in FCE*	Days increase to 90 kg
TGE	0.1	4–10	0–0.05	0–3
Epidemic diarrhoea	0.1	4–10	0	?
Aujeszky's disease	0.1–0.2		0.1–0.3	6–14
Parvovirus	–	–	–	–
Enzootic pneumonia	0.2–0.4	10–21	0.05–0.3	3–31
Haemophilus pneumonia	0.1–0.4	7–30	0.1–0.3	4–15
Atrophic rhinitis	0.1–0.2	4–15	0.1–0.2	4–15
Swine dysentery	0.05–0.2	15–20	0.05–0.1	4–8
Streptococcal meningitis	0.05	1–3	0.05	0
Mange	0.1–0.3	7–18	0.05–0.1	3–8
Internal parasites	0.1	7–18	0.1	3–6

* Feed conversion efficiency.

REFERENCES

Bruce, J. M. and Clark, J. J. (1979) *Animal Production,* **28,** part 3
Muirhead, M. R., (1987) The University of Sydney Post Graduate Committee in Veterinary Science. *Pig Production Proc.,* **95,** 637–710

D. H. ROBERTS

Pigs and influenza

INTRODUCTION

THE HIGHLY contagious acute respiratory illness known as influenza appears to have afflicted humans since ancient times. The sudden appearance of epidemics of respiratory disease that persist for a few weeks and disappear equally suddenly is sufficiently characteristic to permit identification of a number of major epidemics in the distant past. These epidemics occurred relatively frequently but at irregular intervals. The epidemics varied in their severity but caused mortality in the elderly. Some epidemics appeared to spread across Russia from Asia.

The 1918–1919 pandemic was particularly severe. The so-called 'Spanish influenza' killed between 20 and 40 million people world-wide; about 0.5% of the population in the USA died. It also altered the course of history. The Chief of Staff of the Imperial Germany Army blamed the failure of the Marne offensive on influenza rather than the influx of fresh American troops. All armies in Europe were hard hit by this outbreak; in fact 80% of the US Army's war deaths were due to influenza (Kaplan and Webster, 1977).'

A new disease was seen in pigs in the USA during the 1918–1919 influenza epidemic in humans. The disease in pigs had many clinical and pathological similarities to influenza in humans and was given the name swine influenza. The severity of the 1918–1919 pandemic greatly accelerated the search for the causative agent of influenza. In 1930 Shope isolated the causative agent from pigs [A/Swine/Iowa/15/30 (H_1N_1)] and Smith and others isolated the agent from humans in 1933 (Shope, 1931; Smith, Andrewes and Laidlaw, 1933).

The influenza virus consists of an internal ribonucleoprotein core or nucleocapsid containing the single stranded viral RNA genome and an outer roughly spherical lipoprotein envelope. The nucleoprotein is enclosed within a matrix protein. These proteins are the major type-specific antigens which form the basis of the classification of influenza viruses into types A, B and C.

All three types of virus infect man but except for occasional reports, infections in other animals are restricted to type A influenza virus (Alexander, 1982). However, influenza C viruses have been isolated from pigs in China (Yuanji *et al.*, 1983).

The single-stranded RNA genome of the virus is made up of eight distinct species of RNA and each segment codes for a virus protein. Viruses of the influenza A type are further divided into subtypes on the basis of their surface envelope antigens, the haemagglutinin (H) and the neuraminidase (N) antigens. The haemagglutinin is responsible for adhesion of the virus to the host cell and induces agglutination of red blood cells. Neuraminidase is an enzyme that allows release of the virus from the cell and facilitates the spread of the virus from the cell to cell.

110

An important property of influenza viruses is their ability to undergo change. Influenza viruses display two kinds of antigenic variation in their H and N antigens. The first kind of change, called antigenic drift, consists of a series of minor alterations of the parent strain of the surface H and N proteins. A strain that has caused all the influenza in humans will often disappear and be replaced by a novel minor variant of the same major serotype. The second variation is called antigenic shift to distinguish an abrupt and major change in the composition of either the H or N anitgens, or both, which, by convention, are designated H_1, H_2, H_3, N_1, N_2 and so forth.

Since 1933, when the first human influenza virus, now designated H_1N_1 was isolated, antigenic drift and antigenic shift have occurred in influenza A viruses. Minor changes (antigenic drift) have been seen in both surface proteins, giving the mutant virus a selective advantage in the otherwise immune host population.

The first major antigenic shift detected after 1933 was recorded in 1957 when a new pandemic strain appeared. The virus was the first of the Asian strains, designated H_2N_2. Both the H and N surface antigens were completely unlike those of the earlier strains. The Asian virus underwent antigenic drift until 1968, when the Hong Kong subtype appeared. The Hong Kong virus possessed a new H protein but the N protein was the same as the Asian strain. The Hong Kong virus, designated H_3N_2, has since shown antigenic drift, producing variants known as the England, Port Chalmers, Scotland and Victoria strains named after the geographic area in which they were first isolated. For example, A/Port Chalmers/1/73 H_3N_2 strains, which caused all the human influenza A in many parts of the world in 1974–1975 season, disappeared. A/Victoria/3/75 H_3N_2 strains were responsible for all the influenza in the same areas in the 1975–1976 season.

In 1977, H_1N_1 strains of influenza A virus returned after an absence of 20 years. These strains possessed antigens of the viruses that caused the 1918–1919 pandemic and continued to be prevalent in the community between 1918 and 1957. This strain was called Russian influenza because it was first reported by the Russians. The reappearance of H_1N_1 strains in 1977 did not result in replacement of H_3N_2 strains of virus and both viruses continue to circulate in the human population.

INFLUENZA VIRUSES IN PIGS

Pigs are susceptible to infection by several different variants of the H_1N_1 and H_3N_2 subtypes of influenza A virus. Influenza in pigs was first observed in the USA during the 1918–1919 human influenza pandemic. The isolation of an influenza virus [A/Swine/Iowa/15/30 (H_1N_1)] by Shope (1931) and retrospective serological studies on humans indicated that the pig virus was antigenically similar to the type A influenza virus responsible for the human pandemic. Since then swine influenza virus has remained in the pig population and has been responsible for one of the most prevalent respiratory diseases in pigs in North America. About 25% of all pigs in the USA that go to slaughter have been infected during their lifetime (Eaterday, 1986).

Classical swine influenza is characterized by a sudden onset of coughing, laboured jerky breathing, fever, anorexia, muscular weakness and a mucous discharge from the eyes and nose. The course of the disease usually varies from 3 to 7 days. Recovery is almost as sudden as the onset.

Viruses of this subtype have been reported to have infected pigs in many countries including Great Britain (Blakemore and Gledhill, 1941). However, some of the early reported isolations were possibly attributable to laboratory contamination (Andrewes and Pereira, 1972). Serological evidence of infection was not apparent in the UK during the years 1939 to 1986.

An outbreak of acute respiratory disease occurred in 1986 in a 400-sow unit in Yorkshire (Roberts, Cartwright and Wibberley, 1987). The outbreak was characterized by respiratory distress, coughing, anorexia, fever, inappetence and loss of condition. The gilts and weaners were affected and the morbidity approached 100%. The inappetence and pyrexia lasted for 4 to 5 days. The animals' recovery was uneventful. An influenza A virus (A/Swine/Weybridge/117316/86) was isolated. The H and N characterization indicated that the virus was similar to H_1N_1 viruses isolated recently from pigs in Europe but distinguishable from classical swine influenza H_1N_1 viruses isolated from pigs in North America. This virus was responsible for a widespread respiratory condition among pigs in England during 1986.

Collaborative studies on H_1N_1 isolates from different countries throughout the world indicate that at least two distinct antigenic variants of these viruses are currently circulating in pigs (Hinshaw *et al.*, 1984). Viruses termed US viruses were isolated from pigs in Hong Kong, Italy, Japan and the USA. Other viruses, termed European viruses, were isolated from pigs in Belgium, France, West Germany, Spain and England. It has been suggested that pigs imported from the USA have served as a source of viruses for pigs in countries such as Italy and Japan. It has also been suggested that the European viruses had a different origin from the US viruses. One potential source could be birds. Recent disease outbreaks in turkeys in France involve viruses very similar to the European porcine viruses and these avian viruses are capable of infecting and replicating in pigs (Hinshaw *et al.*, 1984).

There is widespread evidence of infection of pigs with human (H_3N_2) viruses. A/Hong Kong/68 H_3N_2 - like viruses were first isolated in 1976 from pigs in Taiwan. Subsequently several of the later antigenic variants of human (H_3N_2) viruses have been detected in pigs in almost every country where studies have been done. Antibodies to H_3N_2 influenza A viruses have been found in pigs in Great Britain since 1968 but until 1987 no evidence of clinical disease had ever been reported. Infections in pigs were almost certainly preceded by human infections (Harkness *et al.*, 1972).

In 1987, a particularly severe outbreak of respiratory disease occurred on a large (1600 pigs) finishing unit in Suffolk. A pen of 22 pigs aged about 12 to 13 weeks purchased from a local market eight days previously was the first to show signs of illness. Infection spread rapidly through the unit and within three weeks at least 60% of the pigs had been clinically affected. Initially, the pigs were seen lying about, failing to rise when roused. They were very dull, lethargic and pyrexic, with rectal temperatures of up to 109°F (42.8°C). Anorexia was marked. Pronounced redness of the skin was often present, particularly around the perineal area. Sneezing was not a major feature but many affected pigs had a barking cough. Recovery occurred over a period of about a week as rectal temperatures returned to normal and appetites improved. Seven pigs died during the outbreak.

The direct cost of the outbreak to the farmer was in excess of £3000. This comprised an increased medication cost of £1800 and a further loss of £1200 from deaths and condemnations. In addition, there was the unquantifiable cost of an extra two weeks to slaughter due to loss of growth during the period of inappetence and fever.

An influenza A virus related to the human A/Port Chalmers (H_3N_2) strain was isolated (Pritchard *et al.*, 1987; Wibberley *et al.*, 1988) several years after their disappearance from man. The A/Port Chalmers (H_3N_2) virus circulated in humans between 1973 and 1975.

ZOONOTIC ASPECTS OF PORCINE INFLUENZA VIRUS

Pigs are a substantial reservoir of influenza A virus, especially the H_1N_1 and H_3N_2 subtypes. Continued serological surveillance of elite pig herds in Great Britain in 1987 has revealed that 33% of the serum samples had antibodies to the European porcine influenza virus A/Swine/Weybridge/117316/86 (H_1N_1) and 36% had antibodies to the Port Chalmers-like virus A/Swine/Weybridge 163266/87 (H_3N_2). A total of 5783 serum samples were tested from 307 herds; 117 herds had reactors to the H_1N_1 virus and 196 had reactors to the H_3N_2 virus. Twenty-three percent of the herds had reactors to both H_1N_1 and H_3N_2 viruses. Simultaneous infection of pigs with H_1N_1 and H_3N_2 viruses might result in genetic re-assortment between the viruses and the formation of recombinant viruses. This re-assortment occurred naturally on a farm in Japan and the recombinant H_1N_2 virus caused widespread infection (Sugimura *et al.*, 1980)

The belief that the 1918–1919 epidemic in humans was caused by a virus related to swine influenza (H_1N_1) explains the events occurring in the USA following what became known as the 'Fort Dix Incident' (Alexander, 1982). In 1976 an outbreak of influenza A (H_1N_1) occurred in 500 servicemen at Fort Dix. One man died and the virus isolated was identical to viruses isolated from pigs in the USA. With the 1918–1919 pandemic in mind the US Government appropriated $100 million to produce sufficient vaccine for the entire population of the USA. The vaccination programme was started but eventually abandoned when it became clear that the virus had not spread any further. No direct contact with pigs could be found to account for the Fort Dix outbreak but there is evidence that transmission from pigs to man does occur occasionally. At least 16 outbreaks have been reported but in all these cases the virus has failed to become established in the human population. The number of reported cases are indeed very few when the fact that the virus has been circulating in pigs in the USA since 1918 and Europe since 1976 is taken into consideration.

In 1968, soon after H_3N_2 strains had first appeared in man in Hong Kong they were found to be infecting the local pigs. A similar rapid transfer to pigs has followed human H_3N_2 epidemics in many parts of the world. Nevertheless, back transfer from pigs to man is a possibility. Serological studies of pigs in Great Britain in 1980 and 1982 have provided evidence of infection of pigs with H_1N_1 viruses resembling Russian influenza (A/USSR/98/77) strains which have circulated in humans since 1977 (Roberts *et al.*, 1987).

Parasitism in different host species imposes specific adaptation and different potentialities are developed by the virus in different sorts of hosts. Influenza viruses do not pass to and from man and other animals with complete freedom, but under some conditions such transmission does occur. Porcine influenza viruses constitute some occupational risk to those people close to pigs, but when infection has spread to man in this way, subsequent spread in the human population has been very limited (Hope-Simpson and Golubev, 1987).

REFERENCES

Alexander, D. J. (1982) *J. Roy. Soc. Med.*, **75**, 799–881

Andrewes, C. and Pereira, H. G. (1972) *Viruses of Vertebrates*, 3rd edn, Bailliere Tindall, London, 212 pp.

Blakemore, F. and Gledhill, A. W. (1941) *Vet. Rec.*, **53**, 227–230

Eaterday, B. C. (1986) In *Diseaes of Swine*, 6th edn (eds. A. D. Leman, B. Straw, R. D. Glock *et al.*,) Iowa State University Press, Ames, Iowa, pp. 244–255

Harkness, J. W., Schild, G. C., Lamont, P. H. and Brand, C. M. (1972) *Bull. World Health Organization*, **46**, 709–719

Hinshaw, V. S., Alexander, D. J., Aymard, M. *et al.*, (1984) *Bull. World Health Organization*, **62**, 871–878

Hope-Simpson, R. E. and Golubev, D. B. (1987) *Epidemiology and Infection*, **99**, 5–54

Kaplan, M. M. and Webster, R. G. (1977) *Scientific American*, **237** 88–107

Pritchard, G. C., Dick, I. G. C., Roberts, D. H., Wibberley, G. (1987) *Vet. Rec.*, **121**, 548

Roberts, D. H., Cartwright, S. F. and Wibberley, G. (1987) *Vet. Rec.*, **121**, 53–55

Shope, R. E. (1931) *J. Experimental Med.*, **54**, 349–360

Smith, W., Andrewes, C. H. and Laidlaw, P. P. (1933) *Lancet*, **1**, 66-68

Sugimura, T., Yonemochi, H., Ogawa, T., Tanaka, Y. and Kumagai, T. (1980) *Arch. Virol.*, **66**, 271–274

Wibberley, G., Swallow, C. and Roberts, D. H. (1988) *Br. Vet. J.*, **144**, 196-201

Yuanji, G., Fengen, J., Ping, W., Min, W. and Jiming, Z. (1983) *J. Gen. Virol.*, **64**, 177–182

R. H. C. PENNY and H. J. GUISE

Boar usage and wastage : results of a twenty-six herd survey and limited literature review

INTRODUCTION

IN MODERN pig production, although the board and sow are partners in the reproductive process, the partnership is not an equal one. The impact of the individual boar on unit productivity is much the greater because he exerts his influence through all the sows that are served or inseminated by him.

This may seem a statement of the obvious but, despite his importance within the herd, it is nevertheless a fact that the boar is often the most neglected animal on the farm. Boars are frequently kept in restricted, badly designed accommodation, hygiene may be poor in both his pen and the service area. Boar nutrition has received scant attention, and he is commonly forgotten in routine health procedures, such as vaccination, mange and worm treatments.

In this paper, the results of a 26-herd survey on boar usage and wastage are described alongside a limited literature review.

MATERIALS AND METHODS

A postal questionnaire (backed by telephone discussion) on boar usage and wastage was completed by all 26 members of a pig marketing cooperative (the Group). The total sows (mainly commercial hybrids) and boars, the mean herd size and range, and the sow:board ratio are shown in Tables 1 and 2. Mean herd size was 245 sows and 12.5 boars.

RESULTS

SOW:BOAR RATIO

The sow:boar ratio (boar power) was 19.6:1. However, this figure conceals the true statistic because 13 herds within the survey topped up with artificial insemination (AI).

Accordingly, an attempt was made to estimate the real sow:boar ratio for the Group, by calculating the approximate total number of services or inseminations and making an adjustment in the ratio for the inseminations. Table 3 shows the number of attempted services or inseminations/sow and gilt per oestrus on the Group's farms.

Table 1 SOW:BOAR RATIO

No. herds	Total sows	Mean sows	Total boars	Mean boars	Sow:boar ratio
26	6363	244.7	325*	12.5	19.6:1

* Thirteen herds used some AI, adjusted sow:boar ratio 16.7:1.

Table 2 HERD SIZE

	Total	<100	100–200	200–300	300–400	>400
No. Sows	6363	127	1279	2412	1020	1525
No. Herds	26	2	7	11	3	3

Table 3 ATTEMPTED SERVICES/INSEMINATIONS PER OESTRUS

No. of services/inseminations attempted per oestrus	1	2	3	4
No. of farms	nil	11	14	1

While it has to be admitted that seasonal differences might occur, using percentage figures provided by each unit, some 31 468 services and 5541 inseminations were made, a total of 37 009. If boars had been used in place of the 15% of inseminations, the sow:boar ratio would have been 16.7:1.

NUMBER OF SERVICES/INSEMINATIONS PER OESTRUS

It can be seen from Table 3 that on all farms, two or more services or inseminations were attempted. On 14 farms three attempts were made and in one unit four were tried. All farms were members of the Meat and Livestock Commission (MLC) Pig Recording Scheme and conception rates were generally above the annual mean for all herds in the scheme.

BREEDS OF BOAR IN USE

Large-Whites predominated (77.2%) and Landrace were the least commonly used (Table 4). In answer to the question 'Does breed influence temperament?' there were four replies in the negative and two replies suggesting that good temperament was mainly a question of regular and careful handling. However, 11 replies were in the affirmative. Seven suggested Landrace were of uncertain temperament and low libido, and seven considered Large-Whites to be even tempered or the best boars. Hybrid boars were thought to be aggressive breeders on four units and bad tempered on two.

Table 4 BREEDS OF BOAR IN USE

	Total	Large-White	Landrace	Hybrids
Number of boars	325	251	27	47
%	–	77.2	8.3	15.5

In answer to the question 'Do you detusk your boars?', two replied yes and three occasionally. The breeds of boar kept on the two farms which carried out detusking routinely were Large-White on one and Landrace on the other. The breeds kept on the farms which carried out detusking occasionally were Large-White on two, and Large-White and hybrids on one.

AGE OF BOARS IN USE

In Table 5, the age distribution of the boars on the 26 units is shown: 26.5% were under 1 year old and 27.7% were over 2 years old.

If boars in each age group up to 24 months were placed in the middle of the range (e.g. 6–9 months = 7.5 months), and boars over 24 months were estimated at 30 months, the average age of boars on the farms would be 18.5 months. This figure must be taken as an estimate only.

Table 5 AGES OF BOARS ON FARMS

	Age of boars in months						
	6–9	9–12	12–15	15–18	18–21	21–24	>24
Number of boars	39	47	41	36	32	40	90
%	12.0	14.5	12.6	11.0	9.8	12.3	27.7

ANNUAL CULLING RATE

The total boars culled in the previous 12 months was 136 or 41.8% (Table 6). The reasons given are also set out in this table. Poor libido only accounted for 18.4% of culls, possibly because of the preponderance of Large-White and Hybrid boards, which are both considered to be active breeders. Lameness was reported as the cause in 20.6% of cases. Old age or too heavy accounted for over 50% of culls. Poor grading was listed as a reason for culling on the questionnaire but, somewhat surprisingly, no cull was placed in this category.

Table 6 REASONS FOR CULLING

	Total boars culled	*Culled for*					
		Poor libido	*Poor reproductive performance*	*Lameness*	*Old age*	*Too heavy*	*Other*
No.	136	25	7	28	46	24	6
%	–	18.4	5.1	20.6	33.8	17.6	4.4

BOAR MORTALITY

Eleven boars died in the last year and 24 died in the last three years. The annual mortality rate for the last year was 3.38%. Over the three-year period the mortality averaged 2.46% per annum. The death of a boar on the farm is therefore something of a rarity.

CAUSE OF MORTALITY

Numbers are small, so too much should not be made of the results. The conditions mentioned at least twice were fighting, stress death, and ulcerated or ruptured stomach. Conditions mentioned once only were clostridial infection, ruptured spleen, posterior paralysis due to lead poisoning, haemophilus pleuropneumonia infection (a young boar) and gangrene.

DISEASES IN BOARS AND TREATMENTS

On 18 of the 26 farms, boars had been treated for a variety of conditions. On 11 farms boars had been treated for lameness. On 3 farms all boars had been involved in a medication programme for the control of vaginal discharges in sows and infertility. Boars with pneumonia had been treated on two units, and miscellaneous conditions encountered were ulcers, loss of appetite, injuries and suspected nervous disease.

ERYSIPELAS INFECTION

Because erysipelas infection resulting in possible infertility is a fairly common cause of complaint received by breeding companies soon after sale of a boar, the question was asked 'In your opinion, does erysipelas infection lead to infertility?'. There were four unequivocal replies to 'yes', and three replies of 'probably' or 'possibly'. The other replies were 'no experience on which to judge, or no opinion' (15), and 'no!' (3). One respondent did not answer the question.

DISCUSSION

SOW:BOAR RATIO

This ratio has been falling steadily since the late 1950s when a ratio of 30:1 would have been considered acceptable. The introduction of batch farrowing and the need to service a group of sows on heat around the same time, led to a fall in the ratio to around 25:1. Further changes in husbandry practices associated with increasing intensification and herd size, weekly (continuous) farrowing and the need to sustain reproductive efficiency, have led to further improvements in this ratio to nearer 20:1.

The June 1986 Ministry of Agriculture Fisheries and Food (MAFF) pig census results show a ratio of 20.5:1 if total breeding sows (824 000) plus breeding gilts (79 000) are divided by the boars available for service (44 000). The University of Cambridge Pig Management Scheme closing figures for 1987 give a ratio of 20.6:1, if a similar calculation is made (Ridgeon, 1987).

The figures calculated have all been means, but a low sow:boar ratio is considered an essential ingredient for good herd reproductive efficiency and the best herds tend to have low ratios. However, in the USA sow:boar ratios of 30:1 or more are now being recommended.

NUMBER OF SERVICES PER OESTRUS

The practice of multiple services is also being questioned in the USA, and a single service per oestrus is now being recommended (A. D. Leman, 1987, personal communication). The scientific basis for this controversial change in breeding management is that, although the spermatazoa can live for quite a long time in a partially inactivated state, the ova survive for a very short time only in the fimbria of the fallopian tube. After ovulation, they need to be met by active sperm half-way down the tube (Hunter, 1988). Nevertheless, until many more field results have been published, it would be wise to continue to recommend units to keep ample boars to cover for any emergency, and to attempt to serve sows at roughly 12-hour intervals (in commercial units with different boars) from the time the female stands until she refuses the boar. Certainly the MLC Pig Plan figures for 1987 confirm that 36% of participants relied on two services, 46% two or three, 9% on three or more and only 2% on one (Anon, 1987).

The best way to maintain a boar at maximum reproductive efficiency still seems to be to allow him two, and an older boar possibly three, services a week on a regular basis.

THE WORKING LIFE OF THE BOAR

The reproductive life of boars is strictly limited. An important contributing factor is the rapid turnover of the generations in pig breeding in the quest for better and better growth, feed conversion and carcase quality. Currently the boar's mean working life could be somewhere between one and two years. In the Cambridge Pig Management Scheme, 47.9% of boars wer replaced in the year (Ridgeon, 1987) and in this study, 41.8% were replaced. The authors have some preliminary figures which suggest that Large-White boars have a working life of around two years, whereas for Landrace the figure is around one and a half years or even less. This last mentioned figure may come as little surprise.

In France, Le Denmat and Runavot (1980) studied the working life of 283 boars in 87 herds, with a mean sow population of 86.4 and a sow:boar ratio of 22.1. One in five herds also used some AI. The age of boars in service averaged 615 ± SD 265 days. Cross breds were 56 days older than pure breds. This supports the quite widely held view that cross breds are sexually more vigorous. Of the boars, 55% had been in service for more than 1 year, only 15% for less than 2 years, and the average age at culling was 23 months. One in five boars was culled at less than 13 months.

In a second paper, Le Denmat *et al.*, (1980) published the results of a 293-herd survey. The sow:boar ratio was 19.8:1, the average age of boars in service was 640 days, and only 17% were over 2.5 years. The age at culling for French Large-Whites, French Landrace, other breeds (Belgian Landrace, Pietrain, Hampshire) and cross breds was 768, 729, 735 and 901 days, respectively. Once again, the shorter working life of the Landrace is apparent, compared with the longer working life of the Large-White and the much longer working life of the cross bred. The mean length of breeding life was 1.5 years.

In a review of the causes of reproductive failure of swine, Rasbech (1969) quoted a breeding period for 66 boars of 447 days, with an average piglet production of 2.3/day of function in a district survey in Denmark. In comparison, 24 AI boars had a mean functional period of only 319 days but an output of 7.4 piglets/day of function. Melrose (1966) reported a functional period for boars at four AI centres ranging from as short as 420 days at one centre to as long as 900 at another. The centre with the shortest boar life had the highest disposal rate of boars for further breeding. The practice of AI has advanced and expanded since the report of Melrose (1966) so one might now expect a shorter working life in UK at AI centres.

THE REASONS FOR CULLING BOARS

Le Denmat *el al.*, (1980) reported the main reasons for culling boars from 293 herds as excessive weight or age (31%), reproductive problems (20%), lameness (20%) and other conditions (29%). In our survey, more boars were culled for excess weight or age, but cullings for reproductive problems and lameness were comparable with the French study.

Melrose (1966) analysed the reasons for culling 69 boars from a total of 122 standing at UK AI centres. His results are shown in Table 7. The main reasons were locomotor disorders (15), adverse service behaviour (11), poor service quality (9), disease or injury (8) and low fertility and old age (5). Overall, reproductive inefficiency accounted for 36.2% of culls and Landrace boars were more likely to be culled for this reason.

Rasbech (1969) reported that 40–50% of breeding boars were culled at an early age due to infertility (*impotentia coeundi* or poor semen quality) and the remainder due to factors such as fear of inbreeding, poor progeny, old age and injuries. *Impotentia coeundi* has various causes which include bone and joint disease, erysipelas-induced arthritis and foot lameness, deficient sex drive due to overwork, summer infertility, nutritional deficiencies (mainly of protein, zinc, manganese, copper or Vitamin A, and overfeeding) and systematic diseases, genital disorders such as phimosis, inability to protrude the penis, persistent *frenulum praeputii*, penis haematoma or penis bleeding.

Table 7 REASONS FOR CULLING BOARS AT AI CENTRES (MELROSE, 1966)

Cause	Long-White	Landrace	Other	Total
Low fertility	1	3	1	5
Service behaviour	3	8	–	11
Poor service quality	7	2	–	9
Disease or injury				
Locomotor	9	5	1	15
Old age	5	–	–	5
Small litters	–	1	–	1
Poor progeny	3	–	–	3
Hereditary defects	1	1	–	2
Miscellaneous	7	3	–	10
Total	43	23	3	69
Boars at risk	79	38	5	122

Kuffel (1975), in a paper from the USA on boar management, mentions febrile diseases as the second of the important boar problems. He states that persistent high environmental and body temperatures will affect spermatogenesis and temporary sterility can result, with a recovery time as long as 40–50 days. He gives lameness pride of place as a cause of boar indisposition. Edwards (1977) confirms the increasing importance of lameness in boars to the American producer who is moving from outdoor production 'on dirt' to confinement production on concrete.

The variation that can occur between units in culling for lameness is shown by the observations of Hovorka (1980). Data were obtained on 388 boars at two AI centres in Czechoslovakia from 1972 to 1979. For one 10.3% of culls were for lameness; for the other the figure was 36.4%. It is of interest that the culling rates for boars in the periods January–May, June–October and November–December were 15.8, 71.1 and 13.2% respectively. This suggests a summer problem, although figures by month would have been more meaningful.

FEET

The boar is often the most neglected animal on the farm. He may be housed in a small pen, and forced to stand on a wet, dirty, abrasive floor. His feet can wear excessively, or conversely, overgrow. Foot problems such as white-line lesions, false sand-cracks and heel erosions may lead to perforation of the claw and a sinus at the coronary band (bush-foot). The lateral hind claw is the one most commonly affected and early lesions may be obscured by dirt. The feet must be scrubbed clean, so that a thorough examination can be made of all claws.

Bush-foot lesions are slow to heal. They respond poorly to antibiotics by injection because of the often severe connective tissue reaction surrounding the lesion. Drainage and the application of an astringent, such as 5–10% copper sulphate or fomaldehyde solution often proves more successful. Many years ago, we treated a series of such foot lesions in the sow by amputation of the digit. End results were not as good as with conservative astringent treatment and the recovery period was extended.

PENILE INJURIES AND ABNORMALITIES

These are not uncommon in the boar and they are not always easy to treat. A simplistic approach to haemorrhage from the penis, during or after service, in a young boar is to recommend a 2–3 week period of sexual rest (some clinicians suggest 4 weeks). In many cases, this will allow healing to take place if the injury is not severe, However, when service recommences, bleeding may recur in a proportion of cases. It is these animals which create the difficulty and it may be best to cull the boar at this stage.

Haemorrhage is common in young boars from damage to the glans penis during service. Bite wounds occur and the cavernous bodies may be injured or the tip of the penis may be bitten off. Other less common causes of penile haemorrhage are urethral ulcers and polyps. Bite wounds which involve the urethra may result in fistula formation (Evans and Clark, 1976; King, 1980a: Glossop, 1987).

Ashdown *et al.*, (1981; 1982) studied the angiostructure and venous drainage of the penis of normal boars. They followed this by studying six boars deficient in penile erection and incapable of intromission but able to produce ejaculate containing spermatozoa. Five cases were primary and one secondary. One boar showed an abnormal type of spiral deviation of the penis and five showed abnormal venous drainage of the erectile tissues.

ANAESTHESIA IN PRACTICE

The most reliable method of anaesthesia for the examination of the penis or feet is a combination of azaperone (Stresnil) and metomidate hydrochloride (Hypnodil). Care must be exercised over dose, because penile prolapse may follow the use of azaperone and further self-induced penile damage may result.

THE PREPUTIAL DIVERTICULUM

Boars may urinate or learn to masturbate and ejaculate into diverticulum. Some stockmen 'milk-out' an enlarged diverticulum before service but it is a messy and time-consuming business. Regular culprits should be culled. Surgical removal is performed, almost on a routine basis in some countries, to try to reduce contamination of semen collected at AI Centres (King, 1980b).

TESTICULAR ATROPHY AND ORCHITIS

Degenerative testicular atrophy occurs in boars and is referred to by Arthur *et al.*, (1982) as the commonest porcine testicular disease. It may arise as a result of infections such as erysipelas. It is statements like these that could have led to the quite widely held view, that erysipelas leads to sterility. Rasbech (1969), in his review on the causes of reproductive failure in pigs, states that infections such as erysipelas frequently results in permanent disorders of spermogenic tissue. Reed (1969) is of the opinion that a 5–6 week period of infertility may follow an attack of erysipelas.

These statements about erysipelas infection are interesting. Not all that long ago it was a common belief that orchitis in boars was associated with erysipelas. It has to be admitted that only one case has been seen by the authors that was not at all convincing. However, other veterinarians must hold this view because of the not infrequent cases of farmers complaining to breeding companies of erysipelas infection in recently purchased boars leading to infertility, strongly backed by a veterinary certificate.

It is recognized that a period of temporary infertility may follow an infection in a boar used for natural service or AI, which is treated with some antibiotics. The broad spectrum antibiotics, such as oxytetracycline, seem particularly prone to do this. The question is whether the infertility is due to the infection, the antibiotic or a combination of the two.

Accidental injury, such as testicular trauma or frostbite, may lead to testicular degeneration. This must be differentiated from congenital testicular hypoplasia on the basis of clinical history. Testicular hypoplasia could be hereditary, but in his review of genetically-determined abnormalities of the reproductive system, Bishop (1972) considered the boar to be less frequently affected than the bull. Aspermia or oligospermia are occasionally encountered. They may be temporary or permanent conditions but it could be advisable to treat them as irreversible.

Tumours in pigs, with the exception of lymphosarcoma and melanoma, are uncommon. However, scrotal haemangiomas have been reported in boars of various ages (Munro *et al.*, 1982).

BOAR TEMPERAMENT

This may be an important factor associated with reproductive efficiency because boars may not be able to give a satisfactory service if they are difficult to handle. It is said by female staff on some farms that they have few fears of the Large-White but they don't like Landrace boars. Detusking was not a common practice in our survey, but it is a fairly simple procedure. The equipment needed is a snout-snare, a piece of embryotomy wire 24 inches long, a pair of handles and a piece of wood, like the handle of a pick-axe, to use as a gag. Modern tranquilizers make the task much easier. Removal of both upper and lower tusks is advisable although some operators do not remove the maxillary tusks.

NEEDLE-SHY BOARS

Boars are now encountered that shake their heads vigorously and move backwards and forwards like sows when any attempt is made to handle or inject them, even if they are offered food. Boars are being subjected to more injections and handling in units, with, for example, a suspected leptospirosis or a vaginal discharge problem. A farm was recently visited on which they had given up trying to inject three of their older boars because it was interfering with their desire to serve. These three boars had to be culled.

BOAR MORTALITY

Boar mortality is often included with that for sows, so figures are hard to come by. In the AI boar survey by Melrose (1966), five of the 122 boars at risk (4.1%) died, but the time scale of the survey was not given. Sow mortality in the UK has certainly risen since the days of the survey of the Pig Industry Development Authority in 1964, when the figure was 2.7%.

Guise (1986) in her 26-farm survey, with a mean herd size of 266, reported a mean mortality of 4.8%, with a range of 1.7–12.7%. The current mean figure of MLC Pig Plan herds is 3.9% for home-mixing herds and 3.5% for herds fed compound feeds (Anon. 1987).

In the survey of AI centre boars by Hovorka (1980), emergency slaughter or death accounted for 2.6% and 9.1% of boar wastage respectively. This was over a 7 year period.

Deaths in boars are something of an exceptional occurrence on most pig farms. Conditions such as stress death, fights in which an old boar kills a younger one, and haemorrhage from a gastric ulcer are the more common reasons.

PARBENDAZOLE TOXICITY IN BOARS

The benzimidazoles belong to a range of compounds based on the parent compound thiabendazole. All are claimed to be of very low toxicity. Parbendazole is not now extensively used in the UK, but toxicity in boars was described on three units by Penny and Lloyd-Evans (1981). Since then, a further case has come to our notice in the UK, involving a herd in the survey reported in this paper. Three of nine boars wormed showed symptoms four days after dosing and two died.

Four further outbreaks have been brought to our attention by the Department of Agriculture for Western Australia. Brief summaries of the number affected and the main signs observed are shown in Tables 8 and 9. Some of the benzimidazoles are known to be teratogenic and are thus contra-indicated in early pregnancy. We have not seen any other side effects in pigs.

Table 8 PARBENDAZOLE TOXICITY IN BOARS

		No. dosed	Affected	Interval (days)	Died
1.	LM	12	5	5–6	2
2.	SM	18	6	4–5	1
3.	FB	5	2	5–6	2
4.	VIO	9	3	4	2
5.	PDA	33	4	3–4	–
6.	PDA	26	11	3–4	1
7.	PCU	8	6	4	3
8.	PCU	13	10	4	3
Totals	8	124	47	3–6	14

If there is a lesson to be learned from these reports of parbendazole toxicity it is that, if boars are to receive routine medication, it might be better to treat small numbers at a time, rather than all boars on the farm on the same day.

Table 9 PARBENDAZOLE TOXICITY IN BOARS

	Greenish-yellow diarrhoea	*Dysentery*	*Shock*
1	+++	++	+
2	++	++	+
3	+++	++	+
4	+++	−	+
5	++	?	+
6	++	?	+
7	++	?	+
8	++	?	+

SUMMARY

The results of a survey of boar usage and wastage in a Group of 26 herds, with a total of 6363 sows and 325 boars, are described. The main points considered were sow:boar ratio, number of services per oestrus, breeds of boar in use, age of boars in the herd, annual culling rate and reasons for culling, and annual mortality and the causes of death. The results of this survey are compared with the available literature.

REFERENCES

Anon. (1987) Pig Plan Results for 1987. Meat and Livestock Commission, Bletchley, Bucks, UK

Arthur, G. H., Noakes, D. E. and Pearson, H. (1982) *Veterinary Reproduction and Obstetrics.* Bailliere Tindall, London, 458 pp.

Ashdown, R. R., Barnett, S. W. and Ardalani, G. (1981) Impotence in the boar: Angioarchitecture and venous drainage of the penis in normal boars. *Vet. Rec.,* **109,** 375

Ashdown, R. R., Barnett, S. W. and Ardalani, G. (1982) Impotence in the boar 2: Clinical and anatomical studies on impotent boars. *Vet. Rec.,* **110,** 349

Bishop, M. W. H. (1972) Genetically determined Abnormalities of the Reproductive System. *J. Reproduction and Fertility, Suppl.* **15,** 15–78

Edwards, J. H. (1977) Boar Management. Proceedings American Association of Swine Practitioners Conference. Raleigh, North Carolina, USA, 7–10

Evans, L. E. and Clark, T. L. (1976) Abnormalities and injuries of the boar's penis. In *Proceedings International Pig Veterinary Society Congress* (Ames, Iowa) D12

Glossop, C. (1987) Penile injuries in the boar. *In Practice,* **9,** 211–215

Guise, H. J. (1986) *Cambac – J. Sainsbury Project* Cambac JMA Research Ltd, Wallingford, Oxford, UK pp. 42

Hovorka, J. (1980) The main reasons for culling boars used in artificial insemination. *Veterinarstvi,* **30,** 271

Hunter, R. H. F. (1988) *Pig Vet Soc. Proc.,* in press.

King, R. G. (1980a) Surgical repair of persistent bleeding penis injuries. In *Proceedings International Pig Veterinary Society Congress* (Copenhagen, Denmark) pp 57

King, R. G. (1980b) Surgical Removal of the preputial diverticulum. In *Proceedings International Pig Veterinary Society Congress* (Copenhagen, Denmark) pp. 58

Kuffel, R. (1975) Boar management: A veterinarian's approach. In *Proceedings American Association of Swine Practitioners Conference* (Kansas City) pp. 48–50

Le Denmat, M. and Runavot, J.-P. (1980) *Douze journees de la recherche porcine in France.* French Ministry of Agriculture, Paris, pp. 149–156

Le Denmat, M., Runavot, J.-P. and Albar, J. (1980) Characteristics of the boar population in service with commercial herds. Results of a survey of 293 herds. *Techni-Porc,* **3,** 41–48

Melrose, D. R. (1966) A Review of Progress and of Possible Developments in Artificial Insemination of Pigs. *Vet. Rec.,* **78,** 159–168

Munro, R., Head, K. W. and Munro, H. M. C. (1982) Scrotal haemangiomas in boars. *J. Comp. Pathol.,* **92,** 109

Penny, R. H. C. and Lloyd-Evans, L. P. (1981) Possible toxicity in boars after worming. *Pig Vet. Soc. Proc.,* **7,** 74-76

Rasbech, N. O. (1969) A Review of the Causes of Reproductive Failure in Swine. *Br. Vet. J.,* **125,** 599–616

Reed, H. C. B. (1969) Artificial insemination and fertility of the boar. *Br. Vet. J.,* **125,** 272–280

Ridgeon, R. F. (1987) *Pig Management Scheme Results,* University of Cambridge Agricultural Economics Unit. Cambridge, UK

C. R. LAMB

Aspects of diagnostic imaging in equine pulmonary disease

INTRODUCTION

DIAGNOSTIC IMAGING methods are being used increasingly as aids to the diagnosis of equine pulmonary disease. Prior to 1968 there were few reports of thoracic radiography in the adult horse. However, with high output equipment now installed at most veterinary schools and in some practices, and the advent of 'rare earth' intensifying screens (Koblik, Hornof and O'Brien, 1980), the technique is widely used. Recently, other imaging techniques such as ultrasonography (Rantanen, 1986) and radionuclide imaging (Devous, Theodorakis and Hillidge, 1979; Amis, Pascoe and Hornof, 1984; O'Callaghan, Hornof, Fisher and Raabe 1987; O'Callaghan, Hornof, Fisher and Pascoe, 1987) have been applied to the horse. In general, these techniques provide complementary information, and are often used in combination.

RADIOGRAPHY

Satisfactory thoracic radiographs of foals may be obtained using a portable X-ray machine capable of 20 mA and 90 kV and calcium tungstate screens. However, exposure times are prolonged, so faster rare earth screens are preferred. Small foals should be radiographed in lateral recumbency with the forelimbs pulled cranially to avoid superimposition over the cranial lung field. Use of a grid to reduce scatter is recommended. Thoracic radiography of the standing foal using an air gap instead of a grid has also been described (Martens and Ruoff, 1982).

Radiographic evaluation of the adult equine thorax in the standing position requires three or four overlapping lateral radiographs. The format in the author's hospital follows that described by Farrow (1981a). Using a rare earth film-screen system, exposure factors for a film focus distance of 100 cm vary from 100–110 kV at 12 mA for the caudal lung field to 120 kV at 48 mA for the cranial thorax in a large horse. A high kV technique results in greater latitude on radiographs, improves nodule detection (Kelsey *et al.*, 1982) and increases the margin for error in setting exposure factors, hence reducing retakes. In the adult, considerable magnification of the side of the thorax furthest from the film occurs, blurring out fine structures. Hence, radiographs taken from both left and right may be helpful in demonstrating unilateral lesions. Alternatively, a longer film focus distance such as 200 cm may be used (Feeney *et al.*, 1982), though this requires a four-fold increase in exposure factors.

The inspiratory pause in horses is very brief, so exposures made during the longer expiratory pause may be preferred because they reduce the likelihood of motion blur.

Principles of interpretation of equine thoracic radiographs have been described (Kangstrom, 1968; Farrow, 1981b; Farrow, 1981c; King, 1981). It must be appreciated that interpretation is often limited by the non-specific nature of many radiographic signs. Furthermore, many conditions such as bronchitis, bronchiolitis, chronic obstructive lung disease, or exercise-induced pulmonary hemorrhage (EIPH), often produce radiographs interpreted as normal (Farrow, 1981b). Radiographs should also be interpreted with reference to the history and physical findings in each case. The interpretation of radiographs as normal or incompatible with the clinical signs is an indication for further diagnostic tests. These might include other methods such as ultrasonography or radionuclide imaging (Figure 1) or invasive tissue sampling techniques such as tracheal aspiration of lung biopsy.

Various radiographic patterns are described to aid interpretation. The air space (or alveolar) pattern is characterized by poorly marginated areas of uniform opacity which coalesce, sometimes producing an air bronchogram. Lung consolidation (Figure 2), oedema, haemorrhage, or neoplastic infiltration could result in an air space pattern. In newborn foals, a diffuse air space pattern is seen in conjunction with respiratory distress syndrome due to prematurity and surfactant deficiency (Vaala, 1986). A diffuse air space pattern in adults may result from pulmonary thromboembolism (Kerr, Harkema and O'Brien, 1985).

The so-called interstitial pattern may present as an ill-defined granular opacity which blurs the borders of pulmonary vessels, a fine linear opacity, or as nodules. It is associated with a variety of conditions including pneumonia (viral, bacterial, fungal, or parasitic), bronchiolitis, pulmonary fibrosis, septicaemia, oedema (Figure 3) and, occasionally, pulmonary lymphosarcoma. Rarely, a miliary infiltrate due to tuberculosis may be observed (Mair *et al.*, 1986). Interpretation of such a non-specific pattern usually cannot be made without an appreciation of the history and physical findings in each case. However, certain radiographic signs are more specific. Solitary or multiple nodules, including cavitated lesions with or without gas – fluid interfaces, are usually abscesses (Silverman, Poulos and Suter, 1976). Multiple nodules with slightly 'fluffy' borders are commonly associated with *Rhodococcus equi* pneumonia in foals (Martens, Fiske and Renshaw, 1982; Hillidge, 1986). A localized interstitial infiltrate in the caudodorsal lung field has been associated with EIPH (O'Callaghan and Goulden, 1982; Pascoe *et al.*, 1983; O'Callaghan, Pascoe, O'Brien and Hornof, 1987).

A purely bronchial pattern is unusual on equine thoracic radiographs; bronchial patterns usually occur with some interstitial component. Thickening of the large bronchial walls may appear as paired linear opacities. More often numerous small 2–4 mm) circular opacities, which produce a honeycomb appearance, are observed (Figure 4). They probably indicate thickening of medium-sized airways. Structural changes in the bronchi may be evaluated further by bronchography. Techniques using liquid barium sulphate or insufflation of barium sulphate powder (O'Callaghan and Sanderson, 1982) have been described in horses.

Vascular structures are thought to contribute most to peripheral lung opacity (Sanderson and O'Callaghan, 1983), so changes in their number or calibre are likely to influence the interstitial pattern. Changes in the size, shape and number of visible pulmonary vessels reflect changes in blood flow to the lung. Prominent pulmonary vessels may be seen in horses radiographed soon after exercise in cases of

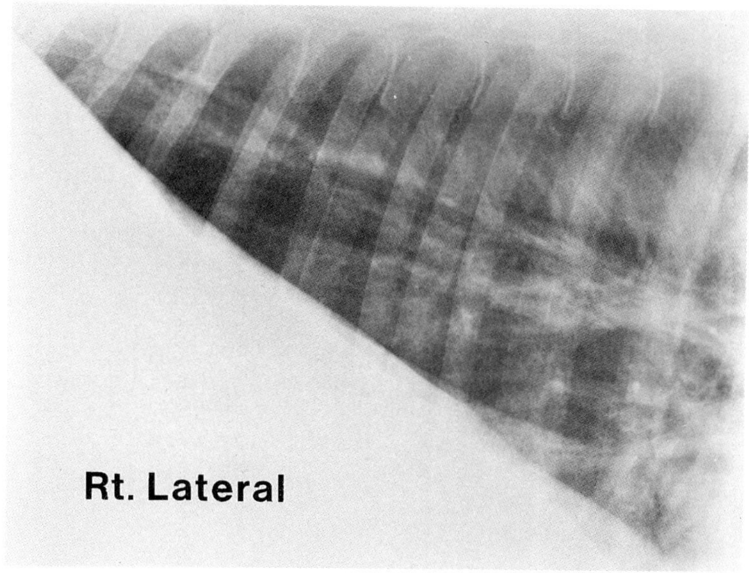

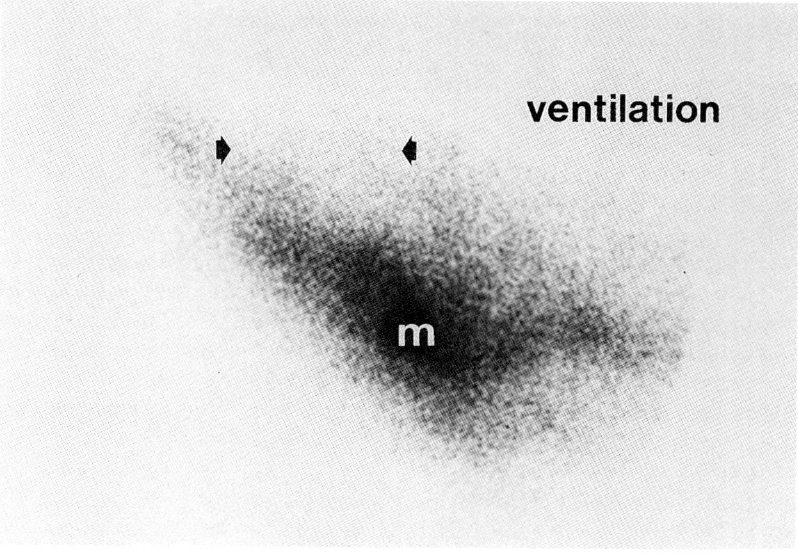

Fig. 1. (a) Right lateral radiograph of a 22-year old pony with chronic 'heaves'. A mild diffuse interstitial pattern is apparent. (b) ^{99m}Tc-DTPA aerosol ventilation scan in the same pony showing a mainly central distribution of aerosol due to turbulence in the large airways. Large peripheral ventilation deficits are also present (between arrows). The focal area of intense activity (m) is a skin marker. Whereas the radiographic signs mainly reflect structural changes in the lung, the ventilation scan gives functional information. (Figure 1b is included by permission of Dr M. W. O'Callaghan).

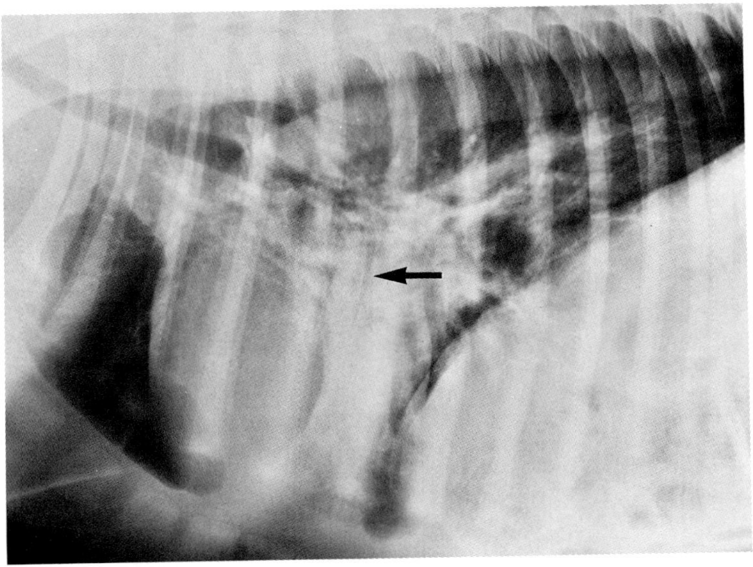

Fig. 2. Lateral radiograph of the thorax of a 4-week old foal with septicaemia. There is a sharply defined area of uniform opacity with air bronchogram (arrow) overlying the caudal aspect of the heart. Radiographic diagnosis: bronchopneumonia.

left-to-right cardiac shunts or mitral insufficiency. Narrowed vessels and relative hyperlucency of the lung field are seen in cases of hypovolaemia and lung hyperinflation.

Pleural fluid tends to obscure the cardiac silhouette and ventral lung field. A gas–fluid interface will not be apparent unless there is concurrent pneumothorax, and so pleural effusion is difficult to distinguish radiographically from ventral consolidation of the lung without air bronchogram. Ultrasonography or thoracentesis should then be considered as adjunct tests. Radiographs taken after pleural drainage may demonstrate previously hidden pulmonary or mediastinal lesions. Pleural effusions of less than 500 ml are not radiographically apparent in the adult horse (Koblik and Hornof, 1985).

Radiography is sometimes useful for evaluating equine mediastinal disease. Pneumomediastinum, a common complication of transtracheal aspiration (Farrow, 1976), may also result from a gas-producing septic process in the mediastinum, extension of pleuropneumonia, tracheal or bronchial rupture or thoracic stake wound. It is recognized radiographically by the ability to see the outer walls of the trachea. The presence of a mediastinal mass may in some cases be demonstrated indirectly by a positive contrast oesophagram (Greet, 1982).

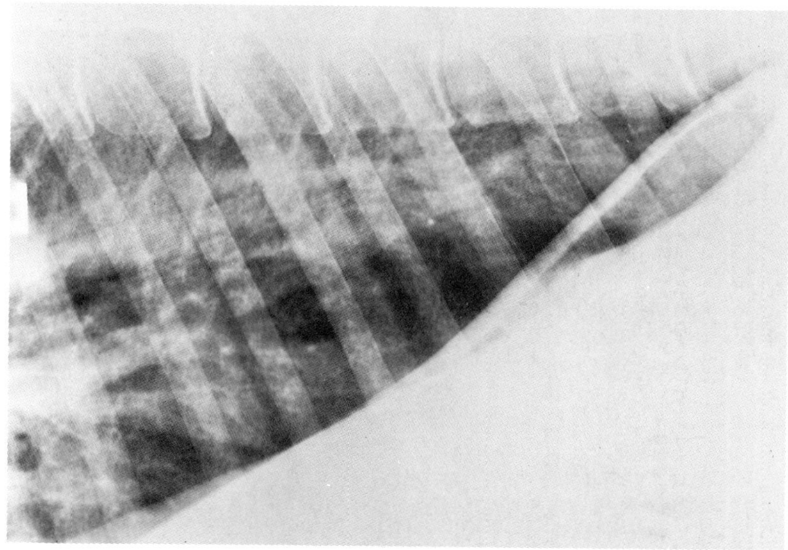

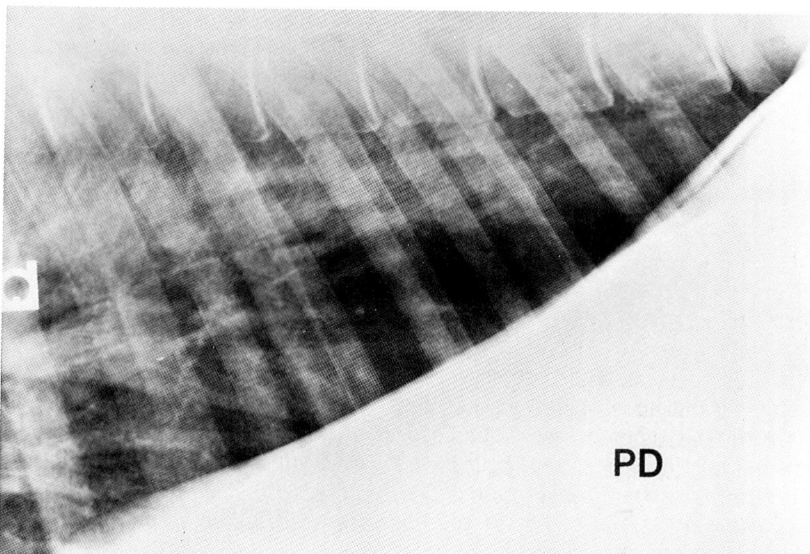

Fig. 3. (a) Lateral radiograph of the caudal thorax of a 21-year old Quarter horse presented with increased respiratory effort and a mucopurulent nasal discharge. A moderate diffuse interstitial pattern is apparent, which blurs vascular structures. Bronchitis/bronchiolitis or bronchopneumonia could produce this appearance. (b) The same horse 2 hours after IV administration of 500 mg Furosemide (Lasix; Hoechst). The interstitial pattern has diminished, improving visualization of the vessels and bronchi. Radiographic interpretation: interstitial pattern reflects pulmonary oedema or vascular recruitment rather than cellular infiltrate; bronchopneumonia less likely than allergic airway disease. Final diagnosis (based on tracheal aspirate cytology, negative culture and response to management changes): 'heaves'.

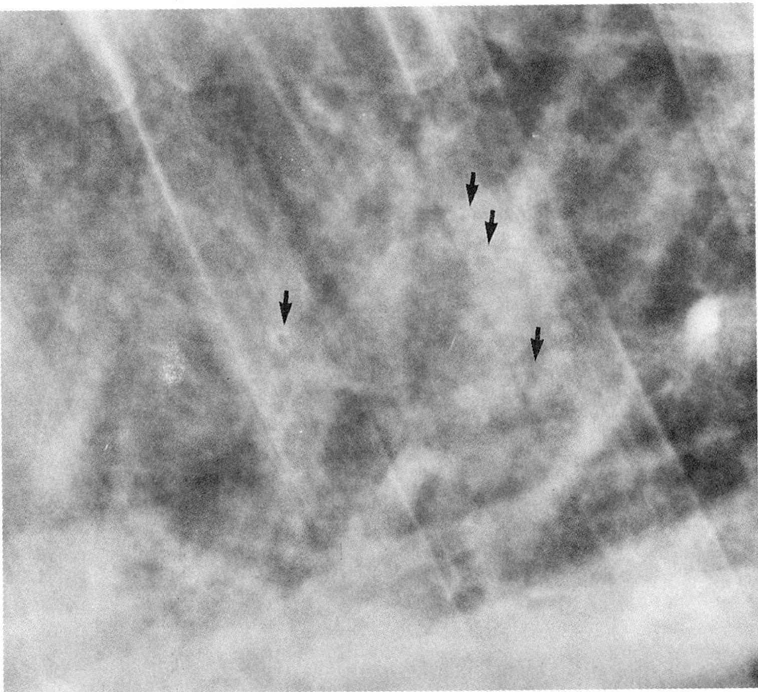

Fig. 4. Detail of a thoracic radiograph of a 12-year old Thoroughbred with increased lung sounds. There is a marked reticular interstitial pattern and numerous thick rings (arrows). Radiographic diagnosis: medium sized airway thickening, probable bronchitis/bronchiolitis. Histologic diagnosis: chronic bronchiolitis.

ULTRASONOGRAPHY

The physical principles of ultrasound applications in animals, interpretation of images and recognition of artifacts have been described (Rantanen and Ewing, 1981; Park *et al.*, 1981). The role of ultrasound in the diagnosis of pulmonary disease is limited, principally because the air-filled lung and ribs reflect a high proportion of the sound waves. Failure of the sound waves to penetrate effectively casts a 'shadow' which hides underlying tissue structure. On the other hand, soft tissues and fluids transmit a greater proportion of the sound wave so that their internal structure is visualized. Pleural fluid (Figure 5) and peripheral lung lesions, such as atelectasis (Figure 6), abscesses and tumours may be imaged (Rantanen, Gage and Paradis, 1981; Mackey, 1983; Rantanen, 1986). An anechoic zone adjacent to the thoracic wall strongly suggests that fluid is present and may be amenable to thoracentesis, but a proportion of cases do not yield fluid (Laing and Filly, 1978). This may be because the fluid is too viscous or consists of clotted blood. The presence of numerous tiny bubbles in the pleural fluid of a horse which has not had thoracentesis has been associated with the presence of a gas-forming bacterial pleuritis.

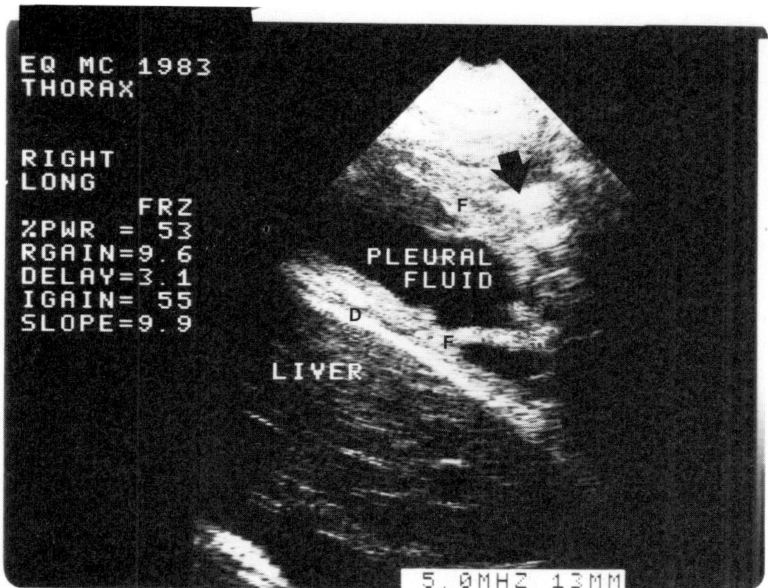

Fig. 5. Longitudinal ultrasonogram of the right caudal thorax showing anechoic (black) pleural fluid trapped by fibrin deposits (F) which also coat the diaphragm (D). The air-filled lung appears as a highly echoic (white) area. Normal liver is present below the diaphragm.

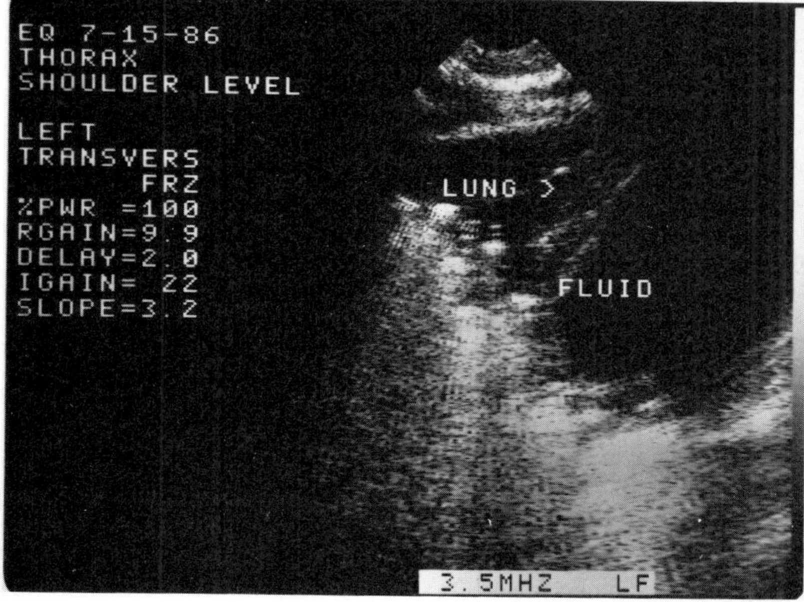

Fig. 6. Transverse ultrasonogram of the left mid-throax demonstrating a large volume of anechoic (black) pleural fluid surrounding collapsed lung.

REFERENCES

Amis, T. C., Pascoe, J. R. and Hornof, W. J. (1984) Topographic distribution of pulmonary ventilation and perfusion in the horse. *Am. J. Vet. Res.*, **45**, 1597–1601

Devous, M. D., Theodorakis, M. C. and Hillidge, C. J. (1979) Scintigraphic evaluation of pulmonary perfusion and ventilation in equine respiratory disease. *Proceedings of the 25th Annual Convention of the American Association of Equine Practitioners*, (Miami Beach, Florida, 1979) pp. 373–374

Farrow, C. S. (1976) Pneumomediastinum in the horse: a complication of transtracheal aspiration. *J. Am. Vet. Rad. Soc.*, **17**, 192–195

Farrow, C. S. (1981a) Radiography of the equine thorax: anatomy and technique. *Vet. Radiol.*, **22**, 62–68

Farrow, C. S. (1981b) Aspects of inflammatory lung disease in the horse. *Vet. Radiol.*, **22**, 107–114

Farrow, C. S. (1981c) Equine thoracic radiology. *J. Am. Vet. Med. Assoc.*, **179**, 776–781

Feeney, D. A., Gordon, B. J., Johnston, G. R., McClanahan, S. L. and Jessen, C. R. (1982) A 200 centimeter focal spot-film distance (FFD) technique for equine thoracic radiography. *Vet. Radiol.*, **23**, 13–19

Greet, T. R. C. (1982) Observations on the potential role of oesophageal radiography in the horse. *Equine Vet. J.*, **14**, 73–79

Hillidge, C. J. (1986) Review of *Corynebacterium (Rhodococcus) equi* lung abscesses in foals: pathogenesis, diagnosis and treatment. *Vet. Rec.*, **119**, 261–264

Kangstrom, L. (1968) The radiological diagnosis of equine pneumonia. *J. Am. Vet. Rad. Soc.*, **9**, 80–88

Kelsey, C. A., Moseley, R. D., Mettler, F. A., Garcia, J. F., Parker T. W. and Briscoe, D. E. (1982) Comparison of nodule detection with 70-kV and 120-kV chest radiographs. *Radiology*, **143**, 609–611

Kerr, L. Y., Harkema, J. R. and O'Brien, T. R. (1985) Radiographic diagnosis. *Vet. Radiol.*, **26**, 123–125

King, G. K. (1981) Equine thoracic radiography. Part II. Radiographic patterns of equine pulmonary and pleural diseases using air-gap rare earth radiography. *Compendium Contin. Educ. Pract. Vet.*, **3**, S283–S287

King, G. K., Martens, R. J. and McCall, V. H. (1981) Equine thoracic radiography. Part I. Air-gap rare earth radiography of the normal equine thorax. *Compendium Contin. Educ. Pract. Vet.*, **3**, S278–S281

Koblik, P. D., Hornof, W. J. and O'Brien, T. R. (1980) Rare earth intensifying screens for veterinary radiography: an evaluation of two systems. *Vet. Radiol.*, **21**, 224–230

Koblik, P. D. and Hornof, W. J. (1985) Diagnostic radiology and nuclear cardiology: their use in assessment of equine cardiovascular disease. *Vet. Clin. North Am. [Equine Practice]*, **1**, 289–309

Laing, F. C. and Filly, R. A. (1978) Problems in the application of ultrasonography for the evaluation of pleural opacities. *Radiology*, **126**, 211–214

Mackey, V. S. (1983) Equine pleuropneumonia: radiology – diagnostic ultrasound – pleuroscopy. In *Proceedings of the 29th Annual Convention of the American Association of Equine Practitioners*, (Las Vegas, Nevada, 1983) pp. 75–80

Mair, T. S., Taylor, F. G. R., Gibbs, C. and Lucke, V. M. (1986) Generalised avian tuberculosis in a horse. *Equine Vet. J.*, **18**, 226–230

Martens, R. J., Fiske, R. A. and Renshaw, H. W. (1982) Experimental subacute foal pneumonia induced by aerosol administration of *Corynebacterium equi*. *Equine Vet. J.*, **14**, 111–116

Martens, R. J. and Ruoff, W. W. (1982) Foal pneumonia: a practical approach to diagnosis and therapy. *Compendium Contin. Educ. Pract. Vet.*, **4**, S361–S373

O'Callaghan, M. W. and Goulden, B. E. (1982) Radiographic changes in the lungs of horses with exercise-induced epistaxis. *NZ Vet. J.*, **30**, 117–118

O'Callaghan, M. W. and Sanderson, G. N. (1982) Clinical bronchography in the horse: development of a method using barium sulphate powder. *Equine Vet. J.*, **14**, 282–289

O'Callaghan, M. W., Hornof, W. J., Fisher, P. and Raabe, O. G. (1987) Ventilation imaging in the horse with ^{99m}Technetium-DTPA radioaerosol. *Equine Vet. J.*, **19**, 19–24

O'Callaghan, M. W., Hornof, W. J., Fisher, P. and Pascoe, J. R. (1987) Exercise- induced pulmonary haemorrhage in the horse: results of a detailed clinical, *post mortem* and imaging study. VII. Ventilation/perfusion Scintigraphy in horses with EIPH *Equine Vet. J.*, **19**, 423–427

O'Callaghan, M. W., Pascoe, J. R., O'Brien, T. R. and Hornof, W. J. (1987) Exercise-induced pulmonary haemorrhage in the horse: results of a detailed clinical, *post mortem* and imaging study. VI. Radiological/pathological correlations. *Equine Vet. J.*, **19**, 419–422

Park, R. D., Nyland, T. G., Lattimer, J. C., Miller, C. W. and Lebel, J. L. (1981) B-mode gray scale ultrasound: imaging artifacts and interpretation principles. *Vet. Radiol.*, **22**, 204–210

Pascoe, J. R., O'Brien, T. R., Wheat, J. D. and Meagher, D. M. (1983) Radiographic aspects of exercise-induced pulmonary hemorrhage in racing horses. *Vet. Radiol.*, **24**, 85–92

Rantanen, N. W. (1981) Ultrasound appearance of normal lung borders and adjacent viscera in the horse. *Vet. Radiol.*, **22**, 217–219

Rantanen, N. W. (1986) Disease of the thorax. *Vet. Clin. North Am. [Equine Practice]* **2**, 49–66

Rantanen, N. W. and Ewing, R. L. (1981) Principles of ultrasound application in animals. *Vet. Radiol.*, **22**, 196–203

Rantanen, N. W., Gage, L. and Paradis, M. R. (1981) Ultrasonography as a diagnostic aid in pleural effusion in horses. *Vet. Radiol.*, **22**, 211–216

Sanderson, G. N. and O'Callaghan, M. W. (1983) Radiographic anatomy of the equine thorax as a basis for radiological interpretation. *NZ Vet. J.*, **31**, 127–130

Silverman, S., Poulos P. W. and Suter, P. F. (1976) Cavitary pulmonary lesions in animals. *J. Am. Vet. Rad. Soc.*, **17**, 134–146

Vaala, W. E. (1986) Diagnosis and treatment of prematurity and neonatal maladjustment syndrome in newborn foals. *Compendium Contin. Educ. Pract. Vet.*, **8**, S211–S224

T. S. MAIR and CHRISTINE GIBBS

The radiographic evaluation of pleural and mediastinal disease in the horse

INTRODUCTION

THE VALUE of radiography in the assessment of chest diseases in man and small animals is well established but in the horse, technical limitations associated with the size of the thorax have tended to preclude its use in general practice. However, with the use of rare earth intensifying screens, high-speed radiographic film and an air gap between the patient and the film, radiographs of diagnostic quality covering much of the adult horse's chest can be obtained using relatively low-powered equipment. The radiographic technique has been described in detail elsewhere in this book (Lamb, 1989).

Radiography, along with other techniques such as ultrasonography (Rantanen *et al.*, 1981; Lamb, 1989), pleuroscopy (Mackey and Wheat, 1985) and oesophagoscopy (Freeman, 1982), is particularly useful in the investigation of pleural and mediastinal diseases. This article describes the radiological features of some of the commoner pleural and mediastinal diseases that are encountered in the horse.

NORMAL ANATOMY

The two pleural cavities (right and left) are lined by the pleura, which consist of a thin layer of connective tissue covered by a single layer of mesothelial cells. In the horse, the two cavities frequently communicate with each other owing to the delicate nature of the caudal mediastinum. Normally the cavities contain only a small amount of fluid which permits frictionless movement of the visceral and parietal surfaces.

The mediastinum is formed by the reflection of the parietal pleura over the heart and other midline structures. It contains the trachea, heart and great vessels, oesophagus, various nerves, thymus, and the sternal, mediastinal and tracheobronchial lymph nodes. Apart from the air-filled trachea, all of the mediastinal structures are of soft tissue density. Only three of them are normally visible radiographically as distinct entities; those include the heart, aorta and caudal vena cava.

PLEURAL EFFUSION

Pleural effusion is defined as the presence of excessive quantities of fluid within the pleural space. The causes are numerous and the types of fluid fall into the general categories of transudate, exudate, haemorrhagic and chylous fluids. In the horse, most effusions are transudative or exudative in nature. Exudative effusions are commonly associated with pleuritis secondary to pneumonia or lung abscesses. Transudative effusions are most often associated with neoplasia. Lymphosarcoma involving the mediastinum is the commonest (Raphel and Beech 1982; Mair, 1987). It is not possible to differentiate between these types of fluid radiographically. Therefore thoracocentesis and fluid analysis are necessary before a definitive diagnosis can be reached. Ultrasonography may also be useful in demonstrating fibrin tags in cases of pleuritis.

The typical radiographic appearance of free pleural fluid is that of an area of homogeneous soft tissue density in the ventral thorax (Figure 1). Clearly defined horizontal gas–fluid interfaces will not be seen unless air is also present in the cavity because lung tissue is partially submerged in surrounding fluid. In some cases of chronic exudative pleuritis, fluid may become encapsulated by fibrous adhesions, with the subsequent development of abscesses in the pleural cavity. In such cases numerous gas-capped fluid levels may be seen radiographically, presumably because of the presence of gas-forming organisms (Colahan and Knight, 1979; Farrow, 1981).

PNEUMOTHORAX

Pneumothorax is the presence of free air or gas within the pleural space. Chest wall trauma is the commonest cause of this condition in the horse, although it may also be induced iatrogenically following thoracocentesis and intra- or trans- thoracic biopsy techniques, or secondarily to pneumomediastinum. The radiographic diagnosis of pneumothorax depends upon the presence of air in the pleural cavity accompanied by partial pulmonary atelectasis (Figure 2). Because the lung is decreased in volume it appears relatively radiopaque when compared with the air-filled pleural space. On a lateral radiograph taken with the horse standing the free pleural air is shown to collect dorsally and the dorsal lung margin to migrate ventrally.

DIAPHRAGMATIC RUPTURE

Diaphragmatic rupture, with subsequent passage of abdominal contents into the chest, is uncommon in the horse when compared with small animals. The cause is usually traumatic, including increased intra-abdominal pressure at parturition (Bristol, 1986). The presenting signs include respiratory distress, or more commonly, colic as a result of intestinal obstruction. Radiography may reveal the presence of intestinal loops within the thorax (Figure 3) or, in more chronic cases, a pleural effusion (Verschooten *et al.*, 1977).

PNEUMOMEDIASTINUM

Pneumomediastinum (the presence of free air within the mediastinum) may occur as a result of rupture of alveoli beneath the visceral pleura in acute lung disease, or secondary to tracheal or oesophageal rupture or dissection of air along the intermuscular fascia of the neck following lacerations in that area. It is also a common sequel to the technique of transtracheal aspiration (Figure 4a) (Farrow, 1976).

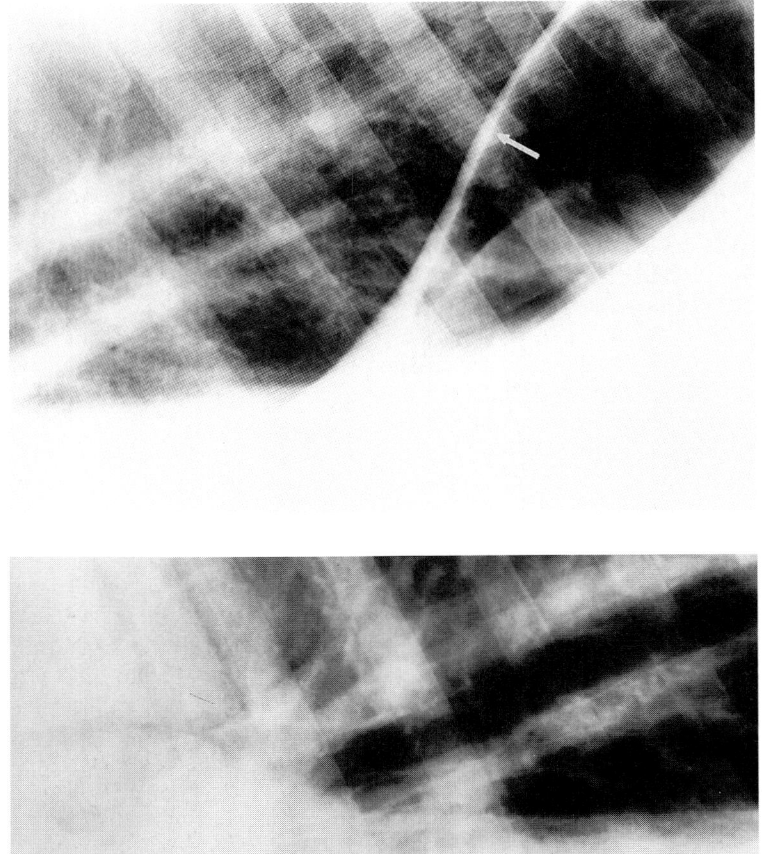

Fig. 1. Pleural fluid (lymphosarcoma) in a 6-year old eventer. Fields 1 (a) and 2 (b) show the absence of aerated lung in the triangular area between the caudal border of heart and diaphragm. At the level of the heart base there is an indistinct interface between lung parenchyma above and a homogenous opacity below which represents the level of free fluid in which the lungs are partially submerged. In (a), the left hemi-diaphragm is shown as a narrow oblique band (arrow) because there is gas in the fundus of the stomach behind it.

Radiographically, gross pneumomediastinum is characterized by the presence of abnormal gas shadows within the soft tissues framing the mediastinal structures which makes their outlines more clearly visible (Figure 4b).

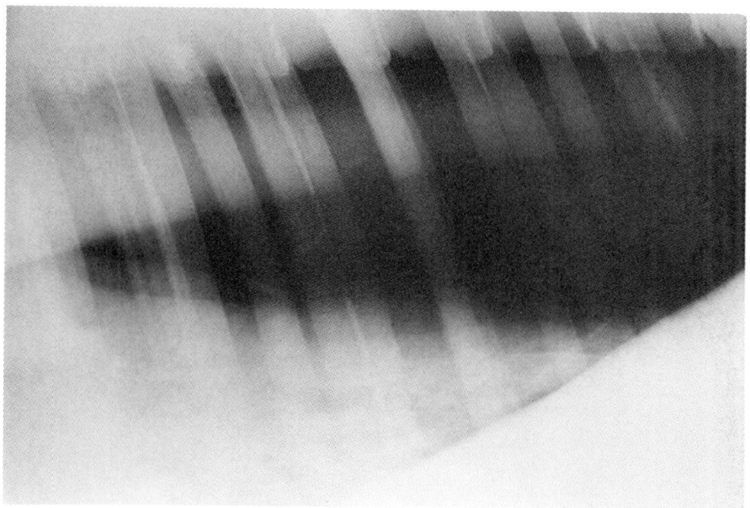

Fig. 2. Pneumothorax (penetrating wound) in a 7 year old Arab gelding. The dorsal
thoracic cavity is uniformly hyperlucent and no pulmonary vascular markings are present,
so that the shadow of the aorta appears exceptionally clear. The dorsal borders of the
partially collapsed caudal lung lobes are clearly visible in a horizontal plane just above the
heart base. As a result of reduced air content the lung parenchyma is more radio dense
than normal and the vascular shadows are crowded together.

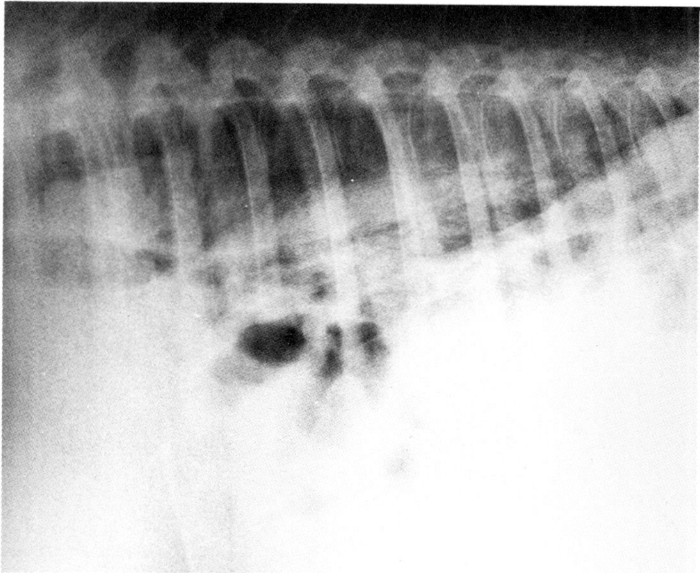

Fig. 3. Ruptured diaphragm in a 2-month old Fjord foal. The dorsal lung fields are
relatively normal but ventrally there is no aerated parenchyma between heart and
diaphragm. In this area and overlying the diaphragm there are several irregularly
shaped radiolucent shadows which represent gas-filled bowel loops in the thorax.

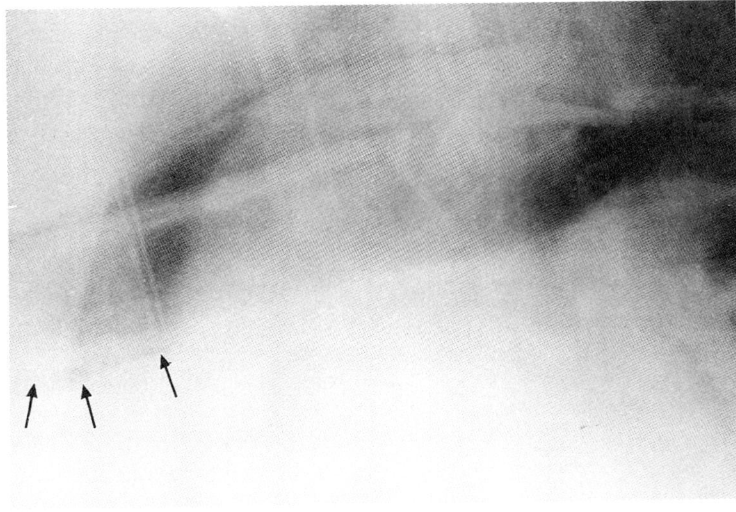

a

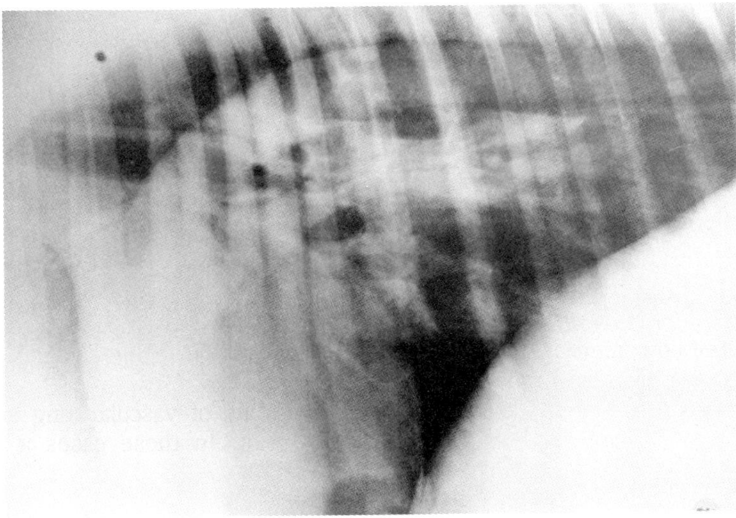

b

Fig. 4.(a) Iatrogenic Pneumomediastinum (following trans-tracheal aspiration) in a 7-year old Cleveland Bay mare. Coned down view of the thoracic trachea and cranial mediastinum is shown. The dorsal margin of the dorsal tracheal wall is clearly delineated and an additional curvilinear streak of air can be seen above it. There is also a small pocket of air ventral to the trachea cranially (arrows). (b) Pneumomediastinum and pneumothorax (cervical oesophageal perforation) in a 4-week old Welsh Cob foal. The dorsal border of the dorsal wall of the trachea, the roots of the great vessels around the heart base and the aorta can all be distinguished more clearly than usual because they are framed by mediastinal air. There is a small pneumothorax. An undulant density interface ventral to the aorta represents the dorsal border of one lung, which is partly collapsed.

MEDIASTINAL MASSES

The thoracic lymph nodes are not normally visible because they are small and of soft tissue density. They therefore merge with adjacent mediastinal structures. However, lymphomegaly involving the cranial mediastinal or tracheobronchial nodes may be sufficient to cause deviation of the distal trachea (Figure 5a). Radiographic evidence of this process is sometimes seen in cases of *Rhodococcus* (Corynebacterium) *equi* pneumonia of foals (Falcon, *et al.*, 1985), and in some neoplastic diseases, particularly lymphosarcoma. Inflammation and calcification of the mediastinal fat may occur in generalized steatitis in foals. In such cases a diffuse soft tissue density will be observed in the cranial chest (Figure 5b).

OESOPHAGEAL DISORDERS

From the thoracic inlet, the oesophagus passes to the right of the midline, crosses the aortic arch and continues caudally towards the diaphragm in the mediastinum, lying ventrally and to the right of the aorta. In the normal empty oesophagus, the longitudinal mucosal folds obliterate the lumen which is therefore not visible radiographically as a distinct structure. Although some oesophageal disorders such as megaoesophagus, radiopaque foreign bodies and impactions with food material may be visible on plain radiographs, the use of contrast agents greatly aids the radiographic examination (Alexander, 1967; Freeman, 1982; Greet, 1982).

Contrast studies of the oesophagus may be performed using agents such as liquid barium sulphate (positive contrast), air (negative contrast), or both (double contrast) (Freeman, 1982). The agents are generally administered as a drench or via a naso-oesophageal tube immediately before the radiograph is taken. Barium sulphate in the normal oesophagus is rapidly cleared by peristalsis, although some will remain briefly in the lumen and outline the mucosal folds (Figure 6), especially at the level of the thoracic inlet and the aortic arch (Bargai, 1972). More detailed investigation of oesophageal function and motility can be performed using fluoroscopy whilst the horse is fed a barium and food mixture. However, this technique requires the use of sophisticated equipment which is not generally available in veterinary practices.

Oesophageal dilatations most commonly occur proximal to chronically obstructed areas. Stricture formation, recurrent food impactions of vascular ring anomalies (Freeman, 1982; Greet, 1982) are possible causes. In these cases a localized oesophageal dilatation is readily detected by positive contrast radiography. If the obstruction occurs at, or caudal to, the thoracic inlet, the distal segment of oesophagus may also become dilated (Freeman, 1982). Generalized megaoesophagus (Figure 7a) may be seen as a primary congenital defect. This is presumably associated with neuromuscular dysfunction (Bowman *et al.*, 1978), or in association with defective upper oesophageal sphincter function in cases of rostral displacement of the palato-pharyngeal arch (Goulden *et al.*, 1976). A variable degree of megaoesophagus and defective oesophageal motility are also known to occur in some cases of grass sickness (Figure 7b). Barium swallow studies can be useful as an aid to diagnosis of this disease (Greet and Whitwell, 1986). Other oesophageal diseases which may be diagnosed by contrast radiography include diverticulum formation, neoplasia, perforation, ulceration and oesophagitis, and congenital atresia (Alexander, 1967; Freeman, 1982; Greet, 1982).

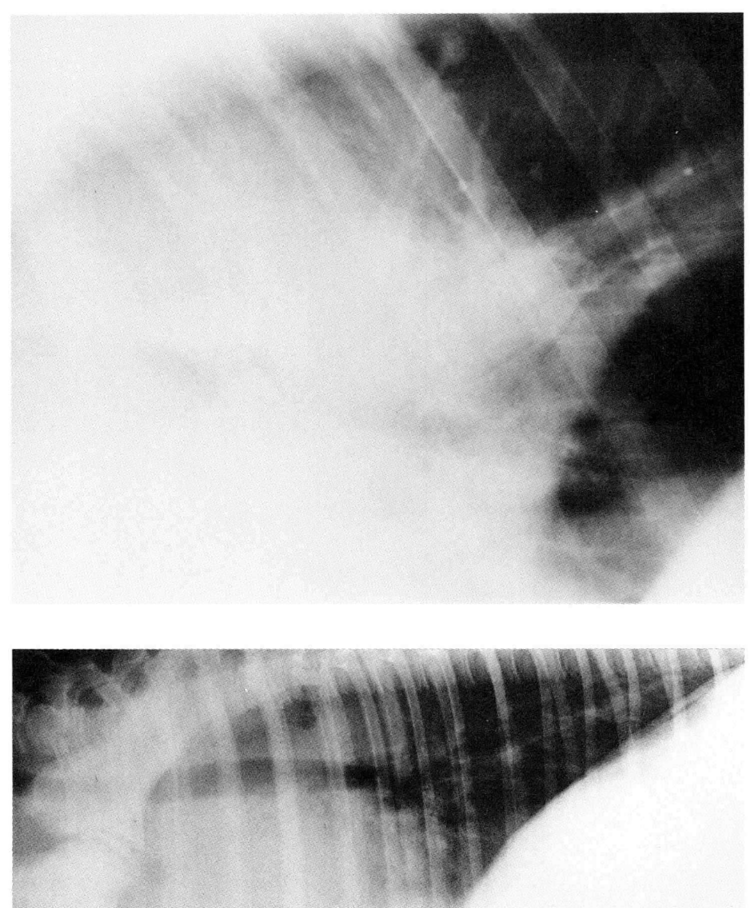

Fig. 5. (a) Peri-hilar mass (streptococcal lymphadenitis) in a 2-year old Hackney pony. The distal trachea narrows abruptly at the carina and there is a diffuse area of increased opacity in the hilar region which merges with the heart base. This appearance is due to gross enlargement of the tracheobronchial lymph nodes. (b) Cranial mediastinal mass (steatitis) in an 8-week old Shetland filly foal. No aerated lung is visible cranial to the heart, indicating increase in volume of the mediastinal contents.

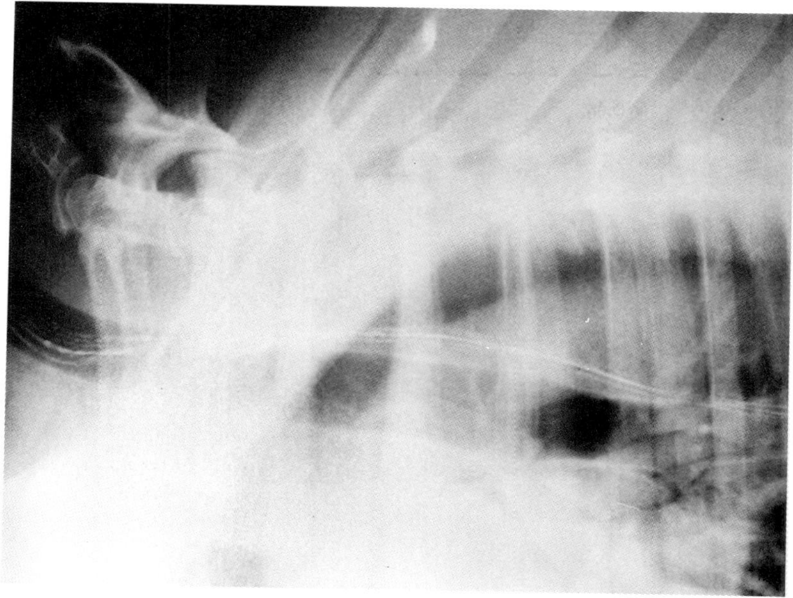

Fig. 6. Normal barium swallow in a 3-year old Welsh Mountain pony. The radiograph was taken 3 minutes after administration of barium sulphate. Outlining of the longitudinal folds is shown.

TRACHEAL DISORDERS

Apart from acquired deviations, abnormalities of the thoracic part of the trachea are not common. However, deformities such as dorsoventral flattening (Carrig *et al.*, 1973) are readily diagnosed radiographically (Figure 8). Radiography would also play a useful role in the investigation of other tracheal disorders such as foreign body obstruction, neoplasia and lacerations or ruptures.

ACKNOWLEDGEMENTS

These studies were performed on X-ray equipment provided in part by a grant from the Horserace Betting Levy Board. We are indebted to Mrs Jeanne Latham and our other radiographers for their technical expertise. T. S. Mair is in receipt of a Wellcome Trust lectureship.

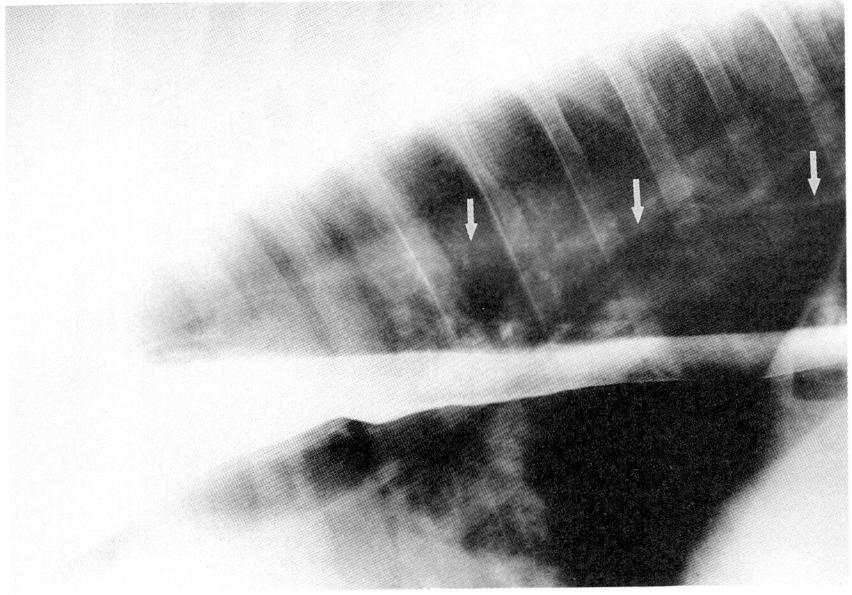

a

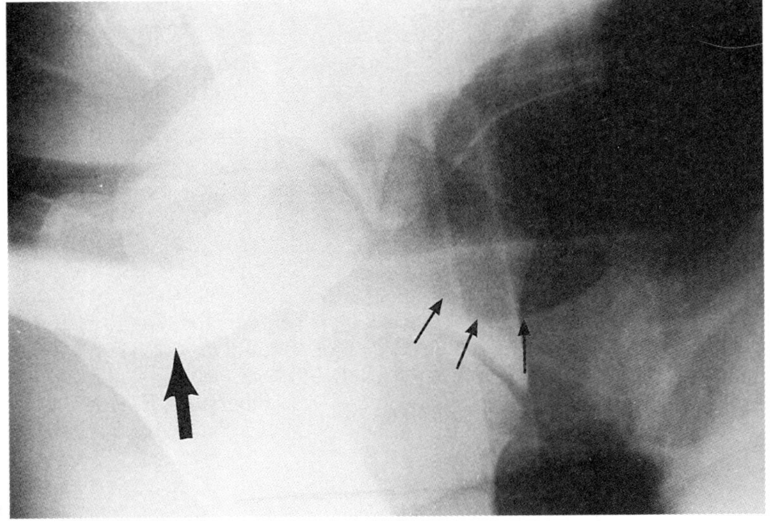

b

Fig. 7. (a) Oesophageal dilatation (megaloesophagus) in a 4-month old thoroughbred colt foal. The barium swallow shows pooling of contrast medium along the entire length of the dilated thoracic oesophagus. The dorsal margin of the contrast column forms a distinct interface with air above it. The dorsal wall of the oesophagus appears as a curvilinear shadow about half way between the contrast column and the thoracic vertebrae (arrows). (b) Oesophageal dilatation (grass sickness) in a 6-year old thoroughbred gelding. The radiograph of the thoracic inlet was taken 10 minutes after administration of barium sulphate via a tube placed in the upper oesophagus. A pool of contrast medium is retained in the most dependent portion of the oesophagus (large arrow). Caudally, at the level of the second and third ribs, an elliptical gas shadow can be seen below the trachea (small arrows), indicating dilatation of the oesophagus in this region also.

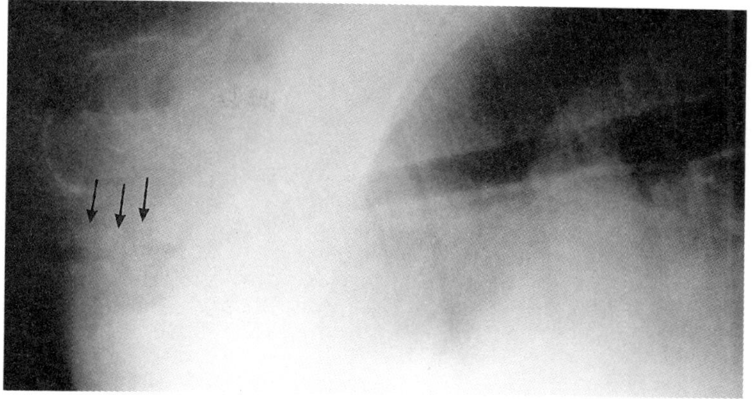

Fig. 8. Tracheal collapse in a 20-year old female donkey. The lower cervical trachea is markedly narrowed with prominent ossification of the cartilage rings (arrows).

REFERENCES

Alexander, J. E. (1967) Radiologic findings in equine choke. *J. Am. Vet. Med. Assoc.*, **151**, 47–53

Bargai, U. (1972) The radiological examination of the digestive system of the horse. *Acta. Radiol. Diag. Stockholm Suppl.*, **319**, 59–61

Bowman, K. F., Vaughan, J. T., Quick, C. B., Hankes, G. H., Redding, R. W., Purohit, R. C., Rumph, P. F., Powers, R. D. and Harper, N. K. (1978) Megaoesophagus in a colt. *J. Am. Vet. Med. Assoc.*, **172**, 334–337

Bristol, D. G. (1986) Diaphragmatic hernias in horses and cattle. *Compend. Contin. Ed.*, **8**, S407–S412

Carrig, C. B., Groenendyk, S. and Seawright, A. A. (1973) Dorsoventral flattening of the trachea in a horse and its attempted surgical correction: A case report. *Vet. Radiol.*, **14**, 32–36

Colahan, P. T. and Knight, H. D. (1979) Drainage of an intrathoracic abscess in a horse via thoracotomy. *J. Am. Vet. Med. Assoc.*, **174**, 1231–1233

Falcon, J., Smith, B. P., O'Brien, T. R., Carlson, G. P. and Biberstein, E. (1985) Clinical and radiographic findings in *Corynebacterium equi* pneumonia of foals. *J. Am. Vet. Med. Assoc.*, **186**, 593–599

Farrow, C. S. (1976) Pneumomediastinum in the horse: a complication of transtracheal aspiration. *Vet. Radiol.*, **17**, 192–195

Farrow, C. S. (1981) Radiographic aspects of inflammatory lung disease in the horse. *Vet. Radiol.*, **22**, 107–114

Freeman, D. E. (1982) In *Equine Medicine and Surgery*. Vol. 1, 3rd edn, (eds R. A. Mansmann, E. S. McAllister and P. W. Pratt) American Veterinary Publications, Santa Barbara, California, pp. 476–497

Goulden, B. E., Anderson, L. J., Davies, A. S. and Barnes, G. R. G. (1976) Rostral displacement of the palatopharyngeal arch: a case report. *Equine Vet. J.*, **8**, 95–98

Greet, T. R. C. (1982) Observations on the potential role of oesophageal radiography in the horse. *Equine Vet. J.*, **14**, 73–79

Greet, T. R. C. and Whitwell, K. E. (1986) Barium swallow as an aid to the diagnosis of grass sickness. *Equine Vet. J.*, **18**, 294–297

Lamb, C. R. (1989) Aspects of diagnostic imaging in equine pulmonary disease. In *The*

Veterinary Annual 29th Issue. (eds C. S. G. Grunsell, M. E. Raw and F. W. G. Hill), Butterworth, London, 127–135

Mackey, V. S. and Wheat, J. D. (1985) Endoscopic examination of the equine thorax. *Equine Vet. J.,* **17,** 140–142

Mair, T. S. (1987) Pleural effusions in the horse. In *The Veterinary Annual* 27th Issue (eds C.S. G. Grunsell, F. W. G. Hill and M-E. Raw) Scientechnia, Bristol 139–146

Rantanen, N. W., Gage, L. and Paradis, M. R. (1981) Ultrasonography as a diagnostic aid in pleural effusion in horses. *Vet. Radiol.,* **22,** 211–216

Raphel, C. F. and Beech, J. (1982) Pleuritis secondary to pneumonia or lung abscessation in 90 horses. *J. Am. Vet. Med. Assoc.,* **181** 808–810

Verschooten, F., Oyaert, W., Muylle, E., DeMoor, A., Steenhaut, M. and Moens, Y. (1977) Diaphragmatic hernia in the horse: four case reports. *Vet. Radiol.,* **18,** 45–50

J. G. LANE

Endoscopy of the equine upper respiratory tract – achievements and challenges

INTRODUCTION

INVESTIGATIONS OF the equine upper respiratory tract have become commonplace in general veterinary practice following the introduction of the flexible fibreoptic endoscope (Cook, 1974a). Rigid rhinolaryngoscopes were available much earlier but had not achieved widespread acceptance because of the limited optical quality of the equipment and the potential hazards to clinicians, horses and the instruments themselves. Flexible endoscopes have facilitated an increase in the range and specificity of diagnosis because the quality of the image is superior and the equipment is well tolerated and safe for the patients. Fibreoptic endoscopes are expensive and there is a tendency for the expectations of clinicians and owners to rise in parallel with the cost of items of equipment or the fees charged to use them. The purpose of this contribution is to weigh the progress which has been made in the accuracy and range of diagnosis against the outstanding limitations of endoscopy in equine rhinolaryngology.

ENDOSCOPIC TECHNIQUE

Endoscopy is usually well accepted by horses and no more restraint than a nose twitch is necessary. This helps to stabilize the head as the instrument is passed into the nasal passages. Fractious animals may be sedated using acepromazine, xylazine or detomidine when structural abnormalities or the source of a nasal discharge are sought. However, the effect of sedatives in the evaluation of subtle functional anomalies of the larynx or palatal arch is contentious. In exceptional circumstances, such as examinations of the mouth, oropharynx and oesophagus, general anaesthesia is indicated to prevent damage to the equipment by biting. Otherwise general anaesthesia is detrimental to effective endoscopy because the postural change produces extensive engorgement of the nasal mucosae and, in recumbency, gravity inhibits the passage of the instrument into the guttural pouches.

The care and maintenance of flexible endoscopes has been discussed elsewhere (Lane, 1981). It is sufficient to repeat here that a number of major hazards may befall these expensive instruments including multiple fibre fracture, leakage of fluids into the coherent (image-carrying) fibre bundle, damage to the objective and eyepiece lenses, detachment of the directional control cables and obstruction of the support

Plate. 1. Normal great ethmoturbinate

Plate. 2. Unilateral purulent discharge from the sinus drainage ostium of a hunter with sinus empyema

Plate. 3. Mycosis on the ventral conchus of a 4-year old Thoroughbred

Plate. 4. Progressive ethmoidal haematoma in an aged pony

Plate. 5. Pharyngeal lymphoid hyperplasia in a 2-year old Thoroughbred

Plate. 6. Mycotic plaque on the medial wall of the right ATD of a partbred gelding

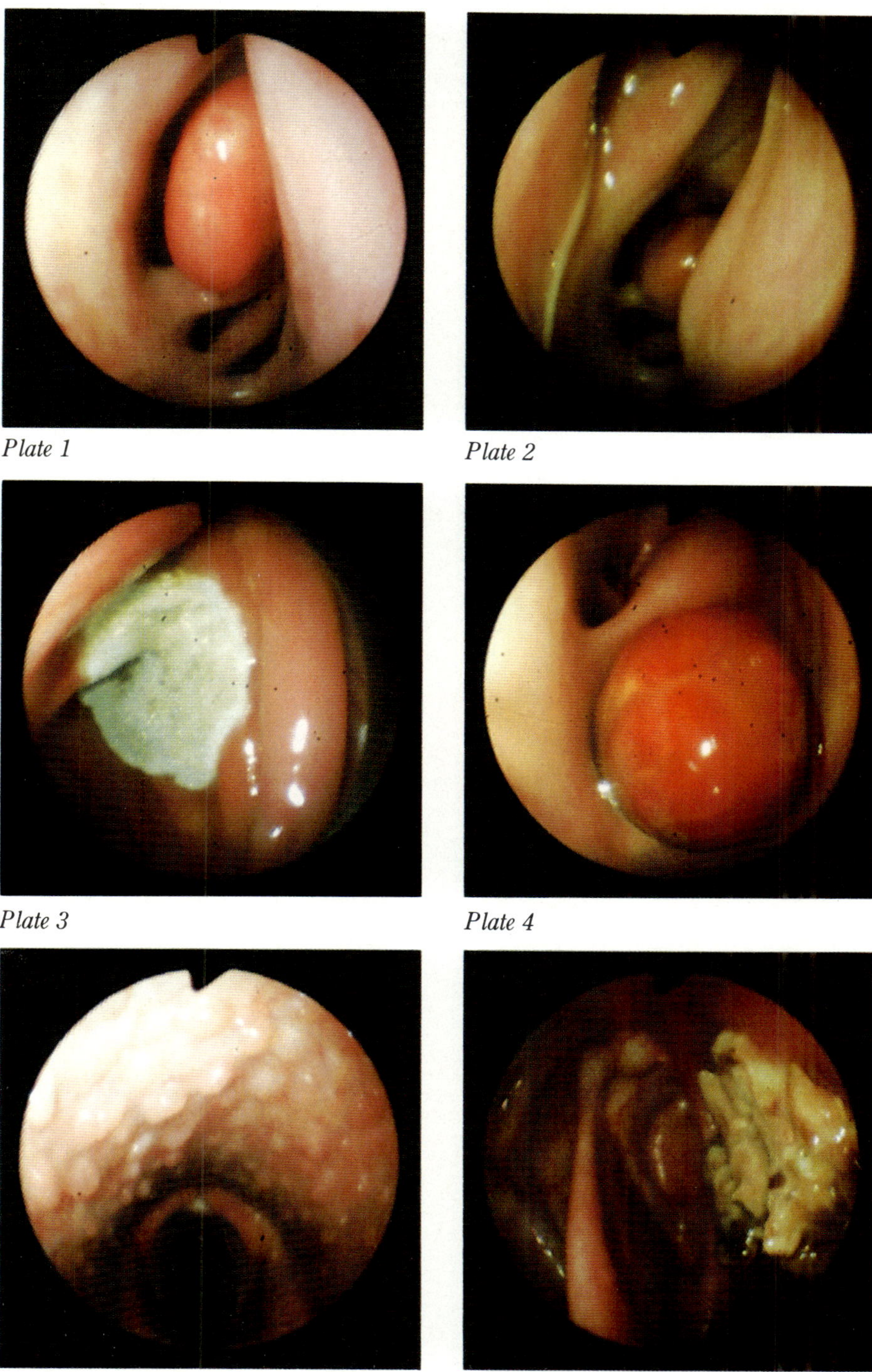

Plate 1

Plate 2

Plate 3

Plate 4

Plate 5

Plate 6

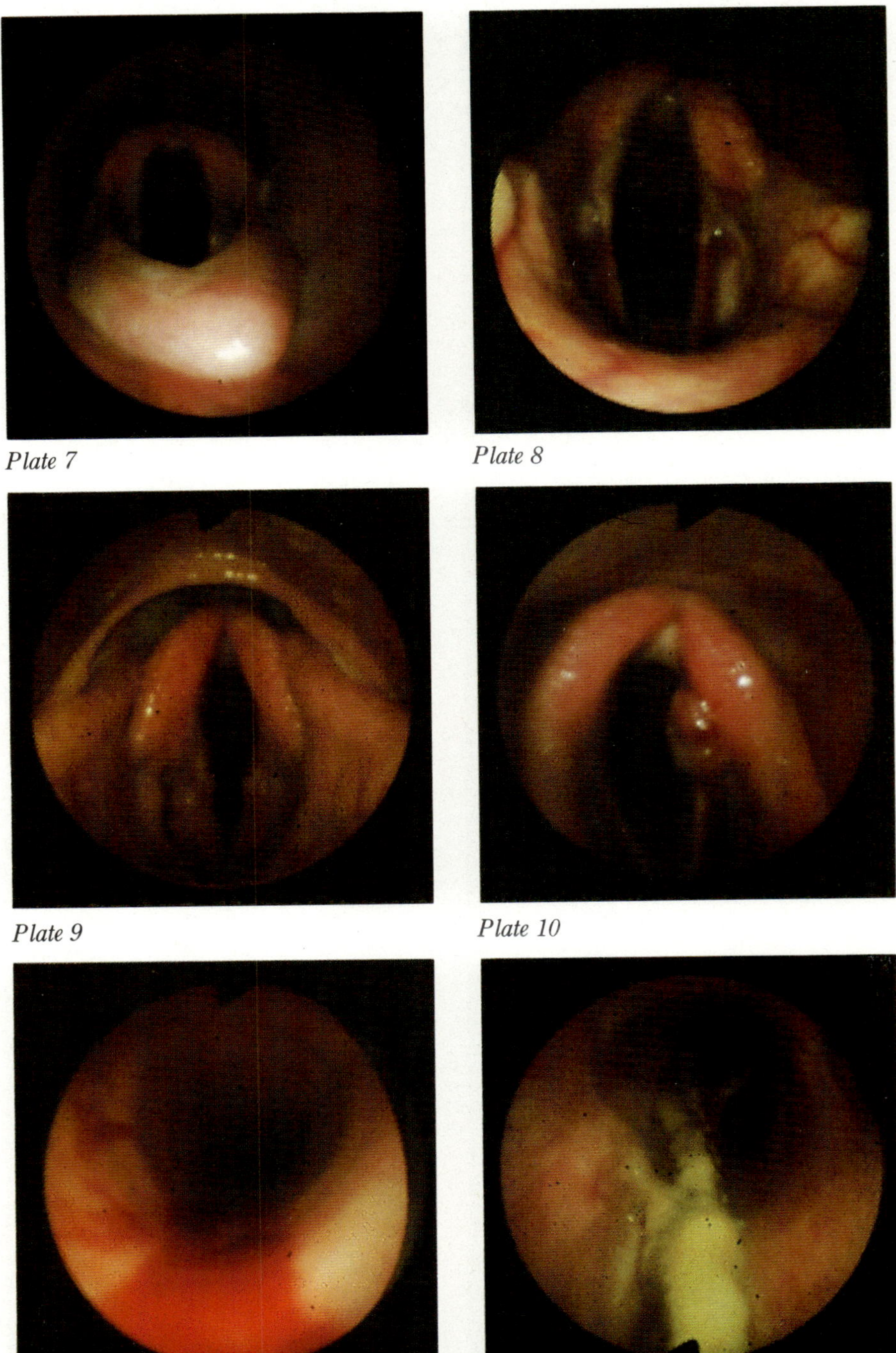

Plate 7

Plate 8

Plate 9

Plate 10

Plate 11

Plate 12

Plate. 7. Entrapment of the epiglottis in a 6-year old gelding. Note that the border of the epiglottis is no longer wrinkled and that the superficial vessels are not visible.

Plate. 8. Laryngeal hemiplegia in a 5-year old gelding. Note that the rima glottidis is asymmetric and that both ventricles have been replaced by scar tissue. The vocal cords are still present.

Plate. 9. Rostral displacement of the palatal arch in a 3-year old Thoroughbred. Note that the entrance to the oesophagus is open.

Plate. 10. Chondritis of the left arytenoid of a jumping pony. Note the axial displacement of the cartilage and the eruption on the medial surface. A contact lesion is present on the right arytenoid.

Plate. 11. Whole blood in the trachea of a 4-year old hurdler 1 hour after vigorous exercise.

Plate. 12. Bramble at the carina of a Thoroughbred yearling.

system channels. These injuries can be avoided and the useful life of the equipment can be extended if routine preventative procedures are adopted. In addition, there is no more effective means to transmit respiratory infections from one horse to another than by the introduction of a contaminated endoscope. Whenever a series of horses are to be subjected to endoscopy per nasum, particularly when they come from different stables, it is neglectful not to cleanse the instrument thoroughly between patients.

NASAL CHAMBERS AND PARANASAL SINUSES

The preferred technique to examine the nasal meati and conchi comprises the introduction of the instrument to the nasopharynx via the ventral meatus followed by inspection of the nasal tissues during slow withdrawal. On retraction from the nasopharynx to the choana, dorsal deviation of the instrument reveals the ethmoid labyrinth and the great ethmoturbinate in particular (Plate 1). Novices may confuse this structure for a polyp or tumour. Close by the sinus drainage ostia open into the caudal middle meatus. A purulent or bloody stream here confirms the origin in some cases of unilateral nasal discharge (Plate 2). An inspection of the conchal mucosal surfaces may reveal lesions such as mycoses (Greet, 1981) (Plate 3) which are usually located close to the sinus ostia.

An assessment of the meati themselves may confirm that the conchi are distended in cases of sinus empyema, cyst (Lane *et al.*, 1987) or neoplasia. Alternatively the spaces rostral to the ethmoturbinates may become occupied by a progressive ethmoidal haematoma (Cook and Littlewort, 1974) which appears as a plum, grey or green mass (Plate 4). Direct inspection of the contents of the frontal and caudal maxillary sinuses can be performed on the standing horse if a trephine hole large enough to introduce the endoscope has been made under local analgesia. In this manner, haematomas of the frontal aspect of the ethmoid labyrinth or intra-antral mycoses may be identified.

The value of endoscopy of the nasal chambers and paranasal sinuses is limited by the restricted access to sites of potential disease. The technique is best used to compliment a thorough clinical and radiological evaluation (Gibbs and Lane, 1987).

NASOPHARYNX

Extensive lymphoid hyperplasia of the walls of the pharyngeal recess and naso-pharynx (Plate 5) is a frequent endoscopic finding in young horses. The term follicular pharyngitis is inappropriate because the occurrence is so high and the enlarged follicles are of doubtful significance (Burrell, 1985). It is suggested that the performance of young animals with marked lymphoid hyperplasia is not compromised but, on the other hand, some clinicians believe that pharyngeal lymphoid hyperplasia (PLH) can be a source of adventitious respiratory noise and that the discomfort of engorged follicles provokes episodic gurgling (Haynes, 1984).

A diagnosis of pharyngeal paralysis as a cause of nasal regurgitation of ingesta is indicated when the pharyngeal walls lack tone, the palatal arch is persistently dorsally displaced and food debris and saliva are present in the lumen. Inspection of the guttural pouches is indicated as mycosis is a likely explanation of this glosso-pharyngeal neuropathy.

AUDITORY TUBE DIVERTICULA (GUTTURAL POUCHES)

It is essential that the endoscope be introduced through the *ventral* nasal meatus if it is later to be passed into the auditory tube diverticula (ATD). The cartilage flap is raised with a wire leader emerging form the biopsy channel of the endoscope and both are advanced into the lumen of the pouch with a longitudinal rotating movement.

Endoscopy is not very helpful in the diagnosis of conditions such as tympany empyema or chondroids. In each case palpation and radiography will be more contributory to a full evaluation. However, pharyngeal compression through ATD distension can be seen endoscopically and this may help in the planning of the anaesthetic regime for surgery. Occasionally inflammation of the wall of the ATD, or diverticulitis, may arise and produce neuropathies more typically associated with mycosis.

ATD mycosis can be a life-threatening condition because of the proximity of major vessels and nerves. Whenever a horse shows spontaneous epistaxis or dysphagia an urgent endoscopic assessment is indicated. Blood or other discharges may be seen flowing from the drainage ostia. Although the identification of a mycotic plaque within the diverticulum (Plate 6) confirms the diagnosis there are practical pitfalls. The stress to the horse of being handled may precipitate a fatal epistaxis (Church *et al.*, 1986). At the very least the presence of a haematoma will obscure visibility although it is usually possible to determine whether the internal maxillary artery is healthy as it runs through the lateral compartment. The possibility of laryngeal hemiplegia or pharyngeal paralysis should be investigated endoscopically before treatment is commenced so that the owner can be appraised of all aspects of the prognosis.

In practice the majority of mycoses arise on the dorso-medial wall of the ADT over the internal carotid artery and proximal ligation of this vessel is a reliable treatment (Church *et al.*, 1986; Greet, 1987). However contrast angiography may be required to identify exceptional cases where another branch of the carotid circulation is diseased (Colles and Cook, 1983).

PALATAL ARCH

Midline defects of the arcus palatopharyngeus are the usual cause of nasal reflux of milk in newborn foals. The anomaly is not easy to diagnose per os in a conscious foal but can be seen without difficulty from the nasal aspect with a slim endoscope.

The primary role of endoscopy in the examination of horses which sustain episodic dorsal displacement of the palatal arch is to eliminate other causes of airway obstruction and to identify factors such as concurrent lower airway disease which may predispose to the dislocation (Haynes, 1984). Owners and trainers often expect the endoscopist to be able to make a positive diagnosis of 'soft palate'. This is not possible, least of all at a pre-purchase examination. The diagnosis is made primarily on the history provided by the rider and, secondarily, by a process of elimination of other possibilities. Almost all horses can be provoked to show momentary dislocation of the palatal arch by stimulation of deglutition. However, critical studies on the significance of the frequency or duration of the displacements have not been reported.

EPIGLOTTIS

Prior to the advent of the fibreoptic endoscope, abnormalities of the equine epiglottis were practically unrecognized. Entrapment of the epiglottis by the glosso-epiglottic and aryepiglottic folds (Plate 7) is more frequently diagnosed in North American (Boles *et al.*, 1978) than in the United Kingdom possibly because of the popularity there of Standardbreds. The signs of epiglottic entrapment are inconsistent and the significance of the findings may be more as a predisposing factor to palatal dislocation than as a primary cause of airway obstruction. The endoscopic diagnosis of entrapment is straightforward provided that the condition is not intermittent and that the enshrouded epiglottis lies above the palatal arch. The stimulation of a series of swallow sequence should provoke entrapment in intermittent cases. Standing lateral radiographs are useful when endoscopy has shown persistent dorsal displacement of the palatal arch as the epiglottis can be checked for size as well as entrapment (Haynes, 1984).

The most common site for pharyngeal cysts is in the subepiglottic mucosa and these lesions are thought to arise from remnants of the thyroglossal duct or following trauma (Koch and Tate, 1978). Endoscopic diagnosis is usually straightforward except when the cyst is hidden by a dorsally displaced palatal arch. Plain lateral radiographs can provide complimentary diagnostic evidence.

LARYNX

The eccentric position of an endoscope in the nasopharynx invariably produces perspective asymmetry of the rima glottidis. Whenever uncertainty exists, the technique should be performed through each nostril in turn. However, in cases of left laryngeal hemiplegia the immobile arytenoid cartilage hangs passively in the airway and the assymetry is obvious (Plate 8). Controversy exists around such terms as partial hemiplegia, hemiparesis and sub-clinical hemiplegia. Some believe that to justify a diagnosis of hemiplegia a horse must produce an audible inspiratory sound at exercise and on endoscopy show no active movement by the left arytenoid cartilage. All other anomalous movements (i.e. asynchrony or transient asymmetry) should be regarded as being within the limits of normality (Baker, 1986). Others believe that most Thoroughbred horses show a degree of left hemiplegia (W. R. Cook, 1985, unpublished data). The wide disparity of views arises through lack of defined parameters to justify a diagnosis of laryngeal hemiplegia. The major challenge for equine laryngologists in the years ahead will be to provide a universally accepted definition of hemiplegia which will reconcile the neuropathological process of the condition with the findings of diagnostic aids such as the endoscope and radiostethoscope. It will also be necessary to correlate the definition with studies of airflow and airway resistance before deciding whether the various surgical techniques which are used for horses with laryngeal hemiplegia are efficacious. In current practice it is wise to subject suspect horses, or those examined prior to sale, to a combination of endoscopic, palpation and exercise tests before reaching a conclusion (Lane, 1987).

Fibreoptic endoscopy has allowed the range of diagnosis of equine laryngeal disorders to be broadened. Rostral displacement of the palatal arch is a term derived from the endoscopic appearance (Plate 9) of a congenital malformation of the derivatives of the fourth branchial arch (Goulden *et al.*, 1976). Affected horses produce stridor at exercise and may be involuntarily aerophagic due to incompetence of the proximal oesophageal sphincter. The diagnosis is best confirmed by radiography which shows rostral displacement of the posterior pillars of the palatal arch and an open oesophagus. Idiopathic laryngeal chondritis (ILC) has been recognized only recently (Haynes *et al.*, 1980). Not only may the signs of the condition be confused with those of hemiplegia but the endoscopic appearance with restricted movement of the affected cartilage may also be confused with ILH in the early stages. Later there is obvious axial displacement of the affected arytenoid and eruptions (Plate 10) from the surface. In the later stages large granulomatous projections might be mistaken for neoplasia.

The 'slap test' which assesses the reflex laryngeal abduction in response to slapping the contralateral thorax, has become an established part of the routine neurological examination of the horse (Greet *et al.*, 1980). It is used to check the integrity of the neural arc through the cervical spinal cord, midbrain and recurrent laryngeal nerve. However the test is as effectively performed by external palpation of the larynx as by endoscopic observation.

TRACHEA AND BRONCHI

The primary objectives of tracheobronchoscopy of horses lie more in the identification and aspiration of discharges arising from the lower respiratory tract (Whitwell and Greet, 1984) than in the diagnosis of structural changes of the conducting airways themselves. It is sufficient to comment here that the widespread use of endoscopes has brought the realization that most often discharges in the horse, especially if they are bilateral and mucoid, arise from the small airways and not from the upper tract. It has also been confirmed that primary lung haemorrhages are almost invariably the source of epistaxis after exercise (Cook, 1974b; Pascoe *et al.*, 1981) (Plate 11).

Mural distortion by congenital collapse or iatrogenic (post-tracheotomy) and traumatic strictures can be viewed from the luminal aspect. However lateral radiographs of the trachea often give a more accurate impression of these obstructions particularly with regard to length. Isolated cases of foreign body inhalation to the region of the carina have been reported (Lane, 1981) and this possibility should be considered whenever a horse presents with an intractible cough together with fetid breath. Brambles are usually involved (Plate 12) and retrieval of the foreign body is also performed under endoscopic observation.

CONCLUSIONS

There can be no doubt that the advantages brought to equine practice by the popularization of flexible endoscopes outweigh the detractions. In the upper respiratory tract, the repertoire and specificity of diagnosis have been increased extensively. The frequency with which new entities are being reported is declining but recent examples include dorsal glottic stenosis (Harrison and Raker, 1988), nasopharyngeal cicatrization (Schumacher and Hanselka, 1987) and parasitic laryngeal papillomatosis (Lane, 1986).

Current outstanding deficiencies for the equine endoscopist arise in the interpretation of anomalous laryngeal motility and assessment of function of the palatal arch.

The recent introduction of the videoendoscope which retains the advantage of flexibility of fibreoptic instruments but with enhanced image production on to a television monitor brings the possibility of improved diagnosis and more detailed analysis of functional disturbances. Nevertheless, even the most advanced instrument must never be regarded as the sole means to diagnosis but rather as an adjunct to complement other techniques such as radiology.

ACKNOWLEDGEMENTS

The colour photographs in this article were made possible by the generous support of KeyMed Ltd.

REFERENCES

Baker, G. J. (1986) Wind examination in yearlings. *Vet. Rec.*, **118**, 133

Boles, C. L., Raker, C. W. and Wheat, J. D. (1978) Epiglottic entrapment by arytenoepiglottic folds. *J. Am. Vet. Med. Assoc.*, **172**, 338–342

Burrell, M. H. (1985) Endoscopic and virological observations on respiratory disease in a group of young Thoroughbreds in training. *Equine Vet. J.*, **17**, 99–103

Church, S., Wyn-Jones, G., Parks, A. H. and Ritchie, H. E. (1986) Treatment of guttural pouch mycosis. *Equine Vet. J.*, **18**, 362–365

Colles, C. M. and Cook, W. R. (1983) Carotid angiography in the horse. *Vet. Rec.*, **113**, 483–489

Cook, W. R. (1974a) Some observations on diseases of the ear, nose and throat in the horse, and endoscopy using a flexible fibreoptic endoscope. *Vet. Rec.*, **94**, 533–541

Cook, W. R. (1974b) Epistaxis in the racehorse. *Equine Vet. J.*, **6**, 45–58

Cook, W. R. and Littlewort, M. C. G. (1974) Progressive haematoma of the ethmoidal region in the horse. *Equine Vet. J.*, **6**, 101–108

Gibbs, C. and Lane, J. G. (1987) Radiographic examination of the facial, nasal and paranasal sinus regions of the horse: II, Radiological findings. *Equine Vet. J.*, **19**, 474–482

Goulden, B. E., Anderson, L. J., Davies, A. S. and Barnes, G. R. G. (1976) Rostral displacement of the palatopharyngeal arch: a case report. *Equine Vet. J.*, **8**, 95–98

Greet, T. R. C. (1981) Nasal aspergillosis in three horses. *Vet. Rec.*, **109**, 487–489

Greet, T. R. C. (1987) Outcome of treatment in 35 cases of guttural pouch mycosis. *Equine Vet. J.*, **19**, 483–487

Greet, T. R. C., Jeffcott, L. B., Whitwell, K. E. and Cook, W. R. (1980) The slap test for laryngeal adductory function in horses with suspected cervical spinal cord damage. *Equine Vet. J.*, **12**, 127–131

Harrison, I. W. and Raker, C. W. (1988) Dorsal glottic stenosis after bilateral arytenoidectomy in two horses. *J. Am. Vet. Med. Assoc.*, **192**, 202–204

Haynes, P. F. (1984) Surgery of the equine respiratory tract. In *The Practice of Large Animal Surgery*. (ed. P. B. Jennings) W. B. Saunders, Philadelphia, pp. 388–487

Haynes, P. F., Snider, T. G., McClure, J. R. and McClure, J. J. (1980) Chronic chondritis of the equine arytenoid cartilage. *J. Am. Vet. Med. Assoc.*, **177**, 1135–1142

Koch, D. B. and Tate, L. P. (1978) Pharyngeal cysts in horses. *J. Am. Vet. Med. Assoc.*, **173**, 858–862

Lane, J. G. (1981) Fibreoptic endoscopy. *Vet. Rec.* (Suppl) *In Prac.*, **3**, 24–30

Lane, J. G. (1986) Parasitic laryngeal papillomatosis in a horse. *Vet. Rec.*, **119**, 591–593

Lane, J. G. (1987) Fibreoptic endoscopy of the equine upper respiratory tract: a commentary on progress. *Equine Vet. J.*, **19**, 495–499

Lane, J. G., Longstaffe, J. A. and Gibbs, C. (1987) Equine paranasal sinus cysts: a report of 15 cases. *Equine Vet. J.*, **19**, 537–544

Pascoe, J. R., Ferraro, G. L., Cannon, J. H., Arthur, R. M. and Wheat, J. D. (1981) Exercise-induced pulmonary haemorrhage in racing Thoroughbreds: A preliminary study. *Am. J. Vet. Res.*, **42**, 703–707

Schumacher, J. and Hanselka, D. V. (1987) Nasopharyngeal cicatrices in horses: 47 cases. *J. Am. Vet. Med. Assoc.*, **191**, 239–242

Whitwell, K. E. and Greet, T. R. C. (1984) Collection and evaluation of tracheobronchial washes in the horse. *Equine Vet. J.*, **16**, 499–508

J. R. HOLMES

Circulatory causes of collapse in the horse

INTRODUCTION

THE WORD 'collapse' is one which is often used to describe a variety of conditions when an animal staggers, falls, remains recumbent for a varying time and may or may not lose consciousness. It can have a variety of causes including fatigue and exhaustion the consequences of which are muscle breakdown (rhabdomyolysis/azoturia), trauma to tendons, ligaments or skeleton (see Smith and Wagner, 1985). It can also have a central nervous system origin. However, by human analogy, the circulatory system is often high on the list of suspect causes.

The conditions under which collapse may occur vary. Collapse is occasionally seen in horses at rest in a field or loose box, during preparation for work and sometimes during work. It is because a rider may be at risk that diagnosis and prognosis assume great importance. Prognosis is even more important than diagnosis. Prognosis is often difficult because rarely is a professional person present when the incident occurs and often recovery and return to apparent normality is rapid.

When investigating possible circulatory causes of collapse it is important to recognize that the finding of cardiac arrhythmia or a murmur in a horse with a very recent history of collapse does not necessarily imply cause and effect. Only by accumulating information on such cases will it be possible to indicate what emphasis should be placed on cardiovascular findings in these cases.

Syncope is defined as a transient loss of consciousness due to inadequate cerebral blood flow. It may be of cardiac origin, usually due to a sudden reduction in cardiac output, or be of vasomotor origin, when loss of vasoconstrictor tone results in a fall in peripheral resistance associated with vasodilation in skeletal muscles and the splanchnic area. The net result in both cases is an abrupt fall in blood pressure. The lowered systemic arterial pressure leads to a lower perfusion pressure and a reduction in blood flow through the tissues. Cerebral blood flow in particular is dependent on perfusion pressure. In addition to the effect on consciousness, cerebral centres involving vasomotor and respiratory regulation may also be affected. Signs include dizziness, loss of vision and unconsciousness.

Theoretically, an abrupt fall in systemic arterial pressure may arise from acute haemorrhage, acute haemopericardium with cardiac compression, from autonomic effects as a result of carotid sinus stimulation, the sudden occurrence during work of arrhythmia, such as atrial fibrillation, the sudden failure of compensation at work in a horse with an existing cardiovascular problem or the sudden development of pump failure. The best example of pump failure is probably rupture of mitral valve chordae.

156

Thrombo-embolism in the coronary circulation sufficient to cause coronary thrombosis which is so frequently observed in humans, appears to be rare in the horse.

The heart consists of two pumps which operate in series. If the two pumps are to be kept in balance without stagnation of blood in the peripheral or pulmonary circulation, their outputs must be matched. Normally about 60% of total blood volume is in the venules and veins which represent capacitance vessels. Increase in this volume due to failure of pump function or vascular bed vasodilatation will have effects similar to exsanguination as far as blood pressure and cerebral blood flow are concerned.

Circulatory failure in the horse may arise suddenly from rupture of major blood vessels, notably the anterior mesenteric artery, as a result of parasite damage. There are also records of rupture of the aorta, the pulmonary artery and the heart chambers. The atria and the thinner walled right ventricle are the chambers at greatest risk. Rupture at these sites or of the intrapericardial aorta lead to haemopericardium and acute failure from cardiac compression. Rupture into the pleural or peritoneal cavities leads to profuse internal haemorrhage and rapid death. In these cases the pathologist may be presented with a chest or abdomen containing a large volume of free blood and it may not always be possible to determine the exact site of the haemorrhage.

COLLAPSE AT REST

The horse is a species with a comparatively slow resting heart rate and the baroreceptor response is particularly important as a means of regulating blood pressure. Thus at rest many normal horses will show first and second degree atrium–ventricle (A–V) block. In some cases two beats may be blocked in sequence. Occasionally up to four sequential missed beats may be encountered. Rhythm generally becomes regular when the heart rate accelerates either as a response to exercise or transiently, due to exicetment. Under these circumstances this disturbance of rhythm is regarded as physiological and of no clinical significance.

Sometimes horses may also show a few missed beats when heart rate slows immediately after a period of exercise. If this irregularity is transient and rhythm becomes and remains regular as heart rate continues to slow, it is likely that this fleeting arrhythmia represents a physiological vagal response associated with the initiation of cardiac deceleration like transient post-exercise sinus arrhythmia .

Occasionally reports are received of horses suddenly collapsing for no apparent reason whilst standing in a loose box or even when free in a field. Often on examination later at rest second degree A–V block is present, particularly if heart rate is slow.

In the horse, the missed beats due to second degree A–V block are usually Mobitz type I with variation in A–V conduction time in conducted beats often with progressive lengthening of conduction time up to each dropped beat. Mobitz type II second degree A–V block, in which the conduction time is fixed, is very rare in horses. In the horse there may sometimes be a mixture of the two types. In humans Mobitz type II A–V block is regarded as indicative of some pathology in the His bundle, which may result in marked bradycardia or abrupt syncopal attacks. It may be a precursor of complete A–V block. The latter is extremely rare in the horse. It is not known whether the occurrence of Mobitz type II A–V block would merit such a guarded prognosis in the horse but combined with a history of collapse such a prognosis would certainly be justified.

The occurrence of frequent type I A–V block at rest following a history of collapse is more difficult to assess. Some horses may experience up to four sequential missed beats without any apparent clinical effect. Even in these horses rhythm almost invariably becomes and remains regular when heart rate accelerates. Thus it is unlikely that these horses would pose a danger actually during work.

In some cases the collapsing episode may be associated with some form of restraint, such as putting on a head collar or bridle, shoeing, grooming or tightening of a girth. Such a situation was described by Cross (1988). A typical senario is one in which, as the girth is tightened, the horse moves backwards, rears and falls and may remain down for a few seconds then struggles to its feet. This is often a quite alarming syndrome to the average owner and it may occur more than once.

It is well recognized in humans that pressure on the carotid sinus by vagal stimulation through the baroreceptor mechanism may result in heart rate slowing, peripheral vascular dilatation and an abrupt fall in systemic arterial pressure which may lead to fainting. There is some evidence that some humans may have an abnormally sensitive carotid sinus. The resulting syncope may result in transient systolic standstill or extreme bradycardia with a fall in blood pressure or a fall in blood pressure without a change in heart rate.

The normal slow resting heart rate of the horse is an index of high vagal tone. Although partial A–V block is common at slow resting rates, usually as a means of regulating blood pressure, and in atrial fibrillation pauses exceeding 8 seconds may be observed with no apparent ill effect, the occurrence of *sudden* vagal stimulation leading to a precipitous fall in systemic arterial pressure could have marked effects. It remains a matter of speculation whether such an explanation can be applied in the horse. It presents an attractive hypothesis especially where handling around the head or where a sudden stretching of the neck may occur. The syncope is generally only transient and the animals often recover before professional help arrives.

COLLAPSE DURING WORK

Occasionally, the very fit horse may experience myocardial failure when under severe stress. Myocardial hypertrophy is a normal response to training. It results in an improved and efficient circulation able to respond to increased work demands. It may also arise as a response to a pathological situation in an attempt to maintain a normal circulation in cases where there is a progressive increase in resistance to flow. However, it can be a mixed blessing. Hypertrophy involves an increase in the size of the myofibrils. A decrease in the surface area of a fibre relative to its volume is unfavourable to its metabolism because it interfers with cell nutrition. Beyond a certain size enlarged myofibrils may lead to a cell hypoxia under stress, resulting in decreased strength in each contractile unit.

Cardiac failure represents a stage in the progressive deterioration of cardiac function, for example, in ischaemic heart disease or where valve function is impaired. Myocardial failure is accompanied by weakening and dilatation of chambers and leads to a reduction in the ejection fraction so that as the condition progresses, cardiac output is reduced and there is a fall in systemic arterial pressure despite compensatory tachycardia. If the pathology progresses slowly, compensation may, at least for some time, maintain the circulation. The most pronounced effects occur if the condition occurs suddenly, particularly if it arises during work.

In the horse the commonest examples of abrupt failure are provided by the sudden development of atrial fibrillation during work or the rupture of mitral valve chordae. Acute decompensation may occur in a horse with an existing cardiac disorder.

Sudden rupture of mitral valve chordae leads to mitral incompetence due to failure of the fluid seal between left atrium and left ventricle, massive regurgitation into the left atrium at systole and a pan-systolic murmur often with a palpable thrill. This interferes with the balance between the two pumps. Pulmonary congestion and oedema rapidly follow. The initial symptoms are predominantly respiratory and the horse may collapse with severe dyspnoea. (Brown *et al.*, 1983; Holmes and Miller, 1984). In fatal cases care is particularly necessary during post-mortem examination to be sure that chordal rupture occurred before death. Where the horse survives, the symptoms may abate within a few days leaving a legacy of a raised resting heart rate and a profound widespread systolic murmur with a palpable thrill. There is often a loud (torrential) third sound along with upward and backward extension of the cardiac area of auscultation associated with left atrial dilatation. This represents the second stage, or stage of compensation, which will be followed by the slow progressive onset of cardiac failure exacerbated by work after varying amounts of time.

Of all the causes of arrhythmia, atrial fibrillation is probably potentially the most serious. It occurs in large horses and may occur suddenly without warning during work in a horse with a previous good performance record. Fundamentally the normal pacemaker in the sinus node is overridden by a perpetual wavefront which meanders continuously through the atrial myocardium. This is set up due to inhomogeneity of excitation and recovery of atrial myocardial fibres, increased by repetition, creating multiple sites of re-entry. These allow an irregular circus movement to persist aided by a large atrial mass with responsive muscle always ahead of the activating wavelets. A number of factors may be involved in the etiology, but focal stretching of the atrial myocardium may be important in those cases which arise during work.

During work, for example on the race course or in the hunting field, the sudden disappearance of the coordinated atrial contraction, which normally completes ventricular filling prior to ventricular contraction, coupled with the disordered rhythm, have immediate effects on stroke volume, cardiac output and arterial pressure. This affects areas of local vasodilatation, particularly the skeletal muscles, and leads to myasthenia and sudden failure to stay in a race. Not only may the horse fail in the race, it may stagger and sometimes collapse (Holmes *et al.*, 1986).

The same situation may occur in the hunting field. Here the horse may appear to recover after a rest and may continue at a slower pace. Examination will reveal marked arrhythmia and an absence of atrial contraction sounds. This arrhythmia will persist at all heart rates, although the characteristic long pauses and flurries of beats are most obvious at slow resting rates. Because some of these cases may be paroxysmal with spontaneous return to sinus rhythm it would be wise to wait for up to 48 hours for this to occur. If the arrhythmia persists beyond this time then treatment with quinidine sulphate should be considered without further delay. If the arrhythmia persists the horse is unsafe to ride.

Occasional premature beats are rarely associated with any symptoms but they may lead to ventricular tachycardia. This consists of a regular rhythm but with bizarre conduction over the ventricles. Electrocardiography is required to establish the diagnosis. Because ectopic beats may occur irregularly and unpredictably, a fairly prolonged and probably repeat examination may be necessary to decide their frequency in any particular case. Although the occasional premature beat is unlikely to be significant, the discovery of premature beats, particularly of ventricular origin, in a horse with a history of recent collapse will certainly emphasize the need for a careful and detailed examination of the circulatory system. When premature beats occur frequently, rest and re-examination in 3–6 months would be advisable.

CONCLUSIONS

In summary, those cases which collapse at rest should be carefully examined both at rest and at work. Circulation may be normal at work and they may pose no hazard to a rider. When collapse occurs at work this presents a much more serious situation. Successful early treatment of atrial fibrillation in cases free of murmurs may return them to work. However, where valve lesions are suspect and there is a history of collapse the prognosis must be grave as far as further work is concerned, even though compensation may occur.

REFERENCES

Brown, C. M., Bell, T. G., Paradis, M. R. and Breeze, R. G. (1983) Rupture of mitral chordae tendineae in two horses. *J. Am. Vet. Med. Ass.*, **182**, 281–283

Cross, E. J. C. (1988) Equine syncope. *Vet. Rec.*, **122**, 215

Holmes, J. R., Henigan, M., Williams, R. B. and Witherington, D. H. (1986) Paroxysmal atrial fibrillation in racehorses. *Equine Vet. J.*, **18**, 37–42

Holmes, J. R. and Miller, P. J. (1984) Three cases of ruptured mitral valve chordae in the horse. *Equine Vet. J.*, **16**, 125–135

Smith, C. A. and Wagner, P. C. (1985) Electrolyte imbalances and metabolic disturbances in endurance horses. *Compendium on Continuing Education for the Practising Veterinarian.* **7**, 575–584

D. C. KNOTTENBELT and F. W. G. HILL

Entrapment of the left colon over the nephro-splenic ligament in the horse: a review of the clinical features and treatment

INTRODUCTION

POSSIBLE DISPLACEMENTS of the equine large intestine of clinical significance have been recorded and reviewed (Kopf, 1982; Hackett, 1983; Huskampf, 1987). Both right and left displacements of the colon are described. In right displacement, the right dorsal colon comes to lie above and to the right of the head of the caecum. An acute colic syndrome ensues which may be even more severe where a complicating torsion occurs in the displaced colon (Huskampf, 1987). Two left displacements are being diagnosed more frequently: an anterior flexion and entrapment on the pelvic flexure over the top of the nephro-splenic ligament, leading to a relatively mild and persistent colic, and perhaps the commonest form of all the displacements, nephro-splenic ligament entrapment. In this displacement the left ventral colon rises up the left abdominal wall and takes the corresponding dorsal colon with it. This results in them becoming entrapped over the nephro-splenic ligament. This paper reviews the clinical features, diagnosis and treatment of the nephro-splenic entrapment.

AETIOLOGY

The precise aetiology of the entrapment of the left colon over the nephro-splenic ligament is unclear. Huskampf (1987) has postulated that it may be the result of the left colon, encouraged by an accumulation of gas, moving up the left abdominal wall (Figure 1a). A distention of the stomach may also displace the spleen ventromedially and create a potential space for the colon between the spleen and adjacent abdominal wall. To support this, two authors (Hackett, 1983; Huskampf, 1987) have described cases of incomplete displacement where the colon is found trapped between the left abdominal wall and spleen.

Prolonged right lateral recumbency may also be an important aetiological factor because two recorded cases were severely lame and had been seen recumbent on their right side for long periods prior to the onset of colic.

161

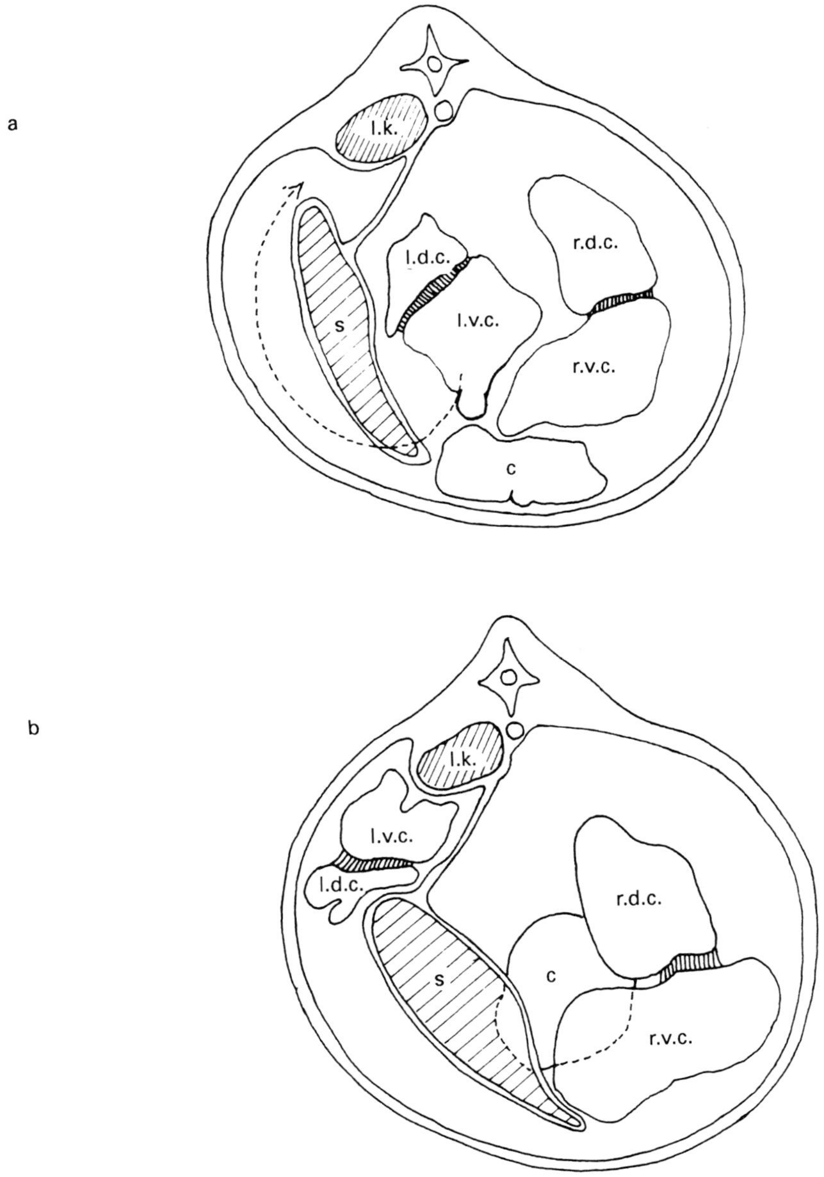

Fig. 1. Cross-section of the abdomen of a horse. (a) Showing the normal anatomical distribution of the large colon; (b) Left colon dorsal displacement. The arrow indicates the route of displacement. Key: r.d.c, right dorsal colon; r.v.c, right ventral colon; l.k, left kidney; r.k., right kidney; l.d.c., left dorsal colon; l.v.c., left ventral colon; c, caecum; s, spleen

ANATOMY

Depending upon the relative size of horse and operator, it is possible to explore up to 40% of the abdomen by rectal palpation (Kopf, 1982). Figure 2a illustrates the normal distribution of the large intestines of the horse in relation to the spleen and pelvic inlet. The value of rectal palpation in order to recognize the usual position of different viscera and organs in the healthy horse cannot be over-emphasized. Such expertise is particularly valuable for the diagnosis of nephro-splenic entrapment.

Rectal palpation cranially and in the mid-line should identify the root of the mesenteric artery. The duodemum may be palpable to the right. Working caudally, the right posterior quadrant gives an impression of emptiness, although the taenia of the caecum may be felt. If a larger gas 'cap' is present, the head of the caecum may be appreciated. The small colon is recognized in the ventral posterior abdomen by the presence of freely moveable faecal balls. At the pelvic inlet, to the left of the mid-line, the pelvic flexure is palpable. By working cranially the spleen may be located well forward against the left abdominal wall. Often the spleen is first appreciated as a 'step' in the abdominal wall which may be gently lifted away from the wall. In following the dorsal border of the spleen upwards and moving to the right the posterior pole of the left kidney is felt. Stretched between these two organs is the nephro-splenic ligament. It is generally possible to insert a flattened hand or fingers into the space formed by the edge of the ligament and the adjacent abdominal wall.

CLINICAL FEATURES AND DIAGNOSIS

Horses of all ages and breeds and of both sexes appear susceptible to nephro-splenic entrapment, although in the series recorded (Table 1) there is a tendency for younger animals to be over-represented. The degree of colic varies with the volume of contents in the colon and the extent of the entrapment (Huskampf, 1987). In rare cases, when the greater portion of the left colon is incarcerated, the colic is severe. More usually there are unrelenting signs of sub-acute colic which may have been present for up to several days and which are unrelieved by symptomatic treatment.

The onset of the colic is insidious and there are intermittent variations in the intensity of the pain, from mild to moderate. When the pain is moderate the animal will go down in sternal recumbency and may even roll. Frequently the pulse is slightly to moderately elevated (50 to 65 beats/min). A tendency for the pulse rate to increase coincides with the episodes of increased abdominal pain. Other vital signs, including capillary refill time, may be either within accepted normal ranges or slightly elevated. Sparce amounts of faeces of normal consistency are voided. Bowel sounds tend to be reduced and the passage of a stomach tube releases very small amounts of gas or nothing at all.

Abdominal paracentesis produces an increased volume of unaltered peritoneal fluid. Blood samples show unaltered haematology and the haematocrit will be elevated only in long-standing cases of entrapment. Blood gas analysis may indicate a mild metabolic acidosis. Rectal palpation, performed with care and method, is usually diagnostic for the disorder. According to Huskampf (1987) the palpable changes are so characteristic as to be definitive and make further diagnostic tests unnecessary. Most frequently taenial bands of the left ventral colon can be felt converging cranially and dorsally on the nephrosplenic space with a medial displacement of the congested spleen away from the left abdominal wall and caudally (Kopf, 1982).

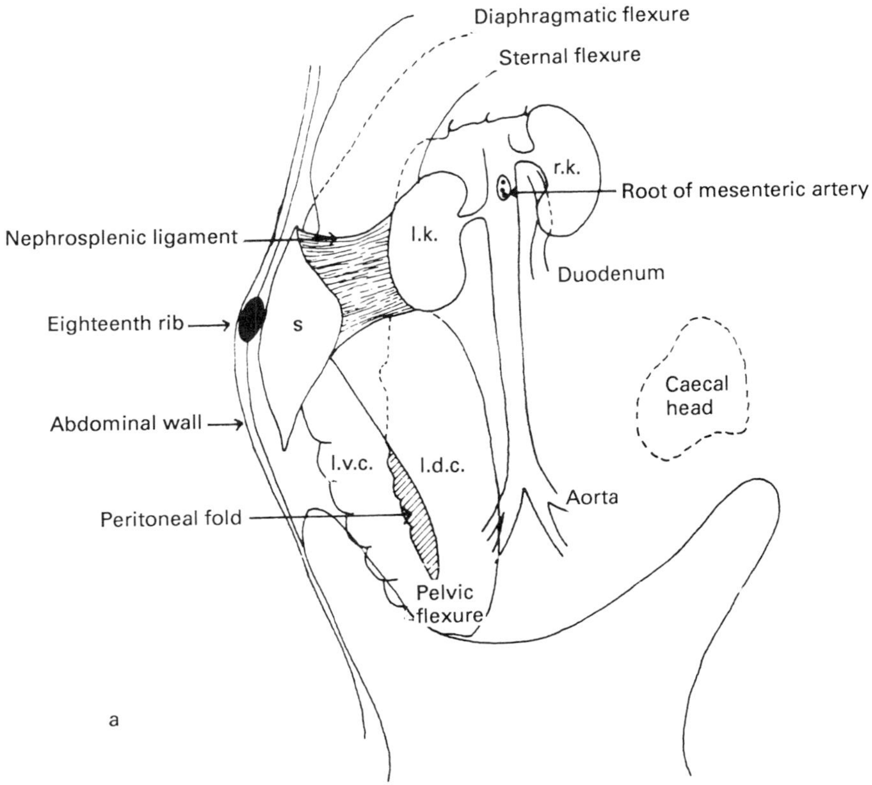

Fig. 2. (a) Diagramatic dorsal view of a horse showing the normal distribution of abdominal organs and (b), left dorsal displacements with taenia of the l.v.c. lying dorsal and converging on the nephrosplenic space. The spleen is partially hidden, engorged and moved medio-ventrally. The caecal head is dilated with gas and the pelvic flexure lies across the pelvic inlet. Key as for Figure 1.

However, the spleen frequently becomes overlain by dilated parts of the left ventral colon and may not be palpable (Figure 2b). The pelvic flexure is normally displaced to the right side of the pelvic inlet. The entrapment results in a varying degree of constriction of the left ventral and dorsal colons. Gas and ingesta accumulate both anterior to the entrapment (in the dorsal colon) and posterior to the constriction (in the ventral colon). These changes, together with palpable converging bands, often seeming to run diagonally from dorsal to left to ventral right across the pelvic inlet. This makes the diagnosis relatively simple.

TREATMENT

Three different approaches have been reported to be successful; waiting and starving, (Bonfig and Huskamp, 1986); rolling the horse in a clockwise direction

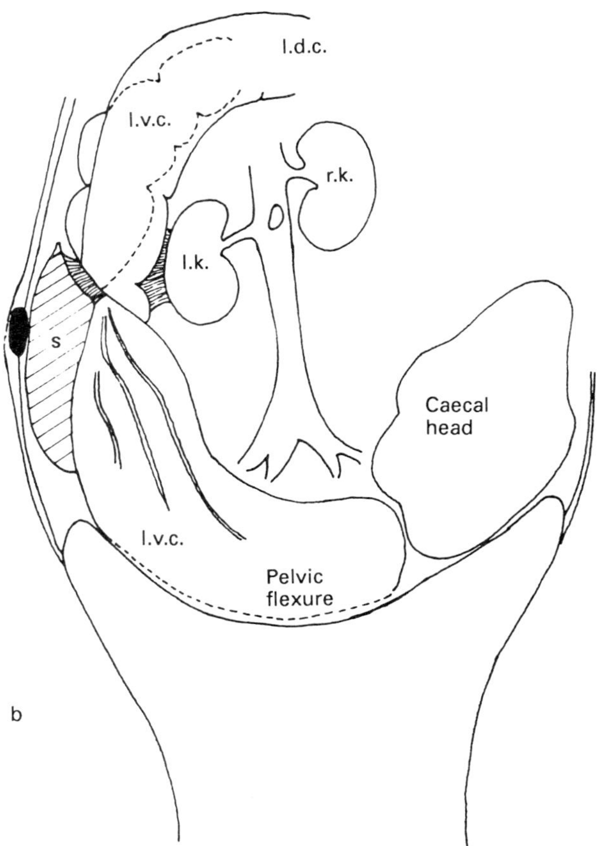

under general anaesthesia (Huskamp, 1987) and surgical laparatomy (Kopf, 1982 and Hackett, 1983).

WAITING AND STARVING

Provided that the disorder is diagnosed early, before the general condition of the horse deteriorates, there is some merit in keeping the animal in a large loose box unrestricted and under observation for 12–24 hours. If the condition remains unrelieved after this time, or sooner, if the condition of the horse warrants, rolling is indicated

ROLLING IN A CLOCKWISE DIRECTION UNDER GENERAL ANAESTHESIA

Details of the rolling technique are:
1. Correct any depletion of imbalance of body fluid and electrolytes
2. Administer general anaesthesia commencing with intravenous Guaphenesin

(GGE) as a 5% solution until the horse is incoordinated and complete the induction with thiopentone sodium, 5 – 9 mg/kg body weight. Ensure that the animal falls to the ground gently. Intubation is carried out, but maintenance gaseous anaesthesia is seldom necessary. The use of GGE is important because adequate muscle relaxation is essential.

3. Place the horse in *right* lateral recumbency for several minutes whilst the abdomen is ballotted deeply, particularly to the left of the mid-line. Good relaxation of the abdominal muscle is important.
4. Whilst continuing to ballot the abdomen, roll the horse slowly onto its back into dorsal recumbency.
5. At this point in the majority of cases rectal palpation will reveal that the displacement has been corrected. If not repeat the procedure.
6. Once corrected lay the horse in left lateral recumbency and allow it to recover from general anaesthesia
7. Following recovery, faeces are passed within 6 hours. Water should be made freely available, but food withheld for 24–36 hours. Further intravenous fluid therapy may be necessary in the first 12 hours.
8. Rectal examinations should be repeated six hourly to confirm that the correction has been maintained.

A conservative approach has much to commend it. Spontaneous resolution has been recorded in many cases immediately following anaesthesia and placement in dorsal recumbency, although occasionally trocharization of the caecum, to relieve gas pressure has been found necessary prior to rolling (Huskamp, 1987).

If the rolling technique fails to correct the displacement, two courses are open dependent upon the preference of the clinician and the general condition of the horse; either waiting 12 hours and repeat rolling or proceeding to surgery immediately and performing a laparotomy.

SURGICAL LAPAROTOMY

Surgery should be reserved for refractory cases which do not respond to rolling. A mid-line laparotomy reposition of the colon may be more difficult than might be anticipated due mainly to the weight of accumulated ingesta in the colon on either side of the entrapment and its voluminous size as a result of gas accumulation and oedema fluids. Colonic decompression may facilitate handling. Repositioning of the spleen avoids manipulating the dilated and oedematous colon. However, where thiopentone sodium alone has been used for the induction of general anaesthesia, the spleen itself can be engorged and very large, making handling difficult. Induction of general anaesthesia using a mixture of xylazine (1.1 mg/kg) and ketamine (2.2 mg/kg) intravenously avoids the complication of an engorged spleen.

Huskamp (1987) prefers a standing laparatomy through the left flank, after first resecting the eighteenth rib because this approach gives good access to the nephrosplenic space, allowing closure to prevent the possibility of recurrence.

Several workers have recorded the management and outcome of a series of cases of left colon entrapment and the details are summarized in Table 1.

Table 1 LEFT COLON ENTRAPMENT OVER THE NEPHRO-SPLENIC LIGAMENT

Author	Number of cases	Age (years) mean and range	Sex Male/Geld/Female	Treatment method	Success %
Huskampf (1982)	78	††	–	Surgery	97
Hackett (1983)	7	5 (1–10)	1 3 3	Surgery	100
Boening and Von Saldern (1986)	17	8–7 (4–12)	2 14 1	Hoist rolling †	88
Reeves et al., (1986)	11	–	–	Surgery	72
Bonfig and Huskampf (1986)	25	–	–	Starvation/rolling/ Surgery	100
Knottenbelt and Hill (unpublished data)	9	2 (1–8)	6 1 2	Surgery (4)	50
				Rolling (5)	100*

* One animal was destroyed after 6 days due to intractable laminitis
† Using power hoist to roll and spin
†† Value not known

PROGNOSIS

Without exception a good response is recorded whichever of the three treatments have been employed. Notwithstanding, the surgical procedure carries the greatest risk, particularly when colonic decompression has been employed with its associated risk of peritonitis. The incidence of recurrence in individual horses has been low.

ACKNOWLEDGEMENT

We should like to thank Dr H. Kalsbeek, Faculty of Veterinary Medicine, RUU, for introducing us to the rolling technique.

REFERENCES

Boening, K. J. and Von Saldern, F. Ch. (1986) Non-surgical treatment of left dorsal displacement of the large colon of horses under anaesthesia. In: *Equine Colic Research, Proceedings of the Second Symnposium,* Vol. 2. (University of Georgia) Veterinary Learning Systems, New Jersey, p. 325

Bonfig, H. and Huskampf, B. (1986) Zur therapie der verlagerung des colon ascendens in den milzierenraum. *Pferdeheilkunde* **2,** 243

Hackett, R. P. (1983) Non-strangulated colonic displacement in horses. *J. Am. Vet. Med. Ass.* **182,** 235

Huskampf, B. (1982) The diagnosis and treatment of acute abdominal conditions in the horse. In: *Proceedings of the Equine Colic Research Symposium.* (University of Georgia) USA. p. 261

Huskampf, B. (1987) Displacement of the large colon. In: *Current Veterinary Therapy in Equine Medicine,* 2nd ed, (ed. N. E. Robnson) Saunders, pp. 60

Kopf, N. (1982) Rectal findings in horses with intestinal obstruction. In: *Proceedings of the Equine Colic Research Symposium,* (University of Georgia) USA pp. 236

Reeves, M. J., Hilbert, B. J. and Morris, R. S. (1986) A retrospective study of 320 colic cases, referred to a veterinary teaching hospital. In: *Equine Colic Research, Proceedings of the Second Symposium,* Vol 2 (University of Georgia) Veterinary Learning Systems, New Jersey, pp. 24

P. J. N. PINSENT

Grass sickness of horses (grass disease: equine dysautonomia)

INTRODUCTION

GRASS SICKNESS is one of the most obscure, and certainly one of the most depressing, diseases which affect our domestic livestock. Despite the deaths of many thousands of horses and nearly eighty years of study and investigation, we are still unsure of the etiological and predisposing factors involved in this disease, which leads to a distressing, painful, and often lengthy illness and almost invariably ends in death.

HISTORY AND EPIDEMIOLOGY

Grass sickness was first described in Forfarshire, Scotland in 1909. It then appeared in other parts of the Scottish Lowlands, in southwestern Scotland, including Ayrshire and Lanarkshire, and later in the Scottish Borders. Serious outbreaks of the disease occurred in Cumbria, Lancashire, and North Wales, in the 1920s and 1930s. The Cambrian coast and southwest Wales were the next areas to be affected, followed by the southern Welsh counties, Herefordshire and Radnorshire. For a number of years there seemed to be little or no further spread, save for an area in the southeastern English counties including Kent.

Nevertheless, in recent years, the disease has occurred extensively in the southwest. It may now safely be said that, although the areas of highest incidence remain as described, there have been cases in almost every part of England, Wales, and Scotland. Ireland appears to have remained practically free of the disease. Outside the British Isles grass sickness seems to appear largely along the northern and western coasts of Europe. Apart from these areas only occasional cases have been seen.

The disease occurs in horses and ponies and occasionally in donkeys and mules. It affects the sexes equally. It has been reported in all age ranges from 10 months old to more than 20-years old. Nevertheless, there is a clear cut age incidence. The great majority of cases occur between two and seven years of age. There is no special breed susceptibility. The condition is certainly seen more often in ponies and light horses than in Thoroughbreds but this may be because it is practically always the grazing animal that is affected. Cases have been reported in part stabled or fully stabled animals and even in pit ponies underground, but the incidence is very rare. In general, grass sickness is a disease of the grazing horse. Although it has been recognized to occur throughout the year, it is significantly more common in April, June and July and particularly in May.

Grass sickness occurs on any type of pasture but is probably more common during spells of fine weather when the grass is dry. Many breeders in the grass sickness areas believe that certain fields, which often seem to be low-lying paddocks along streams in some way predispose. However, it may, of course, be that these are the fields routinely used for grazing during the critical months. Many breeders believe that there is a familial incidence but this is difficult to substantiate in pony studs where it is always likely that members of the same family will be grazing on the possibly dangerous fields during these critical months.

Nevertheless, some breeders do claim a lowered disease incidence when so-called 'danger' fields are avoided during the spring months. It is widely believed that the first two months out at pasture in winter-stabled horses are the most dangerous. However, these are usually among the acknowledged danger months from April until June. There is evidence that a change to fresh pasture, and especially the first eight weeks at pasture at different premises, may trigger off the disease.

Some premises have a notoriously high incidence of grass sickness and a new arrival at such premises suffers enhanced risk compared with new arrivals at other premises. There is a markedly higher incidence of grass sickness during some years. The incidence from area to area varies so greatly that the overall average annual incidence for the country as a whole cannot be accurately estimated.

The mortality rate is practically 100%. Very rarely, a chronic case may recover, or at least, survive. Unfortunately, such cases seldom thrive. They accommodate to some extent but remain thin and lethargic for what remains of their lives. There is, however, a suggestion that there is a varying degree of subclinical disease in the grazing population and that only a minimal proportion of these cases develop to show clinical picture *is* suggestive. However, it must be admitted that the pathognomonic histological lesions of the disease are found only in animals with suggestive clinical symptoms. Unfortunately, the histological procedures and interpretations are time consuming and require considerable specialist experience, so are rarely carried out unless the clinical picture *is* suggestive. Because the autonomic lesions are the only pathognomonic lesions of the disease, no case, however suggestive, can be considered confirmed unless the animal dies and histology is performed. Thus the diagnosis of surviving chronic cases is only subjective.

CLINICAL SIGNS

It is traditional to classify cases of grass sickness as peracute, acute, subacute, or chronic. In fact, peracute and acute forms of the disease are basically similar. The only real difference is a matter of duration. Subacute and chronic forms are also basically similar. The marked clinical division is between the acute forms and the chronic forms. It is therefore more logical to divide cases into acute or chronic categories.

ACUTE CASES

In acute cases there is usually a sudden onset of the disease. However, some cases exhibit a history of a transient 'colic' attack three weeks previously and have then been vaguely unwell until a further colic attack occurs and merges into the clinical picture of acute grass disease. Temperature is in the normal range, but the pulse rate is characteristically 70–80 beats per minute, and may be higher.

Oesophageal mobility is impaired. This interferes with the swallowing mechanism causing water and slimy green grassy fluid material to appear at the nostrils. In a few cases swallowing is not impaired. This may be due to variations in the distribution of lesions in the autonomic ganglia. This may confuse the diagnosis because an abnormal swallowing function is a common characteristic of grass sickness.

There may be forcible regurgitation of water and slime-coated grass down the nostrils, the anti-peristaltic movement causing considerable discomfort. The stomach and small intestine are markedly distended with slimy green fluid, to as much as three times their normal volume. The distention is often readily detectable in the left flank. There is complete bowel stasis with atony from the oesophagus to the rectum, and tympany can often be detected on percussion. The rectum is empty, the mucous membrane is dry and small pieces of blackish faeces are adherent to it. The colon contains firm impactive material, palpable on rectal examination, but it never becomes grossly distended as in subacute impaction of the pelvic flexure, and the corrugations in its walls are not obliterated.

Urine is dark, scanty, and concentrated. Patchy sweating occurs over much of the flank, and muscular tremors are also present. There is intermittent low grade abdominal pain, and very rapid weight loss as the tissues dehydrate. All blood components save calcium and chloride become concentrated due to anhydraemia.

PCV, blood, urea, and blood glucose levels are very high. Chloride and calcium levels are low. The white cell picture is variable. Death is invariable in one to four days.

It is interesting that in grass sickness, as opposed to feline dysautonomia, the pupil only appears to dilate in occasional cases.

CHRONIC CASES

Patients survive from four days to three weeks or even longer and become slowly, sometimes almost imperceptibly, ill. However, pain may be more noticeable than in the acute cases. Sweating occurs behind the elbow, in front of the stifle, and beneath the base of the tail which is held clamped down between the hind legs. There are tremors in the flank and behind the elbow. The back is arched, and there is a tendency for all four feet to remain fairly close together, giving an 'elephant on a tub' appearance. Rapid and massive dehydration and loss of flesh occur. The abdominal floor may be tucked up to such an extent that in long standing cases it is possible to feel the spine through the ventral abdomen. The advanced case resembles an emaciated greyhound. Few or no faeces pass and any that do are small, black and hard. A few cases pass scanty cow-like faeces. The pulse rate in more severe cases may be as high as 60–70 beats per minute. However, very chronic cases may show a normal pulse rate.

There is no regurgitation but swallowing is difficult. Eating is slow and laborious and abdominal pain is more marked after eating. The whole length of the gut, as well as the stomach, is empty save for some hard dry impactive material in the colon. Later, snoring, a drooping penis and an aberrant appetite appear. The spleen is often enlarged and the posterior edge palpable on rectal examination as a vertical structure close to the abdominal wall on the left side.

The blood urea becomes even higher, but PCV and glucose levels may be more or less normal.

PATHOLOGY

Gross pathological lesions in grass sickness tend to be variable and non-specific. There may be noticeable oesophageal dilatation, and oesophageal ulceration may well be present. The ulcers are often distributed in linear fashion and may involve the full depth of the mucosa.

In the more acute cases there may be congested areas distributed sporadically along the gut. A few cases show slight degrees of hepatic fatty change.

Nevertheless, macroscopic signs are of no real significance in diagnosis, which ultimately depends upon the detection of histological neuropathological changes. There may be affected areas with severe neuron degeneration amongst the myenteric (Auerbach's) and the submucous (Meissner's) alimentary plexuses. The following peripheral ganglia are usually affected:
1. The coeliaco-mesenteric ganglion.
2. The thoracic sympathetic chain.
3. The stellate ganglion.
4. The anterior cervical ganglion.
5. The ciliary ganglion.
Within the spinal cord, the dorsal root ganglion, the intermediolateral nucleus and, in some cases, the ventral horn may be affected. Certain brain stem nuclei and the gasserian ganglion may also be involved.

AETIOLOGY

There are still no clear cut indications as to aetiology. The apparent spread of the disease throughout the United Kingdom and its increasing incidence in new areas, might suggest an infective agent. Gilmour's work (1973; 1975; 1976; 1977) showed that serum from cases of acute grass sickness inoculated into healthy horses could produce typical lesions in the coeliac and mesenteric ganglia although no clinical signs developed. Nevertheless, the histology does not suggest an inflammatory etiology. A neurotoxic agent of some sort seems more likely. The toxins of botulism and clostridial enterotoxaemias have been suggested in the past, but later dismissed. As yet, no further progress has been made.

DIAGNOSIS AND DIFFERENTIAL DIAGNOSIS

Ultimately diagnosis still depends on the demonstration of the characteristic neuronal changes in the autonomic ganglia, of which the coeliac is the most conveniently sited at post-mortem examination. Even laparotomy, with its tedious routine, grave risks, and economic cost, is not always clear cut. However, the diagnosis should be determined as quickly as possible so that sufferers can be destroyed without delay. Acute grass sickness cases must be differentiated from acute colics, including gastric dilatation and high gut obstruction as well as from botulism, rhabdomyolysis, hyperlipaemia, and acute strongylosis. It must also be distinguished from oesophageal obstruction, pharyngeal paraylis, pharyngitis, and other forms of dysphagia. Chronic grass sickness requires differentiation from the chronic wasting diseases such as chronic liver damage, the malabsorption syndromes produced by diffuse small intestinal lymphosarcoma or granulomatous enteritis and long standing chronic strongylosis. It must be rememberd that the most chronic grass sickness cases may have a pulse rate just within normal limits and they may not show appreciable dysphagia but merely slow swallowing.

DIAGNOSTIC TESTS

Possible diagnostic tests include;

1. The detection of loss of gut peptides on immunocytochemical examination of rectal biopsy tissue. Unfortunately, there is much less loss from the rectum than from the ileum and large colon, which are not available for biopsy.
2. Measurement of plasma catecholamine levels. These are higher in horses with grass sickness than in normal horses and those with obstructive colic. However, the assay is difficult and time consuming.
3. Radiography using barium sulphate swallows. Greet and Whitwell (1986) demonstrated that grass sickness cases show delay in the passage of barium sulphate down the oesophagus. Marked oesophageal incoordination is visible on lateral radiography, especially when image intensification techniques are used. Obviously, the method requires radiographical skills and equipment not always available to the practitioner in the grass sickness areas. In any case, the signs are much less obvious in the more chronic cases. Endoscopic examination for ulcerative lesions at the lower end of the oesophagus, which are often a feature of grass sickness, may also be helpful. However, the lesions are not always easy to see. In addition such ulceration may be confusing in cases where a stomach tube has been passed several times.

TREATMENT

There is no useful treatment. An acute case may be eased by emptying the stomach and giving intravenous fluids but this gives temporary alleviation only. Parasympathomimetics have been tried without success. Theoretically, peptide therapy might be helpful but it is, for various reasons impracticable.

On humane grounds euthanasia, without delay, is the only logical course to take. This course of action emphasizes the need for a reasonably cheap, simple, and above all, accurate diagnostic test.

It is hoped that advances in the understanding of grass sickness will be assisted by research into human and feline dysautonomias. However, dysautonomias cause grave problems in any affected species.

RECOMMENDED FURTHER READING

Bishop, A. E., Hodson, N. P., Major, J. H., Probert, L., Yeats, J., Edwards, G. B., Wright J. A., Bloom, S. R. and Polak, J. M. (1984) The regulatory peptide system in equine grass sickness. *Experimentia*, **40**, 801–806

Gilmour, J. S. (1973) Microscopic lesions of the nervous system in grass sickness of the horse. *Res. Vet. Sci.*, **15**, 197–200

Gilmour, J. S. (1975) Autonomic lesions in grass sickness of the horse. *Neuropathology and Appl. Neurobiol.* **1**, 39–47

Gilmour, J. S. (1976) Autonomic lesions in grass sickness of the horse *Neuropathol. Appl. Neurobiol.*, **2**, 389–394

Gilmour, J. (1977) Experimental studies of neurotoxic activity in blood fractions from acute cases of grass disease. *Res. Vet. Sci.*, **22**, 1–4

Greet, T. R. C. and Whitwell, K. E. (1986) Radiological features of the equine oesophagus in grass sickness–the barium swallow as an aid to diagnosis. *Equine Vet. J.*, **18**, 294–297

Greig, J. R. (1928) Acute grass disease–an interpretation of the clinical symptoms. *Vet. Rec.*, **8**, 31–33

Hodson, N. P., Cawson, R., Edwards, G. B. (1984) Catecholamines in equine grass sickness. *Vet. Rec.*, **115**, 18–19

Hodson, N., Edwards, G. B., Barnett, S. W., Bishop, A. E., Cole, G. A., Probert, L., Bloom, S. R., Polak, J. M. (1982) Grass sickness of horses – changes in the regulatory peptide system of the bowel. *Vet. Rec.*, **110**, 276

R. S. JONES

The use of detomidine as a premedicant and sedative in horses

DETOMIDINE IS an alpha-two agonist, which was developed in Finland by the Farmos Group and is marketed in the United Kingdom by Norden Laboratories as Domosedan. In addition to being an alpha-two agonist it may have weak alpha-one receptor affinity (Vainio, 1985). The sedation and side-effects produced by the drug are a direct result of its pharmacological properties. The distribution and activity of alpha-adrenergic receptors have been reviewed by Lammintausta (1986) with particular reference to the actions of detomidine.

Alpha-2 receptors are found both pre- and post-synaptically in the central nervous system and the periphery. Stimulation of the central pre-synaptic alpha-2 adrenergic receptors inhibits the release of noradrenalin, leading to a decrease in cortical neuronal activity. This effect produces the sedation of the alpha-2 agonists such as detomidine and xylazine. The central depressant effect on the cardiovascular centres results in bradycardia and hypotension. Alpha-2 agonist drugs such as clomidine are used in human subjects as hypotensive agents. After intravenous injection, however, peripheral cardiovascular effects produced by the alpha-adrenergic stimulation at the post synaptic level will produce vasoconstriction and hypertension. The final effect on the cardiovascular system is a balance between both the central and peripheral effects. This varies with the dose route of administration and species (Ruskoahos, 1986).

The cardiovascular effects of detomidine are somewhat dramatic in the horse because doses as low as 20 μ_g/kg will produce severe bradycardia and hypertension. There are marked disturbances in cardiac rhythm and both sino-atrial and atrio-ventricular block have been observed (Vainio, 1985). Bradycardia and heart block appear to be maximal following the administration of 20 µg/kg of detomidine by the intravenous route, but an increase in dose will lead to an increase in the duration of the heart block. However, there is a considerable individual variation in the degree of heart block and its significance is difficult to assess. It is well known that second degree heart block is common in fit, unsedated horses at rest, but sino-atrial block is rare. Heart block does not appear to have any temporary or permanent ill effects but the possibility that detomidine may cause dysrhythmias must always be considered when the drug is to be administered to horses.

The intravenous administration of a dose of detomidine in excess of 20 µg/kg has been shown to produce a marked and prolonged hypertension (Vainio, 1985; Short, Matthews *et al.*, 1986). A dose of 10 µg/kg will produce a bradycardia but the hypertension is transient and 15 minutes after the injection the arterial blood pressure falls to the region of 10% below control.

175

It has been shown that atropine when administered at a dose of 0.01 mg/kg is not effective in controlling the bradycardia (Alitalo, 1986). It has, however, been demonstrated by Short, Stauffer *et al.*, (1986) that the prior administration of 0.02 m/kg of atropine by the intravenous route will prevent both the bradycardia and heart block produced by doses of 20 μg/kg and 40 μg/kg of detomidine.

The respiratory effects of detomidine in horses would appear to be somewhat variable. It is usual to see a slight increase in the respiratory rate in horses. However, the respiratory effect is assessed by variations in arterial blood pH, Pco_2 and Po_2 would appear to be minimal.

The main side-effects of detomidine administration appear to be a result of the peripheral adrenergic stimulation. The side-effects include ataxia, sweating, pilo-erection and increased frequency of micturition (Vainio, 1985). However, Clarke and Taylor (1986) reported that swaying and ataxia were the most common side-effects and that lower dose rates would reduce the incidence of these effects. The sweating seen in some horses might be considered as an impediment to successful clipping but this does not appear to be the case.

The pharmacokinetics of detomidine have been studied in laboratory animals and in horses. The results showed a rapid distribution into the tissues including the brain. There is a rapid first distribution phase with a half-life of a few minutes and a redistribution half-life of 0.5 – 2.5 hours. This appears to be the important factor in the control of both the rapid onset and dose-dependent termination of the clinical effects of detomidine. Excretion in the urine is the major route of elimination, although a small fraction is also excreted in the faeces. No differences in elimination were observed between the intravenous or intramuscular route of administration.

A number of papers have been published on the clinical use of detomidine both as a sedative and as a premedicant in the horse. Vainio (1985) reported on the use of the drug in 108 horses in Finland. The mean age of the animals was 6 years (range 1–17) and the mean body weight was 449 kg (range 150–700). A variety of clinical procedures were carried out in standing horses using doses from 8–250 μg/kg with a mean of 54 μg/kg. The intravenous route was used for administration in the majority of horses (81%) and the intramuscular route in the remainder. Following intravenous injection the sedative effect occurred in 2 minutes and after intramuscular injection in 5 minutes. The major side effect was staggering, which occurred in about 90% of the horses, although the incidence was lower in horses which received the lower doses of the drug. The drug proved to be a useful sedative in horses.

A dose range of 5–30 μg/kg (mean 13) was administered to 114 horses on 126 occasions for sedation by Clarke and Taylor (1986). A variety of breeds and horses were included in the trial and a wide range of procedures were carried out. The weights ranged from 120–950 kg and the ages from a few months to 20 plus years. Lower doses were used as the participating clinicians became familiar with usage of the drug. Doses of 10 g/kg by the intravenous route had a duration of action of 20 minutes and 20 μg/kg produced 50–60 minutes profound sedation. Sedation was classified as poor in 4 of the 126 administrations but it should be pointed out whilst the animal did not exhibit physical signs of sedation no further sedation was required for the procedure to be carried out. The main side effects were ataxia, sweating and bradycardia. Ataxia accompanied deep sedation but was relatively transient in duration with doses of 10 μg/kg.

The use of detomidine in combination with a variety of opiate drugs in horses has been investigated by Paton and Clarke (1987). The main aim of the trial was to investigate the enhancement of the detomidine sedation by an opiate. The opiates investigated were morphine, pethidine, methadone and butorphanol. A dose of either 10 or 20 μg/kg on detomidine was administered intravenously and the opiate was given 5–7 minutes later by the intravenous route. A variety of behavioural and physical responses were used to assess the degree of sedation. The administration of the opiate would appear to improve the sedation produced by detomidine. Pethidine produced various side-effects and should not be administered intravenously. The combination is likely to produce problems in the stability of the horse and it is recommended that detomidine alone should be administered. Only if its sedation effects are inadequate should an opiate be given. The drug of choice is butorphanol at a dose of 0.05 – 0.1 μg/kg.

Detomidine has also been administered as a premedicant before the induction of general anaesthesia in the horse. A report of the use of the drug in 273 horses has been reported by Clarke and Taylor (1987). One horse in which anaesthesia had been induced with ketamine died some 40 minutes later during halothane anaesthesia. This was considered to be due to a severe hypotension due to a relatively high concentration of halothane in the early anaesthetic period. Serious cardiac arrhythmias were observed in two other horses. However, the authors concluded that in general detomidine is an excellent premedicant. However, particular attention should be taken of its long lasting sedative and cardiovascular effects during the subsequent anaesthetic.

The use of a detomidine/ketamine anaesthetic technique has been described in 50 anaesthetics performed on 46 horses (Fisher, 1987). A wide variety of types of horses with a wide age and weight distribution were anaesthetized. All of the horses received an intravenous dose of 20–22 μg/kg of detomidine for sedation and approximately three minutes later anaesthesia was induced with ketamine 2.2 mg/kg. No serious side effects were observed.

REFERENCES

Alitalo, I. (1986) *Acta. Vet. Scand.,* **82,** (Suppl) 193–196
Clarke, K. W. and Taylor, P. M. (1986) *Equine Vet. J.,* **18,** 366–370
Clarke, K. W. and Taylor, P. M. (1987) *J. Ass. Vet. Anaesth.,* **14,** 29–32
Fisher, R. J. (1987) *J. Ass. Vet. Anaesth.,* **14,** 33–43
Lammintausta, R. (1986) *Acta. Vet. Scand.,* **82,** (Suppl) 11–16
Paton, B. S. and Clarke, K. W. (1987) *J. Ass. Vet. Anaesth.,* **14,** 44–52
Ruskoahos, H. (1986) *Acta. Vet. Scand.,* **82,** (Suppl) 17–28
Short, C. E., Matthews, N., Harvey, R. and Tyner, C. L. (1986) *Act. Vet. Scand.,* **82,** (Suppl) 139–159
Short, C. E., Stauffer, J. L., Goldberg, G. and Vainio, O. (1986) *Acta. Vet. Scand.,* **27,** 548–559
Vainio, O. (1985) Academic Dissertation, Helsinki

E. GREGORY MACEWEN

Therapy and prognosis for canine multiple myeloma

INTRODUCTION

MULTIPLE MYELOMA, plasma cell neoplasms and primary (Waldenstrom's) macroglobulinaemia represent less than one fifth of canine malignant tumours (Priester, 1980). The aetiology of multiple myeloma is unknown. In humans multiple myeloma has been associated with chronic administration of antigens for desensitization of allergies (Bergsagel and Rider, 1985). In rodent models, chronic irritation and inflammation can be associated with monoclonal immunoglobulin spikes (Bergsagel and Rider, 1985).

PATHOLOGICAL FEATURES AND BIOLOGICAL BEHAVIOUR

Plasma cells are produced mainly in haematopoietic bone marrow, lymph nodes, spleen, submucosa of the upper airway passages, and the gastrointestinal tract. Most plasma cell neoplasms form multiple tumors in bone and cause a generalized increase in marrow plasma cells. These neoplasms rarely present as solid tumors in bone or in extramedullary sites. Extramedullary plasmacytomas have been reported in the gastrointestinal tract in dogs (MacEwen, Patnaik, Johnson *et al.*, 1984). Less commonly, they have been seen in the spleen or lymph nodes and the skin. It is possible for them to occur in any site.

Solitary plasmacytomas of bone appear to be uncommon and may represent an early stage of multiple myeloma. Solitary plasmacytoma which were nonsecretory (did not secrete immunoglobulin) have also been reported in the dog (MacEwen, Patnaik, Hurvitz *et al.*, 1984)

Extramedullary plasmacytomas tend to stay localized to the regional area in which they are found. They rarely metastasize to the bone (MacEwen, Patnaik, Johnson *et al.*, 1984; MacEwen and Hurvitz, 1977; Matus and Heifer, 1985; Matus, Heifer, MacEwen *et al.*, 1988). On the other hand, solitary bony plasma cell tumors tend to spread quite rapidly to other bones and become a more generalized disease as seen in multiple myeloma (MacEwen, Patnaik, Hurvitz *et al.*, 1984; Matus and Heifer, 1985).

The disease manifestations of plasma cell neoplasms are exceedingly variable. These tumours can appear in almost any site. The symptoms caused by the tumour must be added to those resulting from the monoclonal immunoglobulin (M-protein) produced by the neoplasm. Dogs may present with signs of bone pain or fracture when osteolytic lesions are present (MacEwen and Hurvitz, 1977; Matus and Heifer,

178

1985). Other classical features of this disease include the hyperviscosity syndrome, hypercalcaemia and renal failure (MacEwen and Hurvitz, 1977; Matus and Heifer, 1985). Hypercalcaemia develops as a result of increased bone resorption stimulated by the release of an osteoclast-activating factor (OFA) or other substances produced by the myeloma cells (Mundy *et al.*, 1974). Bone lesions are usually seen in about 50% of the dogs presenting for plasma cell myeloma (Matus, Heifer, MacEwen *et al.*, 1988).

Renal abnormalities will be seen in approximately one-third of the patients with plasma cell myeloma (Matus, Heifer, MacEwen *et al.* 1988). Many factors contribute to the development of this renal failure. In animals with hypercalcaemia, excessive amounts of calcium may interfere with renal function. However, the important renal lesions specifically related to plasma cell myeloma are myeloma cast formation and diffuse renal tissue precipitation of M-proteins, especially light chains.

The hyperviscosity syndrome develops when the size, shape, and concentration of the serum M-protein causes a marked increase in serum viscosity (Bergsagel and Rider, 1985; MacEwen and Hurvitz, 1977; Matus and Heifer, 1985). The hyperviscosity syndrome is seen most commonly in macroglobulinemia (IgM) and plasma cell myeloma due to IgA. The IgA may polymerize in the serum, thus producing a very high molecular weight protein aggregate. IgG has also been shown to produce hyperviscosity syndrome, although this is quite unusual (Thrall, 1981). The clinical features of hyperviscosity syndrome are essentially related to hypervolaemia. The hyperviscosity syndrome may manifest as either a bleeding diathesis, cerebral dysfunction, or congestive heart failure. Funduscopic abnormalities show characteristic retinal haemorrhage and/or detachment. Venous dilation with sacculation and tortuosity are commonly apparent in the hyperviscosity syndrome. Approximately 20% of the dogs with monoclonal gammopathies will present the hyperviscosity syndrome (Matus, Heifer, MacEwen *et al.*, 1988).

In dogs with plasma cell myeloma, mild leukopaenia and anaemia are not uncommon findings. These are due to bone marrow replacement with tumor cells. Abnormal plasma cells circulating in the peripheral blood are quite uncommon and are usually seen in around 10% of the cases (Matus, Heifer, MacEwen *et al.*, 1988).

MACROGLOBULINAEMIA

Macroglobulinaemia can be seen with lymphoplasmacytic neoplasms, and B-lymphocyte neoplasms such as chronic lymphocytic leukaemia (MacEwen *et al.*, 1977; Braund *et al.*, 1978). Animals with macroglobulinaemia usually have hepatosplenomegaly and lymphadenopathy. It would be extremely rare to see osteolyte bone lesions. Due to the high molecular weight of IgM (900 000) is it more common to see the hyperviscosity syndrome. Cryoglobulinaemia has also been reported in dogs with macroglobulinaemia (Hurvitz *et al.*, 1977; Braund *et al.*, 1979)

DIAGNOSIS AND TREATMENT

The diagnosis of a plasma cell neoplasm requires the demonstration of uncontrolled growth of a plasma cell clone. Evidence of uncontrolled growth is provided by the invasion of normal tissue by plasma cells causing osteolytic bone lesions or plasmocytomas in extra skeletal sites. A progressive increase in the amount of serum M-protein (myeloma protein) or light chain proteinuria provides additional evidence of uncontrolled growth.

Specifically each dog should undergo the following evaluation:

1. Serum and urine electrophonesis to demonstrate a monoclonal immunoglobulin (in the serum) or light chains (in the urine).
2. A radiographic skeletal survey to demonstrate an evidence of osteoporosis or osteolysis.
3. Bone marrow aspirations to look for an increase in number or clustering of plasma cells.

In addition, the clinical evaluation of an animal with suspected plasma cell tumor should also include a CBC, platelet count and chemistry profile. Particular attention should be paid to renal function and calcium levels.

It is relatively easy to differentiate the B-lymphocyte neoplasm associated with an IgM protein because the animals will have other features diagnostic of chronic lymphocytic leukaemia or diffuse lymphocytic lymphomas (MacEwen *et al.*, 1977; Braund *et al.*, 1978).

Animals with plasma cell tumors should be considered to be immunological cripples. The infections seen in myeloma infected animals are associated with bone marrow suppression and immunosuppressive factors associated with the disease itself (Jacobson and Zolla-Pazner, 1986). An important aspect in the treatment of myeloma is prompt and urgent investigation and treatment of any febrile episode. Appropriate bacterial cultures and sensitivity should be taken and serious infections should be treated by bactericidal antibiotic therapy.

Renal function must be closely monitored and treated vigorously if abnormalities do occur. Medical management should include establishment of hydration and renal perfusion with maintenance of adequate glomerular filtration.

Another major concern which can require immediate treatment is hypercalcaemia. The treatment of hypercalcaemia should include the use of sodium chloride hydration in combination with furosemide which causes a calcium diuresis. Prednisone therapy is indicated as an aid to calcium diuresis and will decrease intestinal absorption and inhibit osteoclast activation. In addition to these supportive measures to lower calcium, chemotherapy should be initiated to control tumour cell progression.

Bony lysis and generalized osteoporosis may predispose an animal to a pathological fracture. Whenever possible it is most desirable to treat these bony lesions with either localized radiation therapy or combination chemotherapy.

The hyperviscosity syndrome may also be present but, fortunately, most animals do not require emergency intervention to treat the condition. In some select cases, either because of severe neurological impairment or haemorrhagic diathesis, plasmapheresis may be required to lower the serum viscosity (Matus *et al.*, 1983). However, the initiation of chemotherapy will usually improve the viscosity in a matter of a few weeks.

The most effective way to manage plasma cell tumors is by the use of chemotherapy (Matus and Hurvitz, 1977; Matus and Heifer, 1985; Matus, Heifer, MacEwen *et al.*, 1988). Successful chemotherapy relieves bone pain, reduces myeloma cell mass, initiates skeletal healing, and lowers the level of serum immunoglobulin. Chemotherapy has also been shown to improve and lengthen survival time (Matus, Heifer, MacEwen *et al.*, 1988). The agents which have received the most attention in treating multiple myeloma are the alkalating agents, melphalan and cyclophosphamide. The addition of prednisone to alkalating agents will also increase their effectiveness. Although no optimal dose schedule has been devised, melphalan has been used quite extensively in the dog at a dose of 0.1 mg/kg of body weight, per os, SID for 10 days, then 0.05 mg/kg per os SID continuously. Cyclophosphamide can be used both as an intravenous bolus at 200-300 mg/m^2 I.V. once weekly, or given as a low dose, per os at 50 mg/m^2 per day for 4 days per week. Prednisone is usually administered at a dose of 0.5 mg/kg SID per os for 10 days, then 0.5 mg/kg on alternate days for 60 days then stopped.

One side effect of melphalan is bone marrow suppression, particularly platelet suppression. It is recommended that if this happens, cyclophosphamide should be substituted for malphalan. Chlorambucil is another alkalating agent which has been used quite successfully in treating macroglobulinaemia (MacEwen and Hurvitz, 1977; MacEwen et al., 1977; Hurvitz et al., 1977). The dose of chlorambucil is 0.2 mg/kg SID per os daily. Chlorambucil is a very safe alkalating agent with almost no clinical signs of toxicity noted at that dose level.

PROGNOSIS

In a recent study of 37 dogs treated with either melphalan, with or without cyclophosphamide and prednisone, the median survival time was 540 days (Matus, Heifer et al., 1988). In this study a complete response was noted in 43% (16 of 37 dogs).

Hypercalcaemia, light chains of myeloma protein in the urine, and extensive bony lesions have been associated with poor prognosis. Sex, the type of monoclonal Ig class, increased serum viscosity, and azotemia did not correlate significantly with prognosis, although a trend toward increased survival time was apparent in the nonazotemic group (Matus, Heifer, MacEwen et al., 1988).

Although chemotherapy will not cure this disease it will significantly prolong survival time. The vast majority of dogs tolerate the therapy very well with minimal side effects. Treated dogs tend to improve clinically and experience a good quality survival.

The response to therapy must be evaluated in terms of the clinical signs monitoring specific laboratory changes and radiographic findings. Monoclonal spikes will usually decrease to less than 50% of the initial value within 6–8 weeks. As the therapy progresses, the immunoglobulin spike will eventually disappear.

Although the experience with treating macroglobulinaemia is not as large. The prognosis should be good as those with multiple myeloma.

REFERENCES

Bergsagel, D. E. and Rider, W. D. (1985) Plasma cell neoplasms. In *Cancer Principles and Practice of Oncology* (eds J. R. DeVita, S. Hellman and S. A. Rosenberg) Lippincott, PA pp. 1753–1795

Braund, K. G., Everett, R. M., Albert, R. N., *et al.*, (1978) Neurologic manifestation of monoclonal IgM gammopathy associated with lymphocytic leukemia in a dog. *J. Am. Vet. Med. Assoc.*, **172**, 1407–1410

Braund, K. G., Everett, R. M., Bartels, J. E. *et al.*, (1977) Neurologic manifestations of IgM multiple myeloma associated with cryoglobulinemia in a dog. *J. Am. Vet. Med. Assoc.*, **174**, 1321–1325

Hurvitz, A. I., MacEwen, E. G., Middaugh, C. R. *et al.* (1977) Monoclonal cryoglobulinemia with macroglobinemia in a dog. *J. Am. Vet. Med. Assoc.,* **170,** 511–513

Jacobson, D. R., Zolla-Pazner, S. (1986) Immunosuppression and infection of multiple myeloma. *Seminars in Oncology,* **13,** 282–290

MacEwen, E. G. and Hurvitz A.I., (1977): Diagnosis and management of monoclonal gamminopathies. *Vet Clin NA* **7**: 119–131

MacEwen, E. G., Hurvitz, A. I. and Hayes, A. A. (1977) Hyperviscosity syndrome associated with lymphocytic leukemia in three dogs. *J. Am. Vet. Med. Assoc.,* **170,** 1309–1312

MacEwen, E. G., Patnaik, A. K., Hurvitz, A. I. *et al.,* (1984) Non-secretory multiple myeloma in two dogs. *J. Am. Vet. Med. Assoc.* **184,** 1283–1286

MacEwen, E. G., Patnaik, A. K., Johnson, G. F. *et al.,* (1984) Extramedullary plasmacytoma of the gastrointestinal tract in two dogs. *J. Am. Vet. Med. Assoc.,* **184,** 1396–1398

Matus, R. E. and Heifer, C. E. (1985) Immunoglobulin producing tumors. *Vet. Clin. NA.* **15**: 741–753

Matus, R. E., Heifer, C. E., Gordon, B. R. *et al.,* (1983) Plasma plasmapheresis and chemotherapy of hyperviscosity syndrome associated with monoclonal gammophathy in the dog. *J. Am. Vet. Med. Assoc.* **183,** 215–218

Matus, R. E., Heifer, C. E., MacEwen, E. G. *et al.,* (1988) Multiple myeloma in the dog: Prognostic factors and review of 60 cases. *J. Am. Vet. Med. Assoc.,* in press.

Mundy, G. R., Raisz, L. G., Cooper, R. A. *et al* (1974) Evidence for the secretion of an osteoclast stimulating factor myeloma. *New England J. Med.,* **291,** 1041–1046

Priester, W. A. (1980) The occurrence of tumors in domestic animals. *National Cancer Institute Monograph 54,* Dept. of Health and Human Services, Bethesda, MD, pp. 36

Thrall, M. A. (1981) Lymphoproliferative disorders. *Vet. Clin. NA (Small An Pract)* **11,** 321–347

C. J. L. LITTLE

Otitis media in the dog: a review

INTRODUCTION

THE TYMPANIC or middle ear cavity (MEC) is an air space within the petrous temporal bone of the skull. Together with the tympanic membrane and the ossicles it functions to receive and conduct airborne vibrations from the external ear to the cochlea (Brooks, 1976). The MEC is lined by a modified respiratory mucosa which is continuous with that of the auditory (eustachian) tube and nasopharynx (Sade, 1979). The epithelium contains both ciliated and secretory cells but the greater part is formed of a low cuboidal or squamous pavement epithelium. The lamina propria of this mucosa is sparse. Simple tubular glands are found within the MEC of normal dogs but these are restricted to areas where the lamina propria is more abundant, particularly around the aural ostium of the auditory tube (Little, 1988).

ANATOMY

The anatomy of the canine MEC has been described in detail (Getty, 1964). From the clinical perspective it is important to recall that the facial nerve passes through the middle ear and that sympathetic nerve fibres forming the cariticotympanic plexus are also found there. The facial nerve innervates the muscles of facial expression, whilst the sympathetic fibres negotiate the MEC *en route* from the cranial cervical ganglion to the eye (McClure, 1964; Neer, 1984). The organs of hearing and balance, which are the structures of the inner ear, are housed in the dense bone of the pyramid. They are separated from the MEC by the thin but resilient membrane of the round window (Paparella *et al.*, 1980).

OTITIS MEDIA

Otitis externa, colloquially known as ear canker, is recognized as an important and common condition in the dog (Lane, 1982). However, inflammation of the middle ear cavity, otitis media, has long been known to occur in dogs (Scott, 1897; Guard, 1923), and Spreull (1964) claimed that it may be found in up to 50% of dogs with chronic otitis externa. Smeak and Dehoff (1986) reported that it was present at the time of surgery in 85% of 39 ears with chronic 'end-stage' external ear disease. However, there are no data indicating the prevalence of this condition in the canine population as a whole.

The pathogenesis of otitis media in the dog is still not fully understood and has been identified as a priority for research (Edney, 1987). In other species, including the rat, guinea-pig, rabbit, pig, sheep, cattle and human, inflammation of the MEC is usually associated with respiratory disease and presumed dysfunction of the auditory tube (Olson and McClure, 1968; Wagner *et al.*, 1976; Flatt *et al.*, 1977; Sade, 1979; Olson, 1981; Jensen *et al.*, 1982; Jensen *et al.*, 1983; Boot and Walvoort, 1986; Friedmann, 1986). In other words, there is an ascending infection from the nasopharynx to the middle ear. It has been conjectured that ascending infection may also be important in the dog (Moltzen, 1961; Lane, 1976) but recent research (Little, 1988) has not supported the hypothesis. It is now widely acknowledged that otitis media in the dog most commonly occurs secondary to otitis externa (Ott, 1964; Spreull, 1964; Parker *et al.*, 1976; Neer and Howard, 1982; Venker-van Haagen, 1983; Harvey, 1985).

The mechanism by which inflammation proceeds from the external to the middle ear, across the tympanic membrane, is not clear. Meynard (1961) proposed that otitis externa could lead to perforation of the tympanic membrane and subsequent otitis media. This putative mechanism has been tacitly accepted by others (Spreull, 1964; Ott, 1964; Fraser *et al.*, 1970; Lane, 1976) but Wilcock (1985) stated that the canine ear drum is resistant to inflammatory lysis. Venker-van Haagen (1983) has asserted that spontaneous rupture occurs only rarely in dogs. This agrees with the findings of pathological studies which have shown thickening of the tympanic membrane in dogs with concurrent otitis externa and media (Little, 1988). However, it is conceivable that spontaneous perforations of the ear drum may occur which then heal. The tympanic membrane shows remarkable regenerative properties even in the presence of suppurative otitis media (Rogers and Snow, 1968; Johnson and Hawke, 1987).

PATHOLOGY

The histopathological changes in the inflammed middle ear cavity of the dog are similar to those which have been induced experimentally in several species by electrocauterization or ligation of the auditory tube (Sade, 1979; Tojo *et al.*, 1985). They also resemble the changes which are found in spontaneous otitis media in other species (Olson and McClure, 1968; Flatt *et al.*, 1977; Sade, 1979; Friedmann, 1986). Epithelial hyperplasia occurs and the lamina propria is transformed into a loose, vascular and oedematous granulation tissue (Figure 1). In some instances, areas of dense mature connective tissue and new bone are found. An inflammatory cell infiltrate consisting of lymphoid cells and polymorphonuclear leukocytes is usually present. Occasionally, lymphoid follicles with germinal centres are found. Gland-like structures, which may be cystic and can contain cholesterol clefts, are often seen within the granulation tissue (Little, 1988). Cholesteatoma may accompany otitis media in the dog (Little, 1988) but the precise origin of this cystic structure, which contains keratin, is in some doubt. The condition resembles cholesteatoma in people and in the mongolian gerbil (*Meriones unguiculatus*) (Sade, 1979; Chole *et al.*, 1981; Friedmann, 1986).

CLINICAL FINDINGS

The consensus view is that the presentation and clinical signs of otitis media are similar to those of otitis externa (Ott, 1964; Spreull, 1964; Fraser *et al.*, 1970; Venker-van Haagen, 1983; Harvey, 1985; Lane and Little, 1986).

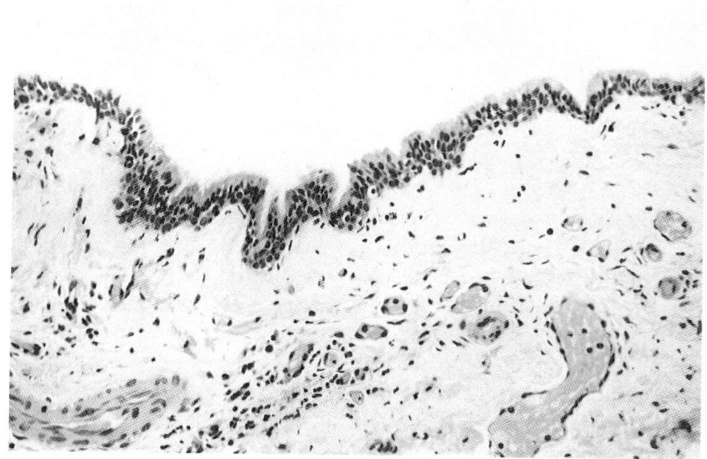

Fig. 1. Granulation tissue from the middle ear cavity of a dog with otitis media. The covering epithelium is pseudostratified and ciliated.

The author has carried out a study of dogs with chronic aural disease referred to a second opinion clinic (Little, 1988). Eighty-two dogs with persistent otitis were investigated in detail. Otitis externa was present in all dogs and a total of 124 ears were affected. The presence of otitis media was confirmed by histopathological examination in 61 ears from 41 dogs. The history and clinical signs in those animals with otitis media did not differ substantially from those exhibited by dogs with otitis externa alone. Headshaking, otorrhoea and scratching or pawing at the ear(s) were the most common signs recognized. Signs associated with aural pain (including discomfort on aural massage, during eating and when the mouth was opened, changes in temperament and flagrant aggression) were more common in dogs with otitis media but these were also exhibited by a substantial minority of the dogs where otitis externa alone was diagnosed. Obvious stricture or stenosis of the external ear canal was more often present in those animals which had otitis media than in those with otitis externa alone. The findings of this study did not support the claim (Lane, 1982) that transitory head-tilt and slow head-shaking are good indicators of otitis media.

Neurological abnormalities referrable to the inner ear (otitis interna) or facial nerve were found in only 5 (12%) of the 41 dogs with confirmed otitis media. The detailed results of this study supported a subjective impression that the severity of the otitis externa was more marked in those dogs which were also shown to have otitis media (Little, 1988).

DIAGNOSTIC AIDS

The structures comprising the middle ear of the dog are quite inaccessible so that direct examination is difficult. Many authors (Moltzen, 1961; Ott, 1964; Neer and Howard, 1982) recommend visual inspection of the ear drum using an otoscope as the primary diagnostic aid to the identification of otitis media. However, it has been shown that in dogs with chronic aural disease the narrowing of the ear canal and ottorhoea that accompanies otitis externa hamper this investigation (Spreull, 1964; Little, 1988). Otoscopy under general anaesthesia remains a valuable technique for the evaluation of the integument of the ear canal (Lane, 1982) but it is of limited value in assessing the integrity of the tympanic membrane and the condition of the middle ear.

Palpation of the tympanic membrane with a blunt probe or needle has been advocated as a reliable means of evaluating the integrity of the ear drum (Spreull, 1964; Fraser *et al.*, 1970; Lane, 1982). Experimental work in cadavers has shown that such procedures are very inaccurate and may provoke iatrogenic perforations (Little, 1988). Moreover, the rationale for using this technique is in doubt because in spite of anecdotal reports there is little objective evidence that perforations of the tympanic membrane often accompany middle ear disease.

Radiography of the external and middle ears can provide valuable diagnostic information (Farrow, 1985; Tojo *et al.*, 1985; Douglas *et al.*, 1987). Ventro–dorsal and open-mouth projections are particularly informative although other views have also been advocated. Narrowing of the air shadow of the ear canal and ossification of the aural cartilages are often present in animals with chronic otitis externa. Where such changes are severe they may provide an index to the presence of middle ear disease (Little, 1988). However, disease of the middle ear has been found in the absence of demonstrable radiological abnormalities (Farrow, 1985; Little, 1988).

TREATMENT

The treatment of middle ear disease in the past using such techniques as repeated flushing of the middle ear with saline or medication (Moltzen, 1961; Spreull, 1964; Lane, 1982; Neer and Howard, 1982) has proved difficult to evaluate precisely because diagnosis has often been based on subjective assessments and, in the absence of histopathological evidence, there have been no universally accepted criteria for the diagnosis of otitis media. These difficulties have been confounded by the presence of inflammation in the external ear canal which is probably the primary seat of disease in most instances (Lane and Little, 1986; Little, 1988). Surgical procedures which aim to ablate the entire ear canal, including the osseous portion, and allow bulla osteotomy by a lateral approach, have been widely adopted during recent years (Ott, 1974; Harvey, 1985; Mason *et al.*, 1988). These techniques are surgically demanding. They require a good working knowledge of aural anatomy in view of the possible complications which include facial nerve paralysis and trauma to the inner ear (Mason *et al.*, 1988). Long term evaluation of such techniques are awaited but preliminary results are encouraging (Lane, 1986; Mason *et al.*, 1988). Ablation of the ear is obviously a radical procedure. Less invasive treatment regimes should be adopted where possible.

FURTHER RESEARCH

Recently aural diseases in companion animals have been investigated using a variety of objective non-invasive techniques including brainstem auditory evoked potentials (Kay *et al.*, 1984), respiratory audiometry (Bradford *et al.*, 1973) and acoustic impedance audiometry (Penrod and Coulter, 1980; Forsythe, 1985; Osguthorpe, 1986; Sims *et al.*, 1986; Little, 1988). These techniques offer powerful research tools but are also of direct relevance to the understanding of the pathophysiology and management of these diseases. Tympanometry, for example, a branch of acoustic impedance audiometry, has been shown to provide an accurate technique for the evaluation of the integrity and stiffness of the tympanic membrane and may become as useful in veterinary ENT as it is in human otolaryngology (Little, 1988). In view of the high incidence of ear disease in small animals and the possible implications of these conditions for comparative medicine, further research is urgently needed.

REFERENCES

Boot, R. and Walvoort, H. P. (1986) *Lab Anim.* **20**, 242–248

Bradford, L. J., McKinley, J. H., Rousey, C. L., Klein, D. E. (1973) *Am. J. Vet. Res.*, **34**, 1183–1187

Brooks, D. N. (1976) in *Scientific Foundations of Otolaryngology* (eds R. Hinchcliffe and D. Harrison), Heinemann, London, pp. 281–290

Chole, R. A., Henry, K. R., McGinn, M. D. (1981) *Am. J. Otol.*, **2**, 204–210

Douglas, S. W., Herrtage, M. E., Williamson, H. D. (1987) in *Principles of Veterinary Radiology*, 4th ed, Balliere Tindall, London, pp. 191–192

Edney, A. T. B. (1987) *Vet. Rec.*, **120**, 319–320

Farrow, C. S. (1985) *Mod. Vet. Pract.* **66**, 871–874

Flatt, R. E., Deyoung, D. W., Hogle, R. M. (1977) *Lab. Anim. Sci.*, **27**, 343–347

Forsythe, W. B. (1985) *Am. J. Vet. Res.*, **46**, 1351–1353

Fraser, G., Gregor, W. W., Mackenzie, C. P., Spreull, J. S. A., Withers, A. R. (1970) *J. Small Animal Pract.*, **10**, 725–754

Friedmann, I. (1986) In *Systemic Pathology* 3rd ed, Vol. 1, Churchill Livingstone, London, pp.256–284

Getty, R. (1964) In *Anatomy of the Dog* (eds M. E. Miller, G. C. Christensen and H. E. Evans), W. B. Saunders, Philadelphia, pp. 847–863

Guard, W. F. (1923) *Vet. Med.*, **18**, 317–323

Harvey, C. E. (1985) In *Textbook of Small Animal Surgery* (ed. D. H. Slatter), W. B. Saunders, Philadelphia, pp. 1915–1923

Jensen, R., Pierson, R. E., Weibel, J. L., Tucker, J. O., Swift, B. L. (1982) *J. Am. Vet. Med. Assoc.*, **181**, 805–807

Jensen, R., Maki, L. R., Lauermann, L. H., Raths, W. R., Swift, B. L., Flack, D. E., Hoff, R. L., Hancock, H. A., Tucker, J. O., Horton, D. P., Weibel, J. L. (1983) *J. Am. Vet. Med. Assoc.*, **182**, 967–972

Johnson, A. and Hawke, M. (1987) *Acta Otolaryngol.*, **103**, 81–86

Kay, R., Palmer, A. C., Taylor, P. M. (1984) *Vet. Rec.*, **114**, 81–84

Lane, J. G. (1976) *Vet. Ann.*, **16**, 160–166

Lane, J. G. (1982) In *ENT and Oral Surgery of the Dog and Cat* John Wright, Bristol, pp. 257–278

Lane, J. G. (1986) In *The Complete Manual of Ear Care* Solvay Veterinary Inc/Veterinary Learning System, USA, pp.67–82

Lane, J. G. and Little, C. J. L. (1986) *J. Small Animal Pract.*, **27**, 247–254

Little, C. J. L. (1988) *PhD Thesis.* University of Bristol, UK

Mason, K. L., Harvey, C. E., Orsher, R. J. (1988) *Abstract 2nd IVENTA Ann. Mtg.* (Orlando, Florida)

McClure, R. C. (1964) In *Anatomy of the Dog* (eds. M. E. Miller, G. C. Christensen and H. E. Evans), W. B. Saunders, Philadelphia, pp. 544–571

Meynard, J. A. (1961) *Adv. Small Animal Pract.*, **3**, 62–65

Moltzen, H. (1961) *Adv. Small Animal Pract.*, **3**, 56–61
Neer, M. T. (1984) *Compend. Contin. Educ. Pract. Vet.*, **6**, 740–746
Neer, M. T. and Howard, P. E. (1982) *Compend. Contin. Educ. Pract. Vet.*,**4**, 410–420
Olson, L. D. (1981) *Am. J. Vet. Res.*, **42**, 1433–1440
Olson, L. D. and McClure, E. L. (1968) *Lab. Anim. Care*, **18**, 478–485
Osguthorpe, J. D. (1986) *Laryngoscope*, **96**, 1366–1377
Ott, R. L. (1964) *Mod. Vet. Pract.*, **45**, 39–42
Ott, R. L. (1974) In *Canine Surgery*, 2nd Archibald edn, American Veterinary Publications,
    Santa Barbara pp. 263–260
Paparella, M. M., Goycoolea, M. V., Meyerhoff, W. L. (1980) *Ann. Otol. Rhinol. Laryngol.
    (Suppl)*, **68**, 249–253
Parker, A. J., Schiller, A. G., Cusick, P. K. (1976) *J. Am. Vet. Med. Assoc.*, **168**, 931–933
Penrod, J. P. and Coulter, D. B. (1980) *J. Am. Hosp. Ass.*, **16**, 941–948
Rogers, K. A. and Snow, J. B. (1968) *Ann. Otol. Rhinol. Laryngol.*, **77**, 66–71
Sade, J. (1979) In *Secretory Otitis Media and its Sequelae. Monographs in Clinical Otolaryngo-
    logy 1,* Churchill Livingstone, New York, pp. 317
Scott, W. M. (1897) *The Veterinarian*, **LXX-XLIII** Fourth Series, 498–503
Sims, M. H., Weigel, J. P., Moore, R. E. (1986) *Am. J. Vet. Res.*, **47**, 1022–1031
Smeak, D. D. and DeHoff, W. D. (1986) *Vet. Surg.*, **15**, 161–170
Spreull, J. S. A. (1964) J. *Small Animal Pract.*, **5**, 107–152
Tojo, M., Matsuda, H., Fukui, K., Sasai, H., Baba, E. (1985) *J. Small Animal Pract.*, **26**,
    81–89
Venker-van Haagen A. J. (1983) In *Current Veterinary Therapy; Small Animal Practice VIII*
    (ed. R. W. Kirk), W. B. Saunders, Philadelphia pp. 47–52
Wagner, J. E., Owens, D. R., Kusewitt, D. F., Corley, E. A. (1976) *Lab. Anim. Sci.*, **26**,
    902–907
Wilcock, B. P. (1985) In *Pathology of Domestic Animals,* (eds K. V. F. Jubb, P. C. Kennedy
and N. Palmer), Academic Press, Orlando, pp. 339–406

PHILLIPPA PATON

Ethylene glycol poisoning in small animals

INTRODUCTION

CERTAIN FEATURES peculiar to small animals, the dog in particular, render them more susceptible to the ingestion of noxious agents. These include the instinct to hunt, lack of alimentary finesse, scavenging tendencies and avariciousness. Of more importance, with particular reference to the cat, is the poorly developed ability of organs to detoxify and eliminate these agents, often with fatal results.

Ethylene glycol, a dihydric alcohol widely distributed in the environment, is reported to be one of the most common causes of poisoning in the USA. Sources include anti-freeze, detergents, pharmaceuticals, polish, flavourings, cosmetics, de-icers and tobacco. Unfortunately due to its palability, dogs drink it readily. A lethal dose is 2-6 ml/kg. Its toxicity varies greatly with rapidity of intake, the concomitant intake of food and individual susceptibility. Early diagnosis is made difficult due to an inadequate history, the nonspecific clinical signs and its rapid metabolism and excretion. Thus it is associated with a high death rate due to delay in presentation and therapy.

PATHOGENESIS

In the absence of food, ethylene glycol is rapidly absorbed from the gastro-intestinal tract and initial signs are seen within an hour. Levels of ethylene glycol in serum and urine peak at three and six hours, respectively. Ethylene glycol is metabolized in the liver by alcohol and aldehyde dehydrogenases. These produce anions that are responsible for a major metabolic normochloraemic acidosis (see Figure 1). It exerts effects similar to ethanol on the central nervous system, decreasing serotonin metabolism and amine concentration.

Excretion is mainly via the kidney where significant amounts of unchanged ethylene glycol can be detected for up to 48 hours. One of the end products of metabolism, calcium oxalate, is filtered by the glomerulus. Following the reabsorption of water and other substances, this relatively insoluble salt precipitates to form crystals within the tubules.

At the cellular level, this mechanism increases the formation of cytoplasmic reduced NADH:NAD ratio. This results in an increased concentration of lactic acid, that is metabolized by NAD-dependant dehydrogenase. Hyperosmolality occurs because of the small molecular weight and water solubility of ethylene glycol.

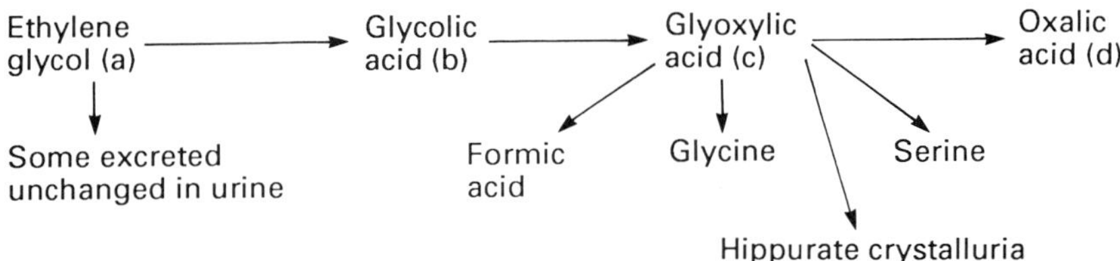

Fig. 1. The metabolism of ethylene glycol. (a) Slow reaction allowing acidosis and nephrosis. (b) Urinary glycolate levels correlate with the clinical signs and mortality. (c) Short $T_{1/2}$ has few toxic effects. (d) This is the ultimate oxidation product. It combines with calcuim to form insoluble calcium oxalate crystals that deposit in renal tubules, brain and other organs.

This rapid rise in serum osmolality should stimulate the release of anti-diuretic hormone but ethylene glycol's ethanol-like effects result in chemical inhibition of its release. Ethylene glycol is not reabsorbed in the collecting ducts of the proximal nephron, thereby promoting an osmotic diuresis. The direct cytotoxic effects of the metabolities, glycolic acid in particular, are responsible for most of the renal tubule epithelial damage.

CLINICAL SIGNS

Due to individual variation in the quantity of ethylene glycol ingested, absorbed and metabolized, clinical signs vary considerably. The main effects of ethylene glycol, due to the direct cytotoxic effects of the metabolites, are seen on the gastrointestinal tract and the urinary, and central nervous systems. In the acute stage vomiting occurs, particularly on an empty stomach. This is because ethylene glycol is both nausea inducing and irritates the gastric mucosa. Vomiting usually prevents coma and death if frequent and complete. However fatal doses are usually retained. Stomach contents may be analysed for the presence of ethylene glycol but this is usually unrewarding.

Dehydration ataxia and weakness develop in the first 12–24 hours. In this form of poisoning animals often appear to recover transiently and then deteriorate. Polydipsia due to the rapid rise in serum osmolality stimulating the thirst centre is a major presenting sign. This is sufficient to lower serum total protein and the PCV, despite a secondary polyuria. Polyuria is the result of volume expansion and osmotic diuresis caused by renal excretion of unchanged ethylene glycol. It is also seen in those animals surviving the acute stage who become unable to concentrate.

Characteristically the cat often develops coffee coloured urine. Tachycardia and tachypnoea develop secondary to the acidosis. There is complete anorexia and with gastrointestinal tract irritation, the passage of semi-soft faeces may be seen. The fall in body temperature is thought to be due to the depressant effects of ethylene glycol. A decreased response to various reflexes, the flexor withdrawal, knuckling and righting reflex is accompanied by fine muscle tremors, particularly around the head and neck. Abdominal tenderness and miosis of the pupils may be seen.

Within twelve hours of ingestion the peracute case shows severe central nervous system depression, coma and terminally convulsions which are thought to be due to uraemia. Milder or more chronic cases where less than lethal amounts have been ingested, or where vomiting has eliminated most of the toxic principal, develop oliguric renal failure. Anorexia and oral ulceration are associated with a rising BUN. Encephalopathy may also be a feature.

DIAGNOSIS

Diagnosis is often difficult in the early stages due to the non-specific clinical signs, rapid metabolism and excretion. Renal azotaemia is not a significant finding of early intoxication but occurs 24–48 hours later. There is haemoconcentration due to clinical dehydration, lymphopenia due to uraemia and neutrophilia. The increase in segmented neutrophils is the result of endogenous steroid release following the central nervous system (CNS) depression and acidosis. Vomiting also augments the conticosteroid release.

Three hours after ingestion the concentration of phosphate in whole blood increases. Inconsistently a hyperglycaemia is due to the inhibition of glycolysis and the Krebs cycle by aldehydes. Concentration of sodium remains unchanged. Potassium increases and both bicarbonate and calcium fall. Hypocalcaemic tetany is unlikely because the metabolism of ethylene gycol keeps serum calcium at normal levels. Elevations in BUN (range 8–200 mmol/l) and creatinine (106–300 μmol/l) occur after the acidotic phase. Blood pH, base excess and P_{O_2} are useful monitors of response to therapy.

Table 1 POST-MORTEM FINDINGS

	Acute	*Chronic*
Gross findings	Inflammation and petechiation of gastric and intestinal mucosa.	Weight loss, dehydrated carcass, gastrointestinal tract haemorrhage.
	Pale swollen kidneys. On a dry weight basis, the kidney may contain >6% calcium oxalate. Uraemic pneumonitis-vascular congestion, pulmonary oedema and fibrin deposition.*	Pale granular kidneys.
Histology	Renal-congested glomeruli, lymphocytic infiltration of the interstitium. Vacuolization, necrosis, and sloughing of renal tubule epithelial cells with casts and irregular deposits of highly birefringent calcium oxalate crystals.	Regenerated tubule epithelium, numerous calcium oxalate crystals in the proximal and distal convoluted tubules and in the small end arteries of the brain and other organs. These do not initiate any tissue reaction.

* This is unrelated to the BUN and completely reversible when fluid therapy stops.

Characteristic urine changes include an acid pH, low specific gravity and proteinuria. On microscopic examination, red blood cells, white blood cells, epithelial cells granular casts and numerous six sided hippurate and insoluable calcium oxalate monohydrate crystals are seen. Ethylene glycol is not detectable in serum or urine after 24–48 hours.

Hippurate crystalluria is the result of an increased transanimation of glyoxalate to glycine. Calcium oxalate in monohydrate form is virtually indistinguishable from hippuric prisms under the light microscope. Electron microscopy, X-ray fluorescence or X-ray diffraction techniques are required to separate the two. Measurement of serum osmolality and the osmolar gap are frequently used as aids to early diagnosis. There are few other conditions in the dog that produce an osmolar gap of more than 100 mosm/kg.

In suspicious cases, or where information is unavailable to the clinician, from either the history, clinical signs or laboratory findings one should look hard for crystals in the urine or do a renal biopsy. Crystalluria is not pathognomic but when it occurs in other conditions, the presenting signs are likely to be different. Similarly, the presence of high levels of glycolic acid in serum, detected by high pressure liquid chromatography is diagnostic.

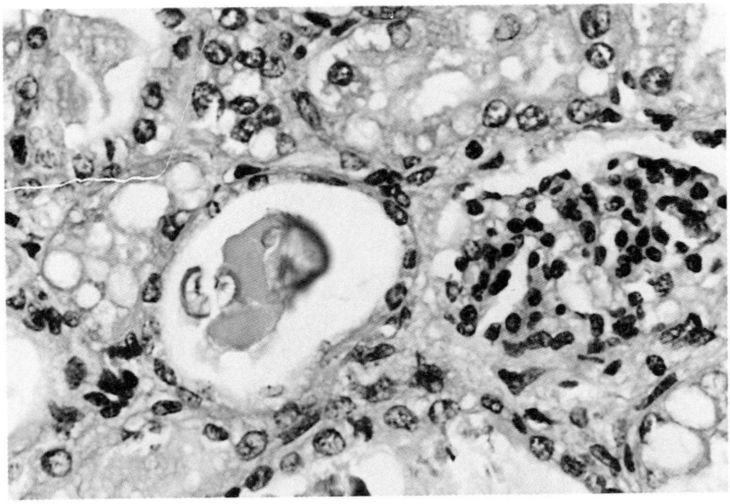

Fig. 2. Photomicrograph (× 400) of a histological section of renal cortex showing a congested glomerulus (right), and numerous degenerating renal tubules. In the centre, a dilated tubule is seen to contain crystals of calcium oxalate

TREATMENT

The immediate requirements are to prevent the further absorption and metabolism of ethylene glycol, to correct the metabolic acidosis and restore a correct fluid balance. If there is any delay such measures are empirical and often ineffective. Ethanol competes with ethylene glycol for the alcohol dehydrogenase enzyme system, thereby decreasing the amount of oxalate formed. Furthermore the solubility of calcium oxalate in urine is improved by various electrolytes and organic compounds, such as lactate citrate and hippurate. Ideally, if urine pH can be maintained above 7.5 with the administration of sodium bicarbonate this effectively increases urine concentrations of sodium and citrate. Alkalizing the urine promotes the combination of calcium and citrate ions, thus decreasing the amount of calcium available for combination with oxalate. Sodium bicarbonate acts also to restore normal blood pH. Both ethanol and bicarbonate must be given within four hours of ingestion of the toxic principal (see Table 2).

Table 2 THERAPEUTIC PROTOCOL FOR THE ADMINISTRATION OF ETHANOL AND SODIUM BICARBONATE

Dog	5.5ml 20% ethanol in saline per kg i.v. 8.0ml 5% $NaHCO_3^-$ per kg i.p.	every 4 hours for 5 treatments and then Q.I.D. for 5.
Cat	5.0 ml/kg ethanol i.p. 6.0 ml/kg HCO_3^- i.p.	every 6 hours for 5 treatments and then Q.I.D. for 5

The disadvantages of such treatment are primarily due to the chemical properties of ethanol and its effects on the CNS where it causes severe depression and coma. Ethanol also stimulates a diuresis further compromising an already dehydrated animal.

Alternatively, compounds inhibiting the alcohol dehydrogenase enzymes can be used. These include alkyldiols, e.g. 1,3, butanediol, pyrazoles such as 4 methyl pyrazole (dogs only), and disulfiram. These compounds are commonly used as food additives. They are relatively nontoxic, do not further depress the CNS or affect renal concentrating ability. 1,3, butanediol must be administered i.v. as an isotonic solution to avoid intravascular haemolysis. It can be given effectively up to 21 hours after ingestion. However, once sufficient numbers of calcium oxalate crystals have been deposited in the renal tubules, it has no therapeutic effects.

Ideally haemodialysis along with ethanol therapy would remove ethylene glycol and its by-products. However, it is rarely available. Peritoneal dialysis operates in a more primitive but similar fashion, and also corrects the uraemia and acidosis. Patients presented early enough (i.e. within 3 hours of ingestion) are treated symptomatically, firstly with emetics, provided coordination, postural and gag reflexes are intact, followed by saline catharctics and activated charcoal preparations. Fluids given to correct the dehydration and acidosis promote the excretion of unchanged ethylene glycol and its breakdown products. CVP or urine output should be monitored to prevent fluid overload.

After hydration is restored or if an oliguric state exists, diuretics and continued controlled fluid administration may relieve the obstruction of tubules by cellular debris and casts. Co-factors pyridoxine and thiamine may be given to divert glyoxylic acid into alternative routes of metabolism that avoid the formation of oxalic acid.

Magnesium may be given to reduce the solubility of calcium oxalate and hence its precipitation. Likewise, the chemical properties of DMSO can be used to advantage. Anticonvulsants are used to control convulsions.

PROGNOSIS

A high death rate is associated with ethylene glycol poisoning due to its rapid metabolism and the delay in presentation and therapy. Because of individual variation in absorption and metabolism, the time interval within which therapy will be successful is difficult to predict. Twelve hours from the time of ingestion is the suggested limit. The treatment itself is not ideal, because an already depressed animal is given another CNS depressant. Similarly, although there may be some regeneration of renal tubular epithelium, a poor response to treatment is seen in anuric cases. A daily decrease in BUN and creatinine levels is a good prognostic sign. Renal oxalosis is often fatal in animals surviving the acidotic phase. Although large numbers of calcium oxalate crystals may be seen in biopsy specimens of dogs that survive, these gradually disappear. Chronic fibrosing renal damage can occur, thus long term dietary management is important.

Because cats succumb to a fraction of the dose lethal for dogs, it is anticipated that many die before reaching home or veterinary attention. Many such fatalities could be avoided by improved awareness of such compounds.

FURTHER READING

Beasley, R. V., Buck, W. B. (1980) Acute ethylene glycol toxicosis: a review. *Vet. Human Toxicol.*, **22**, 255

Beasley, R. V. (1985) Diagnosis and management of ethylene glycol poisoning. *Feline Practice*, **15**, 41

Beckett, S. D., Shields, R. P. (1971) Treatment of acute ethylene glycol toxicosis in the dog. *J. Am. Vet. Med. Assoc.*, **158**, 179

Clarke, E. G. C. (1979) Chapter 17 In *Canine Medicine and Therapeutics*, 1st edn (ed. E. A. Chandler) Blackwell, Oxford

Clarke, M. L., Harvey, D. G., Humphreys, P. J. (1981) In *Veterinary Toxicology*, 2nd edn, Baillier Tindall, London, p. 177

Ettinger, S. J., Feldman, E. C. (1977) Ethylene glycol poisoning in a dog. *Mod. Vet. Pract.*, **58**, 237

Grauer, G. S., Thrall, M. A., Henre, B. A., Grauer, R. M., Hamar, D. W. (1984) Early clinicopathological findings in dogs ingesting ethylene glycol. *J. Am. Vet. Med. Assoc.*, **45**, 2299

Hamlin, R. (1987) Ethylene glycol poisoning in a cat. *Clinical Insight*, **2**, 636

Moriarty, R. W., McDonald, R. H. (1974) The spectrum of ethylene glycol poisoning. *Clin. Toxicol.*, **7**, 583

Sanyer, J. L., Oeheme, S. W., McGavin, M. D. (1973) Systemic treatment of ethylene glycol toxicosis in dogs. *J. Am. Vet. Med. Assoc.*, **34**, 527

Thrall, M. A., Grauer, G. F., Mero, K. N. (1984) Clinicopathologic findings in dogs and cats with ethylene glycol poisoning. *J. Am. Vet. Med. Assoc.* **184**, 37

RUTH DENNIS

Radiology of metabolic bone disease

BONE IS a living tissue which normally has a high degree of metabolic activity and is continually remodelling. This process may be influenced by many circulating substances including minerals, vitamins and hormones, some of which interact.

The subject of metabolic bone disease is complicated by the inconsistent use throughout pathological and clinical literature of the terms osteoporosis, osteomalacia, osteopaenia and osteodystrophy. *Osteoporosis* is a deficiency of osteoid, the organic bone matrix, which means that there is no framework for the deposition of mineral salts. There is therefore, an equal reduction in both osteoid and mineral and so remaining bone is sparse but structurally normal. *Osteomalacia* (literally softening of bones) is a failure of normal mineralization of osteoid, which is present in excessive amounts with a corresponding reduction in the mineral content of bone.

Radiography only demonstrates the mineral content of bone and not the radiolucent osteoid. Thus both osteoporosis and osteomalacia result in decreased radiographic bone density, technically called *osteopaenia*. Differentiation between them can usually only be made histologically. Unfortunately the word osteoporosis rather than osteopaenia is often used as the general term to describe this radiographic appearance.

Osteodystrophy is defined simply as defective formation of bone (Williams and Wilkins, 1972), and appears in the names of several diseases of different aetiologies.

Metabolic bone diseases include both primary bone conditions (e.g., hypertrophic osteodystrophy) and those including bone secondarily (e.g., nutritional secondary hyperparathyroidism). Metabolic disease should be suspected when bone changes are multifocal or diffuse. Solitary lesions are unlikely to be due to metabolic causes.

OSTEOPAENIA (OSTEOPOROSIS)

Osteopaenia is a lesion rather than a specific disease and represents an imbalance between bone production and resorption. Some causes are listed below:
Hyperparathyroidism (primary or secondary)
Pseudohyperparathyroidism (e.g. lymphosarcoma, perianal adenocarcinoma)
Cushing's disease or long-term corticosteroid therapy
Disuse or immobility
Starvation or parasitism
Senility
Hypo- or hyperthyroidism
Diabetes mellitus
Hepatic toxicity
Multiple myeloma

Pituitary dwarfism (growth hormone deficiency)
Oestrogen deficiency
Certain anti-convulsant drugs

Subjective radiographic diagnosis of osteopaenia is difficult, especially if the change is mild or diffuse. Radiography is not a sensitive technique for detecting bone loss because 30–70% of the mineral content of bone may be removed before osteopaenia is detected radiographically. Comparison with previous films of the same animal or with films of a litter mate may be helpful.

Osteopaenia mainly affects bones with a high cancellous component such as vertebrae, flat bones of the skull, scapulae, the ilial wings and the metaphyses of long bones. Resorption of cancellous bone reveals those trabeculae which are most important with respect to weight-bearing stresses. Cortical bone resorption also occurs and results in thinning of the cortices and corollary widening of the medullary cavities. In severe cases the bones are fragile and susceptible to folding or compression fractures with resulting deformity (see section on hyperparathyroidism).

The main radiographic feature of osteopaenia is a reduction in bone density. This must be differentiated from artefactual osteopaenia due to overexposure, excessive scatter or overdevelopment of the film. Differentiation can usually be achieved by comparison with the radiographic density of the adjacent soft tissues. The bones appear 'ghost-like' with wide medullary cavities and thin, shell-like cortices. In the spine, where the change is often most evident, the vertebral end-plates and articular facets are relatively spared, producing marked contrast with the osteopaenic spinous processes, neural arches and vertebral bodies (Figure 1). The trabecular pattern, where still present, is coarse due to increased prominence of remaining trabeculae.

If osteoporosis occurs in young animals due to protein or energy deficiency, characteristic transverse striations or arrest lines may be present in the metaphyses. These are due to intermittent cessation and re-activation of physeal growth.

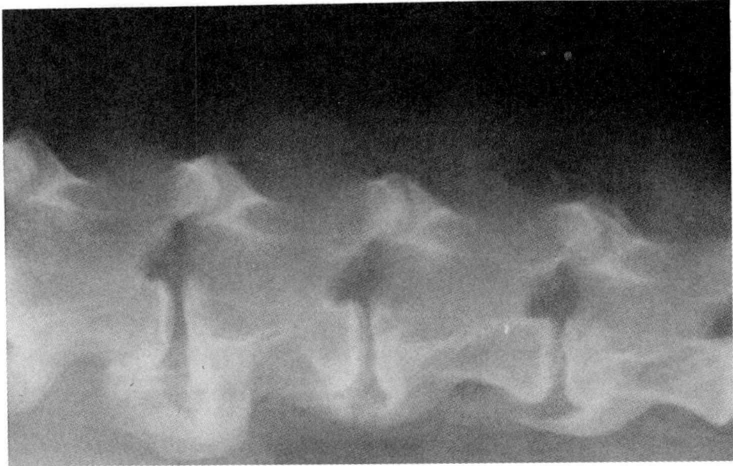

Fig. 1. Mid-lumbar vertebrae of a 9-year old Labrador bitch with osteoporosis due to Cushing's disease. There is a reduction in bone density of the spinous processes, neural arches and vertebral bodies with relative sparing of the articular facets and end plates

DISUSE OSTEOPOROSIS

Disuse osteoporosis is usually confined to a single limb, following paralysis or fracture and immobilization. Marked bone resorption is evident radiographically, especially distal to any fracture site, with epiphyses and carpal and tarsal bones being most severely affected. This condition is common in toy breeds of dogs following non-union of radial and ulnar fractures (Figure 2). Generalized skeletal osteoporosis may also occur following prolonged recumbency or inactivity. Disuse osteoporosis is reversed as the affected part returns to use.

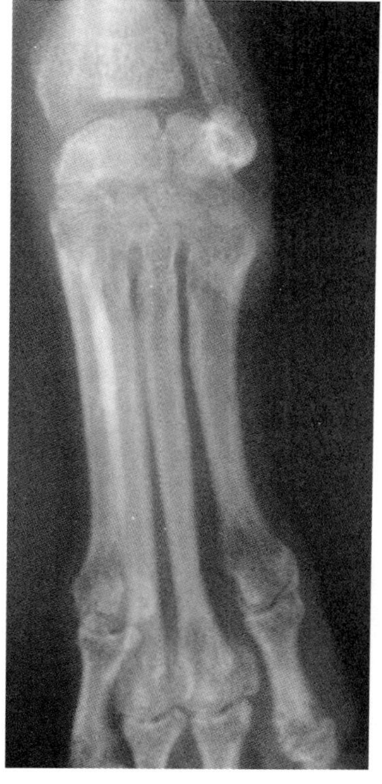

Fig. 2. Lower forelimb of a 13-month old papillon which suffered a non-union of radial and ulnar fractures following an unsuccessful radial pinnning. Disuse osteoporosis is evident in the carpal bones and metacarpal epiphyses, seen as a reduction in bone density with cortical thinning and coarse trabeculation

HYPERPARATHYROIDISM

PRIMARY HYPERPARATHYROIDISM

Primary hyperparathyroidism is a rare condition which occurs when there is functional hyperplasia or neoplasia of the parathyroid gland.

SECONDARY HYPERPARATHYROIDISM

Secondary hyperparathyroidism is more common. It is due to stimulation of the parathyroid glands by nutritional or renal metabolic derangements which result in hypocalcaemia. Nutritional secondary hyperparathyroidism (nutritional/juvenile osteodystrophy or osteoporosis; osteitis fibrosa) is caused by an imbalance between dietary calcium and phosphorus. It is usually seen in small animals fed on high-meat diets. It occurs most often in young animals a few weeks after weaning when skeletal demands are high. The condition is occasionally seen in young horses fed on grain and bran diets which are high in phosphorus and therefore induce hypocalcaemia (synonyms bran disease; Miller's disease; Big Head).

Renal secondary hyperparathyroidism (renal osteodystrophy; renal rickets; rubber jaw) is seen in dogs with chronic renal failure. It predominates in young dogs with congenital renal abnormalities. It is seldom seen in other species. Reduced glomerular filtration rate causes phosphate retention and secondary hypocalcaemia.

All types of hyperparathyroidism cause osteodystrophia fibrosa, a condition of extensive bone resorption and fibro-osseous tissue formation. The changes which occur are similar whatever the cause, although the relative severity in different parts of the skeleton varies. Skull changes predominate in the renal form and in horses. Limb and spinal lesions are more obvious in the nutritional form in small animals.

Radiographically, there is generalized osteopaenia with reduction in bone density, cortical thinning and coarse trabeculation. Growth plates are unaffected. Bone fragility may lead to pathological folding fractures of long bones and compression fractures of vertebrae causing orthopaedic and neurological signs. Pathological fractures are seen as irregular sclerotic bands running transversely or obliquely across affected bones with minimal callus formation (Figures 3 and 4). Long bones may deviate as the fracture sites and vertebrae become shorter than normal. Sternal and rib cage deformities, lordosis and pelvic collapse leading to constipation may also be evident.

Skull bones, particularly maxillae and mandibles, are also affected resulting in a 'moth-eaten' appearance on X-ray. Bone resorption occurs initially around the dental

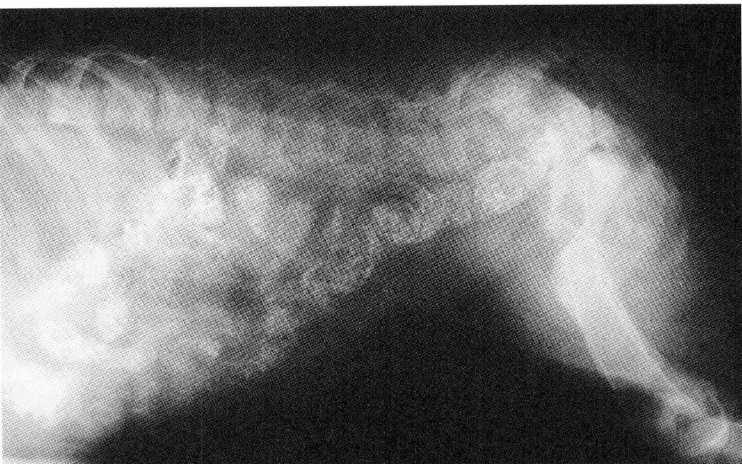

Fig. 3. Lateral abdominal radiograph of a 13 week old Afghan puppy with nutritional secondary hyperparathyroidsim. There is a generalized reduction in bone density compared with the soft tissues. Coritical thinning is evident and there is a deforming folding fracture of one of the femora. Bone meal has been fed to the puppy therapeutically, and is visiable in the gut

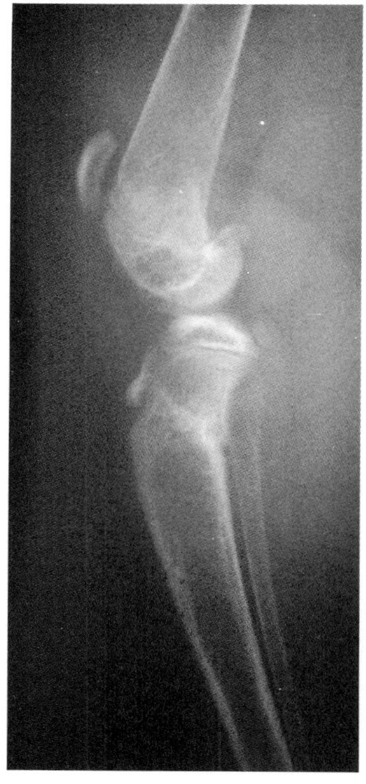

Fig. 4. Lateral stifle radiograph of a 6-month old
Chinchilla cat with nutritional secondary
hyperparathroidism. There is a pathological folding
fracture in the proximal tibia which is seen as an
irregular oblique sclerotic line. Cortical thinning and
coarse trabeculation are also evident

alveoli causing loss of the lamina dura and giving the appearance of floating teeth. The
mandibles become rubbery in texture and facial swelling occurs. In some cases
respiratory difficulty results from obliteration of the nasal cavity by fibrous dysplasia
of the turbinates, which is evident radiographically (Figure 5).

HYPERTROPHIC OSTEODYSTROPHY

Hypertrophic osteodystrophy is also known as metaphyseal osteopathy or juvenile
scurvy and Moller–Barlow's disease. It affects large breeds of dogs between the
ages of three and seven months. Its aetiology is uncertain, but nutritional over-
supplementation may be a major factor. The clinical signs include variable lameness
with metaphyseal heat, pain and swelling, pyrexia, depression, anorexia and weight
loss.

The metaphyses of any appendicular bone may be involved but distal radial, ulnar
and tibial sites are most commonly affected. Occasionally the mandibles, maxillae,
costochondral junctions, scapulae and ilia show changes. Necrosis of metaphyseal
bone occurs. This appears radiographically as an irregular, transverse, radiolucent
band within the metaphysis often with sclerotic borders (Trummelfeldzone, scorbutic
lattice) (Figure 6a) Adjacent growth plates and epiphyses are unaffected. Later in the
disease an irregular collar of mineralization forms around the metaphysis, sometimes

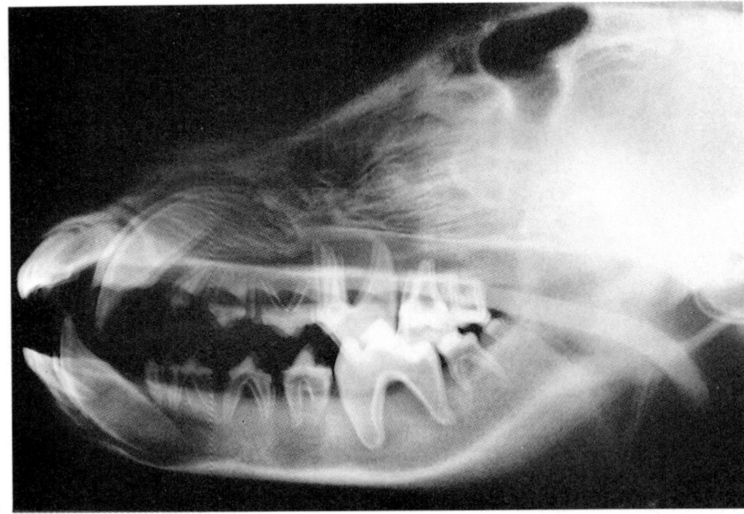

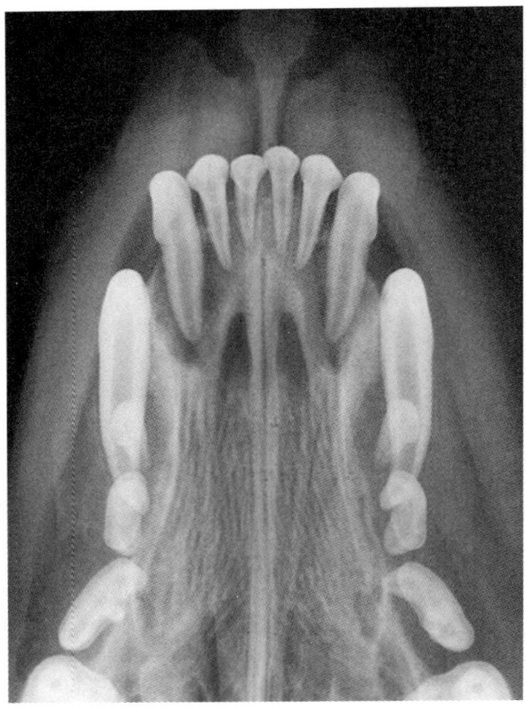

Fig. 5 (a) Later skull radiograph of a 6-month-old Dalmatian with renal secondary hyperparathyroidism. There is generalized bone resorption producing a 'moth-eaten' appearance to the skull bones. Bone loss is particularly evident around the tooth roots. Note the relative prominance of the soft tissues as a result of the bone loss. (b) Intra-oral flm of the upper jaw of a 9-year old Dalmatian with renal secondary hyperparathyroidism. Alvelar bone resorption has resulted in the appearance of 'floating' teeth. The nasal turbinate pattern is blurred due to fibrous change

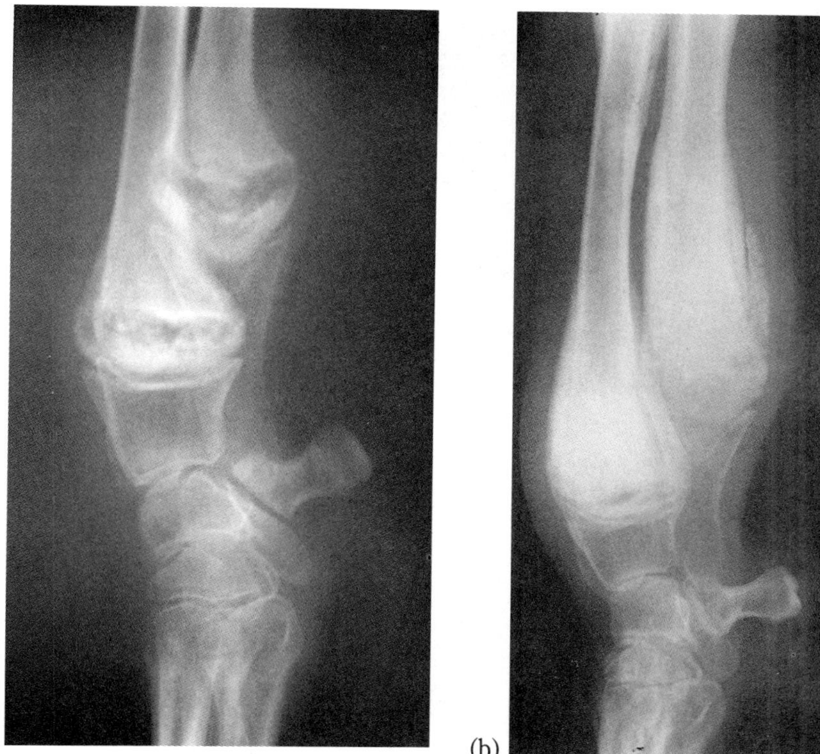

Fig. 6 (a) Distal forearm and carpus of a 15-week old Afghan puppy with hypertrophic osteodystrophy. Irregular radiolucent bands with sclerotic margins are present in the distal radial and ulnar metaphyses. The growth plates are normal. (b) A later stage of hypertrophic osteodystrophy in the distal forearm of a 9-year-old German Shepherd dog. An area of irregular mineralization is visible caudal to the distal ulnar metaphysis. Previous areas of mineralization have remodelled into the cortices of both radius and ulna causing widening of the affected areas and apparent sclerosis due to superimposition. Both (a) and (b) show a degree of osteopaenia in the carpal bones

separated from it by a narrow radiolucent line. This is due to mineralization of associated subperiosteal and extraperiosteal cellular debris and haemorrhage. It subsequently remodels, becoming incorporated into the cortex and often results in metaphyseal widening. Several different areas of mineralization at different stages of remodelling may be seen due to the episodic nature of the disease. Occasionally, diaphyseal cortices may appear thin with bone demineralization, although this may be partly due to disuse osteoporosis (Figure 6b).

The condition is self-limiting and most cases recover. Severe cases may show slowing of physeal growth (especially in the distal ulna) with subsequent angular limb deformities.

RICKETS (JUVENILE OSTEOMALACIA)

Rickets is a disease of young weaned animals and is due to a deficiency of dietary phosphorus or vitamin D. It is now very rare in small animals because of the widespread use of commercial diets. The pathogenesis is a failure of mineralization of cartilage with persistence of growth plate cartilage and epiphyseal collapse. Radiographically, the growth plates are deeper and broader than normal with ragged margination. Metaphyses flare and become mushroom-shaped. Epiphyses are flattened and irregular (Figure 7). The lesions are most prominent in areas of rapid growth, e.g. distal radius and ulna. Long bones show demineralization and may bend or fracture. Retardation of diaphyseal growth leads to a dwarfing in stature, and epiphyseal damage may cause osteoarthrosis. The condition is similar radiographically to the inherited condition of enchondrodystrophy in the English Pointer (Whitbread *et al.*, 1983)

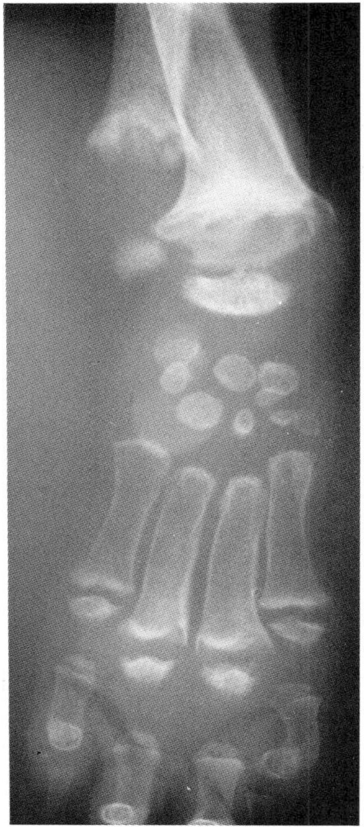

Fig. 7. Craniocaudal view of the lower forelimb of a 4-week old Labrador puppy with rickets. The growth plates are wider than normal and show ragged margination. Metaphyseal flaring and epiphyseal irregularity is also evident

HYPERTROPHIC PULMONARY OSTEOPATHY/OSTEOARTHROPATHY (HPO)

This is also known as Acropachia or Maries disease. HPO is a generalized osteoproductive disorder of the periosteum which is seen in both man and domestic animals in response to the presence of chronic thoracic or occasionally abdominal lesions. Neurogenic and humoral mechanisms have been suggested.

Radiographically spicular, nodular or cauliflower-like periosteal new bone is seen, often at right-angles to the cortex. This produces a characteristic palisade appearance (Figure 8). Later, the new bone may remodel and lamellate. Overlying soft tissue swelling is evident. The changes are bilaterally symmetrical and occur along the shafts of the long bones affecting distal limbs first. In the paws the abaxial surfaces of bones are usually more severely affected than the axial surfaces. The carpal and tarsal bones are usually spared, as are the joints. Occasional involvement of the axial skeleton is seen. The lesions are progressive but rapidly regress if the underlying cause is removed. Differential diagnoses include early bone tumours, osteomyelitis, hypertrophic osteodystrophy, panosteitis and hypervitaminosis A.

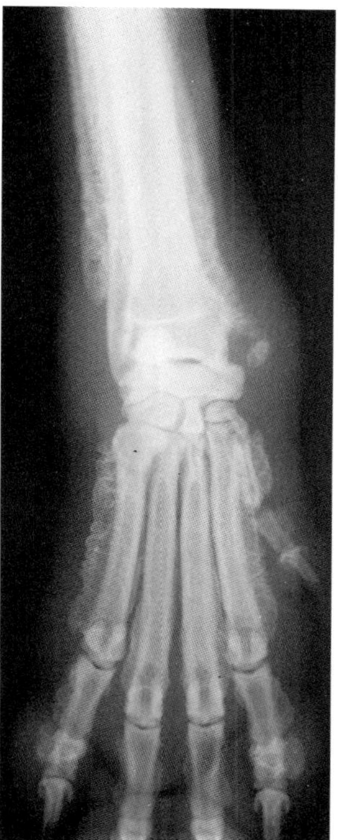

Fig. 8. Lower forelimb of a 7-year-old Labrador with hypertrophic pulmonary osteopathy. Substantial palisading periosteal new bone extends along the shafts of all the long bones. In the foot the new bone is deepest on the abaxial surfaces. Overlying soft tissue swelling is present

HYPERVITAMINOSIS A

Hypervitaminosis A is also known as feline osteodystrophy, osteodystrophy of vitamin A poisoning and deforming cervical spondylosis of the cat. It is usually seen in young adult cats fed a diet rich in liver, although occasionally there is no history of dietary imbalance. The condition has been reported in dogs but is rare.

Excess Vitamin A provokes the formation of periosteal new bone which forms principally on vertebrae and around limb joints and is easily demonstrated radiographically. There is no bone destruction. In the vertebral column characteristic exostoses are seen around the affected area. These may become very large and cause ankylosis of synovial joints. The cervical area is usually most severely affected. (Figure 9). Periosteal reaction and soft tissue calcification (e.g. of the stifle joint fat pad) may occur around limb joints, especially the elbow, hip and stifle. It can cause ankylosis and reduced limb movement. Occasionally the sternum and ribs are affected.

Varying degrees of osteopaenia may be evident radiographically due to disuse or concomitant nutritional secondary hyperparathyroidism. Clinical signs depend on the sites of the lesions and include stiffness, lameness, the adoption of a characteristic kangaroo-like sitting posture, neck pain and cutaneous hyperaesthesia or anaesthesia. Severe cases may be crippled.

Differential diagnoses are spondylosis and mucopolysaccharidosis for the vertebral lesions and osteomata and osteoarthrosis for those in the limbs.

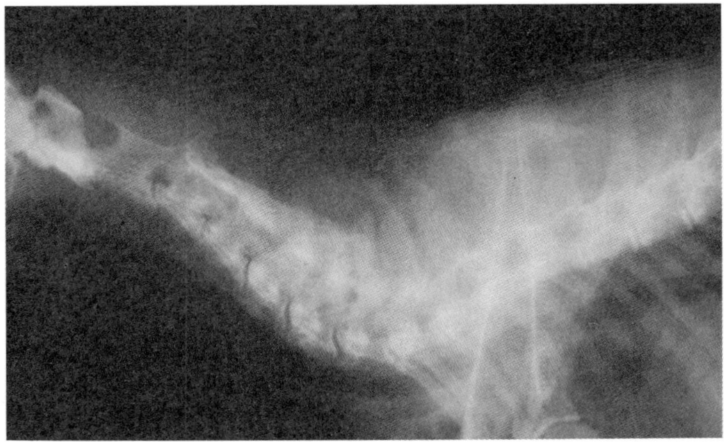

Fig. 9. Hypervitaminosis A in a cat fed on excessive amounts of liver. Deforming exostoses surround the cervical spine causing partial fusion of adjacent vertebrae

MUCOPOLYSACCHARIDOSIS

The mucopolysaccharidoses are a group of lysosomal storage diseases which lead to abnormalities of connective tissue. Two types have been recognized in Siamese and part-Siamese cats. The condition has also been reported as a rare occurrence in dogs. Clinical signs include characteristic flattening of the face, corneal clouding, pectus excavatum, hydrocephalus, posterior ataxia or paresis and generalized skeletal deformities with dwarfism.

Skeletal changes are evident radiographically by six months and consist primarily of spinal changes, with proliferative exostoses causing widening and fusion of vertebral bodies and spinous processes, especially in the cervical spine (Figure 10). Some vertebrae may be short and misshapen with widening of intervertebral spaces, due to epiphyseal dysplasia. The odontoid peg may be hypoplastic. Epiphyseal

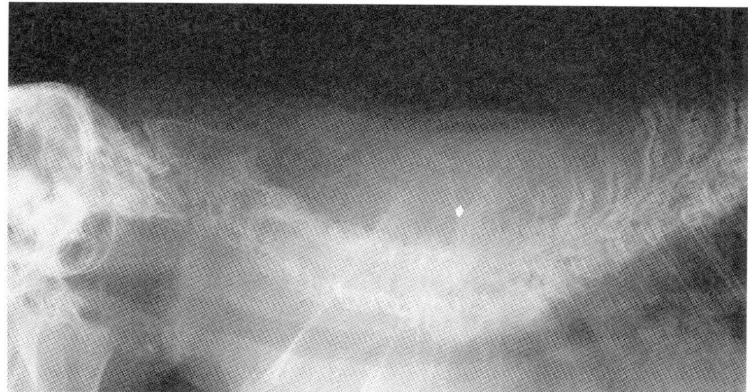

Fig. 10. Mucoploysaccharidosis in a 2-year-old part-Siamese cat. Irregular new bone surrounds cervical and thoracic vertebrae causing ankylosis. The changes are similar to those seen in hypervitaminosis A but are usually more extensive and in this cat involved the whole spine

dysplasia also occurs in the limbs leading to widening and irregularity of epiphyses and osteoarthrosis. Ribs may broaden at the costochondral junctions and hip dysplasia is common. The condition is progressive.

CONGENITAL HYPOTHYROIDISM (CRETINISM)

Congenital hypothyroidism is a rare condition which has been reported in dogs, cats and horses. Boxers appear to be over-represented. Thyroxine deficiency in the immature animal causes retardation in the development of bones forming by endochondral ossification, and affected animals show disproportionate dwarfism. As is humans, the clinical signs are weakness, apathy, mental dullness and myxoedema. A juvenile hair coat persists.

The characteristic radiographic changes include delayed appearance of the limb epiphyses, carpal and tarsal bones. These are irregular and fragmented and produce a stippled appearance. Some ossification centres may be absent and growth plate closure is delayed. Long bones are short and wide with thickened cortices. Epiphyseal dysplasia also occurs in the vertebrae and produces 'beaking' of the end plates (Figure 11). Thoracolumbar kyphosis may be present. Hydrocephalus is sometimes seen.

Affected animals respond well to L-thyroxine supplementation, but the epiphyseal changes lead to residual osteoarthrosis.

PITUITARY DWARFISM

Pituitary dwarfism is caused by a lack of growth hormone. It is encountered in German Shepherd dogs and occasionally in other breeds. It results in proportionate dwarfing with retention of puppy hair. Radiographically, the growth plates show delayed closure and remain open in excess of eighteen months. Generalized

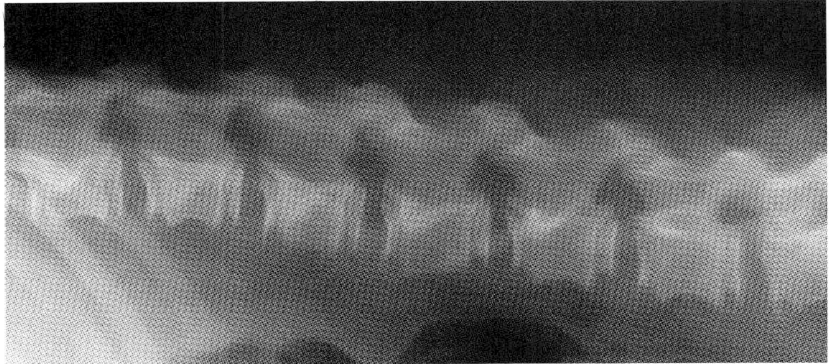

Fig. 11. Lumbar spine of an 8-month-old boxer suffering from congential hypothroidism. Vertebral growth plates have not yet fused and the epiphyses are in completely ossified resulting in ventral spurring

osteopaenia may be evident. There is delayed mineralization of the os penis, which normally occurs at four to five months.

OSTEOGENESIS IMPERFECTA

Osteogenesis imperfecta is an inherited condition of abnormal collagen metabolism and results in bone fragility due to osteoporosis, with multiple fractures. It is one of the most common inherited skeletal disorders in humans but is much less common in domestic animals. Nutritional secondary hyperparathyroidism is sometimes incorrectly given the name osteogenesis imperfecta.

REFERENCES AND FURTHER READING

Ettinger (ed.) (1983) *Textbook of Veterinary International Medicine,* 2nd edition. W. B. Saunders Company, Philadelphia, Chapter 85
Jubb, Kennedy and Palmer (1987) *Pathology of Domestic Animals,* 3rd edition. Academic Press Inc., Chapter 1
Kealy, K. (1987) *Diagnostic Radiology of the Dog and Cat,* 2nd edition. W. B. Saunders Company, Philadelphia
Morgan, Joe P. (1972) *Radiology in Veterinary Orthopaedics,* Lea and Febiger
Newton, C. D. and Nunamaker, D. M. (1985) *Textbook of Small Animal Orthopaedic,* J. B. Lippincott Company
Owens, Jerry M. (1982) *Radiographic Interpretation for the Small Animal Clinician.* Ralston Purina Company
Sumner-Smith (ed.) (1982) *Bone in Clinical Orthopaedics; a Study in Comparative Osteology.* W. B. Saunders Company, Philadelphia
Thrall, W. B. (ed.) (1986) *Textbook of Veterinary Diagnostic Radiology,* W. B. Saunders Company, Philadelphia
Stedman's Medical Dictionary (1972) 22nd edition. Williams and Wilkins Company, Baltimore
Whitbread, T. J., Gill, J. J. B. and Lewis, D. G. (1983) *J. Small Animal Pract.,* **24,** 399–411

CHRISTOPHER MAY

Osteochondrosis in the dog: a review

INTRODUCTION

OSTEOCHONDROSIS WAS originally defined as a generalized skeletal disturbance of either physeal or articular cartilage, caused by defective endochondral ossification (Olsson, 1976). In certain instances, this may result in the development of a dissecting flap of articular cartillage and mild inflammatory changes in the synovial membrane. This presentation is termed osteochondritis dissecans (OCD). This nomenclature is somewhat vague and unhelpful in describing the pathology, but it is now used to describe a range of lesions in which the underlying aetiopathogenesis is poorly understood.

Osteochondrosis is an important cause of lameness in young dogs. It manifests at well recognized sites in certain joints (Table 1). The condition has been recorded in small dogs (Johnson *et al.*, 1980; Bennett, 1984) but it is primarily a problem in medium-sized to large breeds (Hayes *et al.*, 1979). There is a predisposition in males (Vaughan and Jones, 1968; Jones and Vaughan, 1970; Hayes *et al.*, 1979), with a male: female ratio in the range 2:1 to 4:1 (Olsson, 1975b; 1976; Robins, 1978; 1980; Mason *et al.*, 1980; Boudrieau, *et al.*, 1983). Different breeds are associated with different forms of osteochondrosis (Bennett *et al.*, 1981). Bennett (1984) considered that variation in breed postures could be an influencing factor by causing abnormal loading or trauma at particular joints.

The aetiology of osteochondrosis is not yet fully understood. It is probably multifactorial. A genetic capacity for rapid growth and a large mature body weight are important factors and it is likely that trauma plays a role in manifesting the clinical disease, hence the predisposition in large breeds and in males which generally grow more rapidly than females. In the dog, and in other species, there is an association between high caloric intake and an increased risk of developing the disease (Reiland, 1975; Grondalen and Vangen, 1974; Hedhammer *et al.*, 1974). Some experimental studies have implicated hormonal factors (Patsaama *et al.*, 1971), although the concentrations of hormones used in this work were outside the normal physiological range.

PATHOLOGY

Metaphyseal bone growth occurs by the process of endochondral ossification (vascularization followed by ossification of a cartilage precursor) at the physis. Epiphyseal growth occurs similarly by endochondral ossification from the deep layers of the articular cartilage. In osteochondrosis the cartilage is thought to become regionally thickened in response to a localized increase in pressure and/or tension at the predisposition sites (Olsson 1975a; 1975b; 1976; 1977; 1983; Boudrieau *et al.*, 1983). The differentiation of chondrocytes is delayed in these thickened zones and consequently the process of blood vessel penetration and calcification fails. Normal developing cartilage initially receives nutrients by diffusion from the synovial fluid and later from blood vessels in the subchondral bone. Hence, in the thickened areas, chondrocytes become malnourished and may undergo necrosis. The affected zone becomes apparent on radiographs as a lucent defect surrounded by the normal bone density of ossifying chondrocytes. Necrosis of chondrocytes deep in the articular cartilage results in the formation of a horizontal cleft which, with subsequent loading, leads to the development of vertical fissures and the release of degradation products into the joint causing synovial inflammation. In this way a cartilaginous flap is formed. This can fragment to produce a single loose body or several loose bodies within the joint. These 'joint mice' may increase in size and calcify or they can be gradually resorbed from the joint cavity (Olsson, 1975a; 1975b; 1976; 1983; Bennett, 1984). This process will result in secondary degenerative joint disease.

Similar pathology involving a delay in ossification of the cartilage precursor at growth plates may be a factor in separation of the anconeal process and a number of other clinical problems (Tables 1 and 2), which can therefore be attributed to osteochondrosis.

Table 1 OSTEOCHONDROSIS LESIONS OF THE DOG

Joint	*Lesion*
Shoulder	Caudolateral aspect of humeral head
Elbow	Medial condyle of humerus
	Coronoid process of ulna
	Anconeal process of ulna
Stifle	Lateral or medial condyle of femur
Hock	Medial or lateral ridge of tibial tarsal bone

Table 2 OTHERS LESIONS ASSOCIATED WITH OSTEOCHONDROSIS IN THE DOG

Lesion	*Reference*
Distal radius	Butler *et al.*, 1971
Articular processes of cervical vertebrae	Hedhammar *et al.*, 1974
Dorsolateral rim of acetabulum	Olsson, 1976
Slipped proximal femoral epiphysis	Lee, 1976; Bennett, 1984
Medial malleolus of tibia	Rosenblum *et al.*, 1978
Medial epicondyle of humerus	Bennett, 1984
Limb deformity following growth plate involvement	Bennett, 1984
Caudo-medial rim of glenoid	Bennett, 1984
Femoral head	McDonald, 1988

CLINICAL FINDINGS

The disease is typically seen in large breed dogs, particularly males, and the onset of signs usually occurs between four and eight months of age (Vaughan and Jones, 1968). In most dogs there is a gradual onset of lameness in one or more limbs. However, in some cases there is an association with a traumatic episode (Hohn, 1973) and the lameness may be sudden in onset. The severity of lameness is variable, but stiffness after rest is a common feature. The problem is often exacerbated by exercise. In long-standing cases, muscle atrophy may be appreciated and this is particularly evident in the supraspinatus and infraspinatus muscles when the forelimb is affected (Vaughan and Jones, 1968; Leighton, 1971; Hohn, 1973; Robins, 1978).

In certain instances postural abnormalities can be recognized. For example, with OCD of the tibio-tarsal joint there is marked hyperextension of the hock (Alexander *et al.*, 1981). Lesions of the elbow may result in abduction of the foot with the elbow maintained close to the chest when standing (Bennett, 1984; Mason *et al.*, 1980; Boudrieau *et al.*, 1983; Olsson, 1983). However, during the 'swinging leg' phase of the gait, cases with osteochondrosis of the elbow typically show abduction of the joint (Boudrieau *et al.*, 1983).

Pain can usually be elicited by palpation and manipulation of the joint through its range of movement. It may be difficult to differentiate pain in the shoulder and elbow and it is sometimes necessary to radiograph both of these joints to establish which is involved. Reduction in the joint range of motion is not a feature of most cases, although it is recorded in OCD of the hock (Rosenblum *et al.*, 1978; Bennett, 1984), and stifle (Denny and Gibbs, 1980a; Robins, 1970). Crepitus and joint enlargement due to synovial effusion and periarticular soft tissue thickening are common. Clinical signs are not pathognomonic, and osteochondrosis must be confirmed radiographically (Robins, 1978; Bennett *et al.*, 1981).

RADIOGRAPHY

Good quality radiographs are an essential prerequisite to the early diagnosis of osteochondrosis. This usually necessitates general anaesthesia of the dog so that it may be safely and accurately positioned (Robins, 1978; Johnson *et al.*, 1980; Mason *et al.*, 1980; Alexander *et al.*, 1981; Bennett *et al.*, 1981; Olsson, 1983). The condition is frequently bilateral. Hence radiography of the opposite joint is indicated in all cases even when no clinical signs are evident in that limb (Vaughan and Jones, 1968).

SHOULDER

The medio-lateral projection is most useful to demonstrate a loss of the normal contour on the caudal aspect of the humeral head (Figure 1). Typically there is localized rarefaction of the subchondral bone with a varying degree of surrounding sclerosis. However, in early or mild disease, the humeral head may simply appear flattened. In some dogs the lesion is located on the caudo-lateral aspect of the humeral head where it can be difficult to identify radiographically.

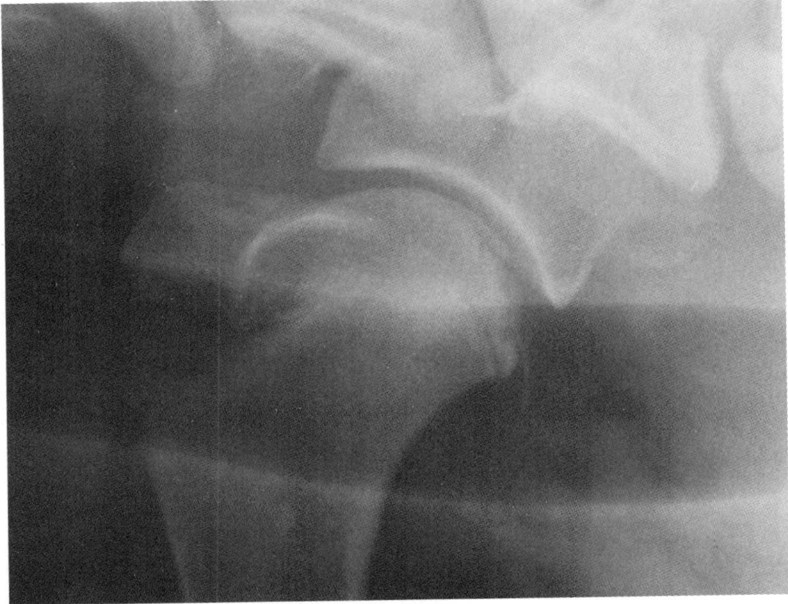

Fig. 1. Lateral radiograph of shoulder showing typical OCD lesion.

If there is calcification of a cartilage flap it is usually seen overlying the defect although it may become detached and frequently lodges in the caudal pouch of the joint capsule where it is readily recognized. Positive contrast arthrography may be useful in some cases to outline a cartilage flap which has not calcified and which cannot be seen on the plain films, or to demonstrate the extent of a lesion prior to surgery (Robins, 1978).

ELBOW

Olsson (1983) advocates radiological investigation in all cases of lameness showing even slight signs from the elbow joint and he considers the medial oblique cranio-caudal view and the fully flexed medio-lateral view essential. Robins (1980) argues that superimposition of bones in the elbow joint makes radiographic interpretation difficult and he proposes that five projections are necessary for routine survey of the elbow.
1. Medio-lateral extended.
2. Medio-lateral flexed.
3. Cranio-caudal.
4. Cranio-caudal medial oblique.
5. Cranio-caudal lateral oblique.
In most cases, two projections (cranio-caudal and medial-lateral flexed) are adequate, but additional views should be considered in difficult cases.

A fragmented coronoid process is not usually visible radiographically and diagnosis is based on the identification of secondary osteophytes (Robins, 1980; Boudrieau *et al.*, 1983; Olsson, 1983; Bennett, 1984). These are most readily seen on the margin of the anconeal process in the flexed medio-lateral position. They are often not present until the dog is seven or eight months old (Figure 2). Many animals will initially present at four or five months of age, when they have no discernible radiographic changes. A repeat examination two months later is indicated in these cases.

Osteochondritis dissecans of the medial humeral condyle is most readily identified on the medial oblique cranio-caudal view as a radiolucent defect resembling that seen in OCD of the shoulder. On a well positioned and exposed radiograph this lesion can be identified in animals only five or six months old. Free calcified bodies are sometimes associated with the lesion and secondary osteophytes will occur. They are most apparent on the anconeal process (Figure 2).

Ununited anconeal process is readily diagnosed on the medio-lateral projection (Figure 3). Union should occur by 18–20 weeks of age. Failure will lead to secondary degenerative changes with subsequent osteophyte formation as outlined for other manifestations of osteochondrosis in the elbow joint.

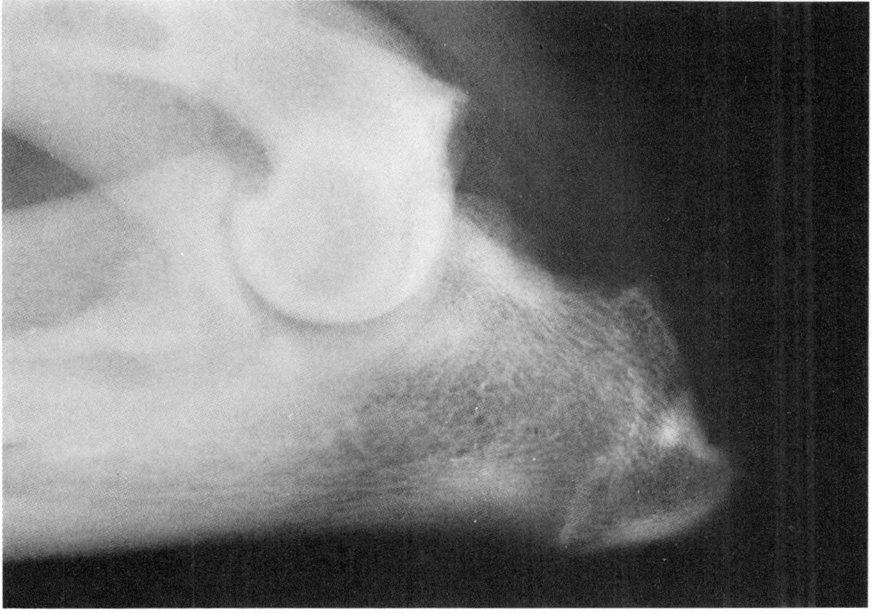

Fig. 2. Flexed lateral radiograph of elbow showing osteophytes on the anconeal process.

STIFLE

OCD of the medial or, more commonly, the lateral condyle of the femur can be difficult to confirm radiographically. A lateral view and a number of cranio-caudal projections with the joint in different degrees of flexion are often necessary (Olsson,

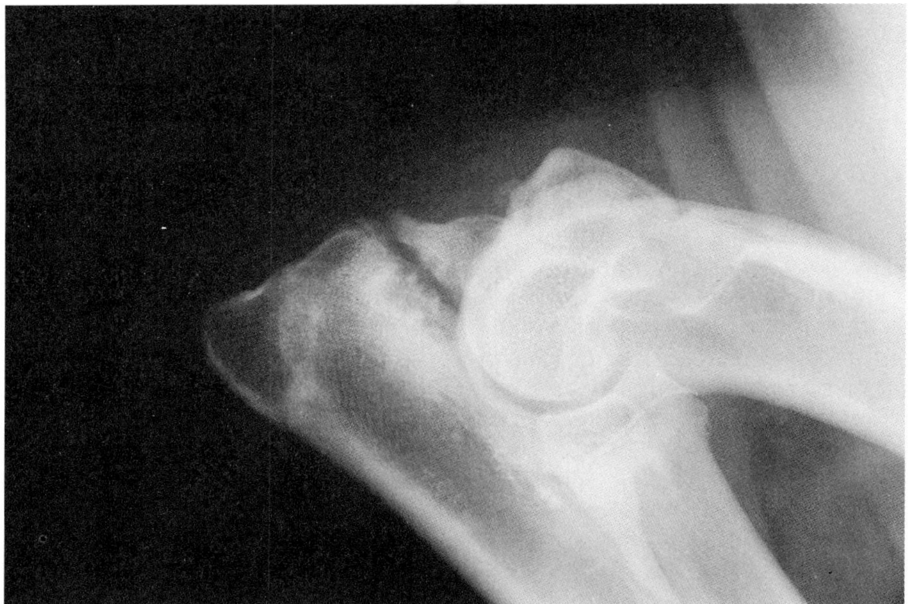

Fig. 3. Flexed lateral radiograph of elbow showing ununited anconeal process.

1977; Bennett, 1984). Denny and Gibbs (1980a) reviewed fourteen cases of stifle osteochondrosis, comprising twenty-two affected joints, in which flattening of the articular margin of affected condyles was an invariable finding on lateral radiographs. They suggest that antero-posterior views are necessary to determine which condyle is affected and are more reliable for the positive identification of subchondral bone defects. However, free mineralized fragments which are an inconsistent feature of stifle osteochondrosis, can be more readily recognized on lateral projections.

In some cases, contrast arthrography may be of use to further define a suspected lesion, or to demonstrate a cartilaginous flap of free radiolucent body (Alexander *et al.*, 1981). Avulsion of the origin of long digital extensor tendon may be difficult to differentiate from osteochondrosis in routine stifle radiographs and a radiolucent defect in the lateral condyle associated with aberrant cranial cruciate ligament attachment may also mimic osteochondrosis radiographically (Dueland *et al.*, 1982).

HOCK

OCD of the medial ridge of the trochlea of the tibial tarsal bone is most readily demonstrated on a cranio-caudal view of the hock (Rosenblum *et al.*, 1978; Bennett, 1984). Early radiographic findings include soft tissue swelling over the medial aspect of the tibiotarsal joint, with an increase in the width of this joint space medially.

Typical osteochondral lesions with or without free mineralized bodies and subchondral bone lysis are seen on the medial ridge of the talus, and/or the medial malleolus of the tibia (Johnson *et al.*, 1980).

Recently, osteochondrosis of the lateral ridge of the tibial tarsal bone has been recognized (unpublished data). This can be demonstrated on lateral views with the joint in full extension and in full flexion, or on a slightly medial oblique cranio-caudal view. Secondary degenerative joint disease, with periarticular osteophyte formation is commonly seen on lateral projections in all cases of osteochondrosis of the hock.

TREATMENT

SHOULDER

OCD of the humeral head should be treated surgically, although lesions without lameness have been shown to heal spontaneously. Olsson (1976) proposes that spontaneous healing will occur even in lame animals if the attached cartilaginous flap is dislodged and subsequently resorbed from the joint cavity. He advocates increasing exercise, with analgesics if necessary, as a means of dislodging the flap.

The main aim of surgery is to remove any free mineralized bodies, which usually lodge in the caudal pouch of the joint capsule. Damaged cartilage surfaces are then curretted to leave bleeding subchondral bone which undergoes fibrocartilaginous repair. Bennett (1984) argues against curretting subchondral defects because these are generally already healing with fibrocartilage. He recommends curetting only diseased cartilage at the periphery of the lesion.

ELBOW

Most cases of OCD of the medial humeral condyle and fragmentation of the coronoid process merit surgery as soon as possible after diagnosis (Denny and Gibbs, 1980b; Tirgari, 1980; Bennett *et al.*, 1981; Olsson, 1983). Some cases with only slight lameness may respond if exercise is regular, controlled and gradually increased over a two month period. There seems little to gain in restricting exercise unless the lameness is severe, in which case treatment should be surgical.

Fragmented coronoid process typically presents as a single free ossicle adjacent to the head of the radius (Figure 4). Occasionally several small fragments are found. In other cases there is fissuring of the articular surface of the coronoid process without complete fragmentation. Free fragments can be removed via a medial elbow exposure (Piermattei and Greeley, 1979; Denny and Gibbs, 1980b) and any fissures are curetted. OCD of the medial humeral condyle is also treated through a medial approach to the elbow joint. Any free fragments are removed and the lesion may be curetted as in the shoulder. Ununited anconeal process should be treated by surgical removal of the ununited portion as early as possible. This is achieved through a lateral approach to the elbow joint (Piermattei and Greeley, 1979).

Prognosis for osteochondrosis of the elbow is generally fair to good, but is poorer when both OCD of the humeral condyle and fragmented coronoid process occur simultaneously. However, degenerative changes will progress whether surgery is undertaken or not. This may present as a clinical problem in later life.

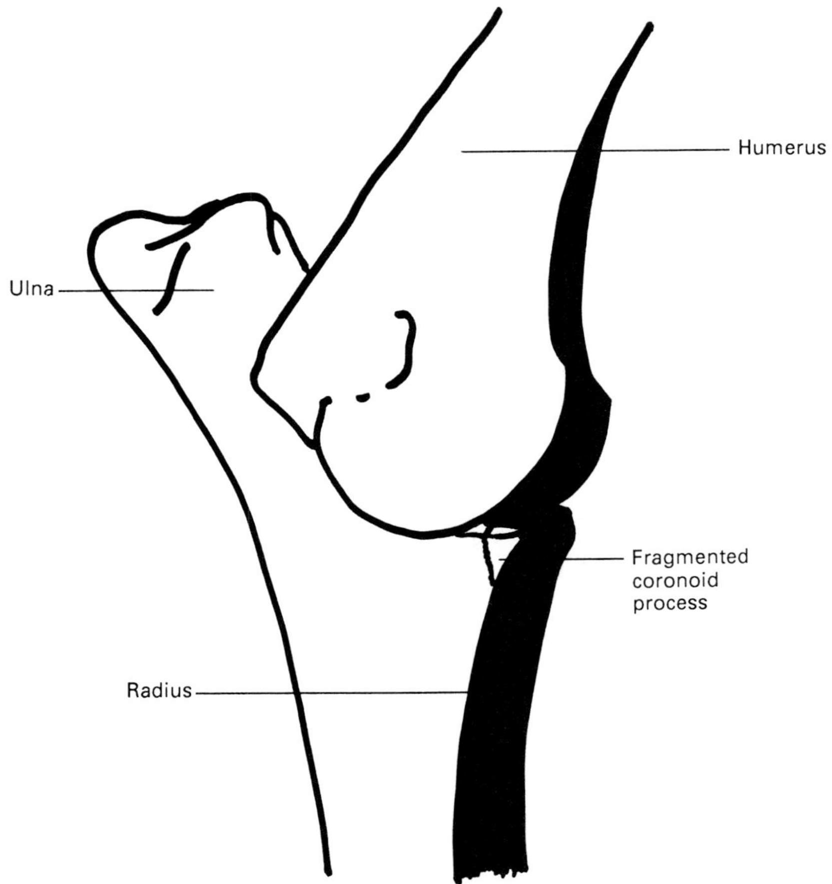

Fig. 4. The location of a fragmented coronoid process. Line drawings of elbow skeleton.

STIFLE

The surgical management of OCD of the stifle is similar to that for the shoulder. Good exposure of the joint is achieved through a lateral parapatellar approach (Piermattei and Greeley, 1979). An alternative to curettage is to re-attach osteochondral fragments using matchstick grafts from cortical bone as small nails (Alexander *et al.*, 1981; Johnson and McTeod, 1977). A limited number of cases treated in this manner had promising functional results with healing of the flap and incorporation of the bone pegs into the defect (Alexander *et al.*, 1981).

HOCK

Osteochondrosis of the medial ridge of the tibial tarsal bone carries a poor prognosis. Secondary degenerative joint disease can lead to severe lameness. Early surgical treatment before the onset of secondary change is therefore indicated in all cases.

Even so, permanent disability is not unusual. A medial approach is made to the trochlear ridge of the tibial tarsal bone (Piermattei and Greeley, 1979) and it is sometimes necessary to section the collateral ligament to gain adequate exposure. Cases of OCD of the lateral ridge of the tibial tarsal are approached by a lateral incision (Piermattei and Greeley, 1979). The lesion may lie cranially or caudally on the ridge, and the approach is modified accordingly with the joint held in flexion or extension to maximize exposure.

In all cases undergoing surgery for osteochondrosis, flushing of the joint with sterile normal saline may help to remove small osteochondral fragments. Post-operatively, a support dressing (Robert–Jones type) is applied for 10–14 days and strict rest is prescribed for 4–6 weeks. A splinted support dressing for up to 3 weeks is useful in dogs undergoing surgery for OCD of the hock. Following the rest period a gradual return to normal exercise is achieved over a further two months.

REFERENCES

Alexander, J. W., Richardson, D. C. and Selcer, B. A. (1981) Osteochondritis dissecans of the elbow, stifle and hock: a review. *J. Am. Animal Hospital Assoc.*, **17**, 51–56

Bennett, D., Duff, S. R. I., Kene, R. O. and Lee, L. (1981) Osteochondritis dissecans and fragmentation of the coronoid process in the elbow joint of the dog *Vet. Rec.*, **109**, 329

Bennett, D. (1984) Joint disease. In *Canine Medicine and Therapeutics*, 2nd edn (ed. E. A. Chandler., J. B. Sutton and D. J. Thompson), Blackwell, Oxford

Boudrieau, R. J., Hohn, R. B. and Bardet, J. F. (1983) Osteochondritis dissecans of the elbow in the dog, *J. Am. Animal Hospital Assoc.*, **19**, 627–635

Butler, H. C., Wallace, L. J. and Ladds, P. W. (1971) Osteochondritis dissecans of the distal end of the radius in a dog. *J. Am. Animal Hospital Assoc.*, **7**, 81–86

Denny, H. R. and Gibbs, C. (1980a) Osteochondritis dissecans of the canine stifle joint. *J. Small Animal Pract.*, **21**, 317–322

Denny, H. R. and Gibbs, C. (1980b) The surgical treatment of osteochondritis dissecans and ununited coronoid process in the canine elbow joint. *J. Small Animal Pract.*, **21**, 323

Dueland, R., Sisson, D. and Evans, H. E. (1982) Aberrant origin of the cranial cruciate ligament mimicking an osteochondral lesion radiographically. A case history report. *Vet. Radiol.*, **23**, 175

Grondalen, T. and Vangen, O. (1974) Osteochondrosis and arthrosis in pigs V. *Acta. Vet. Scand.*, **15**, 61–79

Hayes, H. M., Selby, L. A., Wilson, G. P. *et al.*, (1979) Epidemiological observation of canine elbow disease (emphasis on dysplasia). *J. Am. Animal Hospital Assoc.*, **15**, 449

Hedhammer, A., Win, F. M., Krook, L. *et al* (1974) Overnutrition and skeletal disease. An experimental study in growing Great Dane dogs. *Cornell Veterinarian*, **64**, (Suppl. 5) 83–95

Hohn, R. B. (1973) Osteochondritis dissecans of the humeral head *J. Am. Vet. Med. Assoc.*, **163**, 69

Johnson, K. A., Howlett, C. R., Pettit, G. D. (1980) Osteochondrosis in the hock joints in dogs. *J. Am. Animal Hospital Assoc.*, **16**, 103–113

Johnson, E. W. and McTeod, T. L. (1977) Osteochondral fragments of the distal end of the femur fixed with bone pegs. *J. Bone and Joint Surg.*, **59-A**, 677–679

Jones, D. G. C. and Vaughan, L. C. (1970) The surgical treatment of osteochondrosis dissecans of the humeral head in dogs. *J. Small Animal Pract.*, **11**, 803

Lee, R. (1976) Proximalfemoral epiphyseal seperation in the dog. *J. Small Animal Pract.*, **11**, 669

Leighton, R. L. (1971) Osteochondritis dissecans of the shoulder joint of the dog. *Veterinary Clinics of North America*, **1**, 391–401

McDonald, M. (1988) Osteochondritis dissecans of the femoral head: A case report. *J. Small Animal Pract.*, **29**, 49–54

Mason, T. A., Lavelle, R. B., Skipper, S. C. and Wrigley, W. R. (1980) Osteochondrosis of the elbow joint in young dogs. *J. Small Animal Pract.*, **21**, 641–646

Olsson, S-E. (1975a) Osteochondritis dissecans in the dog. *Proc. Am. Animal Hospital Assoc. Ann M.*, **42**, 360–362

Olsson, S.-E. (1975b) Lameness in the dog. A review of lesions causing osteoanthritiss of the shoulder, elbow, hip, stifle and hock joints. *Proc. Am. Animal Hospital Assoc. Ann. Mtg.*, **42**, 363–369

Olsson, S.-E. (1976) Osteochondrosis: A growing problem to dog breeders. *Gaines Progress,* **Summer,** 1–11

Olsson, S.-E. (1977) Osteochondrosis in the dog. In *Current Veterinary Therapy VI.* (ed. R. W. Kirk), W. B. Saunders, Philadelphia

Olsson, S.-E. (1983) The early diagnosis of fragmented coronoid process and osteochondritis dissecans of the canine elbow joint. *J. Am. Animal Hospital Assoc.*, **19**, 616–626

Paatsama, S. Rokkanen, P., Jussila, J. and Sittnikow, K. (1971) Somatotropin thyrotropin and corticotropin hormone induced changes in the cartilages and bones of the shoulder and knee joint in young dogs. *J. Small Animal Pract.*, **12**, 595–601

Piermattei, D. L. and Greeley, R. G. (1979) *An Atlas of Surgical Approaches to the Bones of the Dog and Cat,* 2nd edn, W. B. Saunders, Philadelphia

Reiland, S. (1975) Osteochondrosis in the pig. *Actuaria Radiologica,* 1–118

Robins, G. M. (1970) A case of osteochondritis dissecans of the stifle joint in a bitch. *J. Small Animal Pract.*, **11**, 813

Robins, G. M. (1978) Osteochondritis dissecans in the dog. *Aust. Vet. J.*, **54**, 272–286

Robins, G. M. (1980) Some aspects of the radiographical examination of the canine elbow joint. *J. Small Animal Pract.*, **21**, 417–428

Rosenblum, G. P., Robins, G. M., Carlisle, C. H. (1978) Osteochondritis dissecans of the tibio-tarsal joint in the dog. *J. Small Animal Pract.*, **19**, 759–767

Smith, C. W. and Stowater, J. L. (1975) Osteochondritis of the canine shoulder joint. A review of 35 cases. *J. Am. Animal Hospital Assoc.*, **11**, 658

Tirgari, M. (1980) Clinical, radiographical and pathological aspects of ununited medial coronoid process of the elbow joint in dogs. *J. Small Animal Pract.*, **21**, 595–608

Vaughan, L. C., Jones, D. G. C. (1968) Osteochondritis dissecans of the head of the humerus in dogs. *J. Small Animal Pract.*, **9**, 283

SERENA BROWNLIE

The primary treatment of heart conditions

INTRODUCTION

DESPITE EXCITING therapeutic advances in the human cardiology field, lack of specialized equipment restricts most small animal practitioners to the palliative treatment of congestive heart failure or arrhythmias. Even so, few veterinary preparations of cardiac drugs are available. Therefore, successful therapy may only be achieved by administering agents which are unlicensed for use in dogs and cats and for which proper dose rates may not have been established. However, good results may be obtained if the owner is prepared to devote time to nursing the animal and experimenting with different tablet regimes. The response of the individual animal is very variable depending on the type and severity of the condition.

Accurate diagnosis is necessary for correct treatment. Common cardiac syndromes are recognized and certain conditions are commoner in some breeds than others. Nevertheless, one must not jump to conclusions; the presence of a murmur may not be significant, and there are other causes of coughing or ascites than heart disease. Careful clinical examination is most important but other diagnostic methods such as electrocardiography, radiography and ultrasound are very useful.

In the treatment of any disease the aim should be to remove the causative factors if possible. For example, arrhythmias often occur secondarily because of hypoxia and electrolyte disturbances. In the brachycephalic breeds, bradyarrhythmias may be controlled by improving the airway surgically. Taurine deficiency has been reported as a cause of feline dilated cardiomyopathy (Pion *et al.*, 1987). Hyperthyroidism has also been noted as a cause of the hypertrophic form of cardiomyopathy in cats (Liu *et al.*, 1982). Signs of right heart failure may occur due to pericardial effusion and may be relieved by drainage of the pericardium. Unfortunately, however, the aetiology of most primary heart diseases is still unknown.

CONGENITAL CARDIAC DEFECTS

In general, a loud murmur accompanied by signs of exercise intolerance, collapse, cyanosis or stunting in an animal less than three years old suggests the presence of a heart defect. Surgical correction is the best treatment, preferably before any signs of failure develop. However, only those defects which may be approached without opening the heart are regularly treated in animals, because very few centres in the world have access to cardiac bypass equipment.

The simplest procedure is ligation of a left to right patent ductus arteriosus (PDA). With good anaesthetic and post operative care, the success rate may be very high (Eyster *et al.*, 1976). Surgery is contra-indicated in cases of right to left PDA with pulmonary hypertension.

Pulmonic stenosis has been treated by pericardial patch grafting (Breznock and Wood, 1976; Clayton-Jones, unpublished data) and by percutaneous balloon valvuloplasty (Bright *et al.*, 1987).

Subaortic stenosis has not been treated in animals without bypass. Valvuloplasty has been used in aortic stenosis in humans (Jackson *et al.*, 1987) and therefore may be a future possibility for animals.

Many cases of ventricular septal defects do not require treatment but in severe cases, pulmonary artery banding has been used as a palliative measure (Eyster *et al.*, 1977). This is much less satisfactory than closure of the defect. Weirich and Blevins (1978) used hypothermia to close septal defects in twelve dogs and one cat, and ten survived surgery. The Blalock – Taussig procedure, i.e. transposition of the subclavian artery to the pulmonary artery, may be used to treat the cyanosis associated with tetralogy of Fallot (Eyster *et al.*, 1977). One attempt at total surgical correction has been reported (Herrtage *et al.*, 1983).

If surgery is impossible, drug treatment for heart failure and exercise restriction are the only options.

VALVULAR INCOMPETENCE

A systolic murmur in the mitral area in a small breed dog of greater than six years, which has dyspnoea and a cough, is suggestive of valvular incompetence. The usual valve affected is the mitral or left atrioventricular valve and incompetence is usually due to the degenerative condition called endocardiosis, though the valve may be congenitally malformed (mitral dysplasia) or damaged by endocarditis. Blood flow backwards through the incompetent valve causes increased left atrial and pulmonary pressure resulting in pulmonary oedema and eventually effects on the right heart. The left ventricle fails first but finally congestive failure ensues. Mitral valves cannot be replaced without bypass, therefore drug treatment of congestive failure is the only option.

The development of a murmur during the course of a febrile illness, especially if accompanied by other signs such as lameness or neck pain, is suspicious of endocarditis. In the dog the usual areas affected are the mitral and aortic valves. It is very helpful if the bacteria responsible can be cultured. Ideally, several blood cultures should be collected when the fever is highest, using sterile precautions. Two culture bottles are used. If the same bacterium is isolated from each it is unlikely to be a contaminant. One of the main reasons for negative cultures is prior administration of antibiotics. If an organism is isolated, a sensitivity test can be performed and an appropriate antibiotic should be administered frequently, and at high dose levels, intravenously if possible, for four to six weeks. If the organisms cannot be cultured, a broad spectrum antibiotic or combination may be chosen. Sisson (1987) recommends an aminoglycoside with penicillin or ampicillin. The prognosis in these cases is very poor, especially if heart failure signs develop, and treatment must be aggressive.

MYOCARDIAL DISEASE

Myocardial disease is frequently diagnosed in cats and in large and giant breed dogs. In both species, this may cause rhythm disturbances, leading to collapsing episodes. These may be treated according to whether they are tachy- or bradyarrhythmias. However, additional signs of cardiac failure are often present, i.e. pulmonary oedema, ascites and hydrothorax. In these cases it is probably wise to treat the failure first, unless the arrhythmia is life threatening.

Tachyarrhythmias may be treated using one of the wide variety of anti-arrhythmic drugs available. The choice is somewhat bewildering. Novotny and Adams (1986) described the range of drugs, their classification and mode of action, and reviewed the information available about dose rates and side effects in dogs. These agents are allotted to one of four classes (See Table 1).

Although many different drugs have been tried in the dog, only propranolol, and occasionally lignocaine, have been used in the cat. Fortunately propranolol is very effective, particularly in hypertrophic cardiomyopathy and hyperthyroidism.

Bradyarrhythmias (See Table 2). Excessive vagal action is common in brachycephalic breeds of dog. This may lead to sinoatrial block. These cases usually respond quite well to parasympatholytic treatment with atropine or glycopyrrolate, either parenterally or orally (See Table 2). Cases with atrio ventricular nodal conduction problems, i.e. first, second and third degree blocks, may not respond. Isoprenaline may be tried with care, (Table 2) but for those which show no improvement, especially third degree blocks, and for most cases with combined brady/ tachyarrhythmias (sick-sinus syndrome) the only successful treatment is pacemaker implantation (Yoshioka *et al.*, 1981; Darke *et al.*, 1985).

CONGESTIVE HEART FAILURE

Heart failure is a progressive inability of the heart to pump blood to meet the demands of the body, first during exercise and later at rest. In compensated heart disease the animal appears normal but it is using up its cardiac reserve.

There are several pathophysiological mechanisms which are initially protective and compensatory but which eventually contribute to deterioration. These are:
1. Increased heart rate. This increases cardiac output but if extreme, it reduces the time available for ventricular filling.
2. Increased ventricular volume. This mechanism increases stroke volume in the normal heart but it requires the myocardium to use more oxygen and create more energy. This is impossible if contractility is reduced by disease or if the distensibility of the heart is affected, for example, by fibrosis. Initially the myocardium responds by hypertrophy and then dilatation.
3. Retention of sodium and water. This is a response to reduced kidney blood flow either caused by neural mechanisms, or the renin – angiotensin – aldosterone system, and increased thirst.
4. Reflex vasoconstriction which increases peripheral resistance and aortic pressure (afterload).

The aims of ideal therapy, therefore, are to decrease heart rate, to improve ventricular filling, to increase contractility, to reduce myocardial oxygen demand if possible, to reduce sodium and water retention and to combat vasoconstriction, without excessive lowering of blood pressure.

Table 1

Class	Drug name	Mode of administration	Uses	Dose rate	Comments and Adverse effects
I A Membrane stabilizing effect. Slow depolarization refractory period prolonged	Quinidine	Oral (i/m, i/v)	Ventricular ectopics Ventricular tachycardia can convert atrial fibrillation – sinus rhythm	6–20 mg/kg BID–TID	Hypotension Can induce arrhythmias especially blocks gastro-intestinal
	Procainamide	Oral	Ventricular arrhythmias	8–20 mg/kg QID (sustained release preps. TID)	As above SLE-like syndrome?
		i/v		6–8 mg/kg over 5 mins – 10–40 μg/kg/min	
	Disopyramide	Oral	Ventricular arrhythmias	6–15 mg/kg TID at least	Short half life. Marked negative inotropic action
I B Slow deplarization and conduction velocity in abnormal cells, not in normal tissue	Lignocaine	i/v	Ventricular arrhythmias especially during anaesthesia	Dog 1–4 mg/kg slowly - 25–75μ/kg/min Cat 0.25-1 mg/kg	Seizures, vomiting (especially cats)
	Phenytoin	Oral	Glycoside-induced arrhythmias	24 mg/kg initially; 3–5 mg/kg TID or QID	Not in cats
	Tocainide	Oral	Ventricular arrhythmias	30 mg/kg TID	Vomiting, excitement
	Mexiletine	Oral	Ventricular arrhythmias	1–2 mg/kg BID or TID	Unknown
	Aprindine	i/v oral	Ventricular arrhythmias	0.1 mg/kg/min 1–2 mg/kg TID	Not available in UK yet. Unknown

I C Do not prolong refractory period. Slow depolarization and conduction	Encainide		Ventricular arrhythmias	?	Not available in UK yet
	Lorcainide		Atrial ectopics		
	Flecainide	Oral		Unknown	
II ß adrenergic blocking agent	Propranolol	Oral	Supraventricular and ventricular arrhythmias. Sinus tachycardia in hyperthyroidism	Dogs 0.1–1 mg/kg TID Cats 2.5–10 mg TID	Negative inotropic action exacerbates bronchospasm
	Atenolol	i/v Oral		0.02 –0.1 mg/kg 0.5–2 mg/kg daily	Selective β-1-blocker
III Prolong action potential and refractory period only	Amiodarone	Oral	Refractory arrhythmias Wolf–Parkinson–White syndrome?	?	Long half life
	Bretylium	i/v	Ventricular arrhythmias chemical reversal in certain cases of ventricular fibrillation?	?	Not with halogenated hydrocarbon anaesthetics?
IV Calcium channel blocking agent	Verapmil	Oral i/v	Supraventricular tachycardia atrial fibrillation? hypertrophic cardiomyopathy?	Dogs 0.5–1.5 mg/kg TID 0.5 mg/kg cats??	Bradycardia, blocks. Severe negative inotropic action. Hospitalize for treatment?

Table 2

Drug name	Mode of administration	Dose rate	Adverse effects
Atropine	i/v, s/c, i/m	0.01–0.02 mg/kg	Dry mouth
	oral	0.02–0.04 mg/kg TID	
Glycopyrrolate	oral	0.01–0.02 mg/kg TID	
Isoprenaline	oral	0.5 mg/kg QID	Not in heart failure arrhythmogenic, hypotensive

Management of the patient calls for exercise reduction, and, in cases of severe decompensation, cage rest. However, there is no point in keeping a dog alive if complete curtailment of exercise makes the animal and the owner miserable. In these cases a balance must be achieved. Low sodium diets are available commercially or may be prepared at home using muscle meat rather than offal, and rice, pasta or mashed potato instead of biscuits. However, such diets are unpalatable. They may be improved by using salt substitute and warming the foods. Because many cardiac patients are losing weight and have reduced appetites anyway, the value of these diets is not as great as has been assumed.

DRUGS USED IN FAILURE TREATMENT (SEE TABLE 3)

DIURETICS

Frusemide is the diuretic most frequently used. It is potent and rapidly acting and can be given parenterally or orally. It inhibits sodium resorption in the kidney tubules and loop of the Henle, even when glomerular filtration is reduced. Hypokalaemia occurs occasionally in cases which have been treated for a long time. Polydipsia and nocturia may be a problem. Giving the drug early in the day is helpful. Care should be taken not to overdose cats because it is possible to dehydrate them, reducing the venous return and precipitating circulatory collapse. Once oedema has stabilized, the dose may be reduced to a maintenance level.

The thiazide diuretics are not so potent and their beneficial effect may be short-lived. Hypokalaemia may occur. Potassium sparing diuretics such as spirono-lactone are expensive and rarely necessary.

CARDIAC GLYCOSIDES

Digoxin and digitoxin used to be the mainstays of cardiac therapy but in human medicine they are now rarely used except to reduce the ventricular rate in atrial fibrillation. They decrease heart rate and increase the force of contraction. The therapeutic dose is very close to the toxic dose. If renal perfusion is poor or there is pre-existing renal disease, digoxin builds up rapidly in the body. Digitoxin is metabolized mostly by the liver and may be safer in these cases. The signs of toxicity are anorexia, vomiting and the development of electrocardiographic abnormalities of any type, especially first degree atrioventricular (AV) block and AV dissociation.

Table 3

Class	Drug name	Mode of administration	Dose rate	Comments and adverse effects
Diuretic	Frusemide	oral, i/v	Dogs 2–3 mg/kg BID Cats 1–2 mg/kg BID	Hypokalaemia May cause dehydration
	Hydrochlorothiazide	oral	2–4 mg/kg BID	Hypokalaemia
	Spironolactone	oral	Dogs 2 mg/kg/day	Potassium sparing
Cardiac glycosides	Digoxin	oral	Dogs 0.01 mg/kg BID max. Cats 0.005 mg/kg lean bodyweight daily or every other day	Tablets safer than elixir
	Digitoxin	oral	0.06 mg/kg BID	
Vasodilator	Hydralazine	oral	Dogs 0.5–2 mg/kg BID	
	Glyceryl trinitrate	cutaneous 2%	Dogs 1/4–1/2 inch paste QID	Hypotension: start with low dose and gradually increase
	Prazosin	oral	Dogs 0.5–2 mg *per dog* BID or TID	
	Captopril	oral	Dogs and cats 1–2 mg/kg BID or TID	
Sympathomimetic	Dobutamine	i/v	Dogs 1–2 µg/kg/min gradually increasing to 3–7 µg/kg/min Cats max. 4µg/kg/min.	Arrhythmias, seizures
Bronchodilator	Aminophylline	oral	5–10 mg/kg	

Rapid digitalization is rarely used now. It is probably safer, especially with older patients, large breed dogs and cats, to start with a low dose and increase it gradually.

VASODILATORS

These drugs are gaining widespread acceptance in heart failure. These are four types:

1. Arteriolar dilators, e.g. hydralazine. This was shown to decrese coughing and heart rate in dogs with left side failure (Hamlin and Kittleson, 1982). However, the same authors in another study in 1983 found that heart rate increased in some dogs (Kitteson and Hamlin, 1983). Stroke volume also increased with no change in preload or contractility; therefore a decrease in afterload was likely. They recommend administering the drug twice daily in incremental doses until an effective dose is reached, to reduce the hypotensive effects.
2. Glyceryl trinitrate. Nitrates relax the venous smooth muscle resulting in preload reduction. They also have minor arterial effects at higher doses. The drug is well absorbed through the skin, which is convenient, provided the owner wears gloves. Because the effects are difficult to predict, the drug is usually used in intensive care situations in acute heart failure.
3. Prazosin. This is an alpha-adrenergic blocker with dilating effects on arteries and veins. No controlled studies have been reported but Atwell (1979) used the drug in four dogs with congestive heart failure and noted marked improvement in all cases. Hypotension is the main side effect.
4. Captopril. This drug inhibits the conversion of angiotensin I to angiotensin II. Its effects were reviewed by Allen *et al.* (1987). It causes vasodilatation and reduces plasma volume in heart failure. It is eliminated by the kidneys and there is conflicting evidence regarding its use in dogs with renal disease. In humans, renal dysfuction, neutropenia, hyperkalaemia, gut disturbances and altered taste sensation have been reported. Complete anorexia is a problem in certain dogs but the dramatic clinical improvement obtained in some refractory cases of heart failure in dogs and cats is encouraging.

OTHER DRUGS

Positive inotropic agents such as the sympathomimetic drugs dopamine and dobutamine and the phosphodiesterase inhibitors amrinone and milrinone are still under investigation in animals. Dobutamine given by intravenous infusion may be useful in emergency treatment of myocardial failure (Keene, 1987).

Theophylline derivatives such as aminophylline and etamiphylline, are of limited effectiveness as cardiac stimulants but are useful where bronchodilation is required, as in cases with combined chronic valvular and airway disease.

REFERENCES

Allen, T. A., Wilke, W. L. and Feltman, M. J. (1987) Captopril and enalapril: angiotensin - converting enzyme inhibitors. *J. Am. Vet. Med. Assoc.*, **190**, 94–96
Atwell, R. B. (1979) The use of alpha-blockade in the treatment of congestive heart failure associated with dirofilariasis and mitral valvular incompetence. *Vet. Rec.*, **104**, 114–117

Breznock, E. M. and Wood, G. L. (1976) A patch-graft technique for correction of pulmonic stenosis in dogs. *J. Am. Vet. Med. Assoc.,* **169,** 1090–1094

Bright, J. M., Jennings, J., Toal, R. and Hood, M. E. (1987) Percutaneous balloon valvuloplasty for treatment of pulmonic stenosis in a dog. *J. Am. Vet. Med. Assoc.,* **191,** 995–996

Darke, P. G. G., Been, M. and Marks, A. (1985) Use of a programmable 'physiologic' cardiac pacemaker in a dog with total atrio-ventricular block (with some comments on complications associated with cardiac pacemakers). *J. Small Animal Pract.,* **26,** 295–303

Eyster, G. E., Braden, T. D., Appleford, M., Johnston, J., Chaffe, A. and Schwegler, S. (1977) Surgical management of tetralogy of Fallot. *J. Small Animal Pract.,* **18,** 387–394

Eyster, G. E., Eyster, J. T., Cords, G. B. and Johnston, J. (1976) Patent ductus arteriosus in the dog; characteristics of occurrence and results of surgery in one hundred consecutive cases. *J. Am. Vet. Med. Assoc.,* **168,** 435–438

Eyster, G. E., Whipple, R. D., Anderson, L. K., Evans, A. T. and O'Handley, P. (1977) Pulmonary artery banding for ventricular septal defect in dogs and cats. *J. Am. Vet. Med. Assoc.,* **170,** 434–438

Hamlin, R. L. and Kittleson, M. D. (1982) Clinical experience with hydralazine for treatment of otherwise intractable cough in dogs with apparent left side heart failure. *J. Am. Vet. Med. Assoc.,* **180,** 1327–1329

Herrtage, M. E., Hall, L. W. and English, T. A. H. (1983) Surgical correction of the tetralogy of Fallot in a dog. *J. Small Animal Pract.,* **24,** 51–62

Jackson, G., Thomas, S., Monaghan, M., Forsyth, A., Jewitt, D. (1987) Inoperable aortic stenosis in the elderly: benefit from percutaneous transluminal valvuloplasty. *Br. Med. J.,* **294,** 83–86

Keene, B. W. (1987) Cardiovascular drugs In *Contemporary Issues in Small Animal Practice – Cardiology.* (ed. J. D. Bonagura) Churchill Livingstone, New York pp. 46.

Kittleson, M. D. and Hamlin, R. L. (1983) Hydralazine pharmacodynamics in the dog. *Am. J. Vet. Res.,* **44,** 1501–1505

Liu, S. K., Peterson, M. E. and Fox, P. R. (1982) Hypertrophic cardiomyopathy and hyperthyroidism in the cat. *J. Am. Vet. Med. Assoc.,* **185,** 52–57

Novotny, M. J. and Adams, H. R. (1986) New perspectives in cardiology. Recent advances in antiarrhythmic drug therapy. *J. Am. Vet. Med. Assoc.,* **189,** 533–539

Pion, P. D., Kittleson, M. D., Rogers, Q. R. and Morris, J. G. (1987) Myocardial failure in cats associated with low plasma taurine: a reversible cardiomyopathy. *Science,* **237,** 764–768

Sisson, D. (1987) Acquired valvular heart disease in dogs and cats. In *Contemporary Issues in Small Animal Practice–Cardiology* (ed. J. D. Bonagura) Churchill Livingstone, New York p. 106

Weirich, W. E. and Blevins, W. E. (1978) Ventral septal defect repair. *Vet. Surg.,* **7,** 2–7

Yoshioka, M. M., Tilley, L. P., Harvey, H. J., Wayne, E. S., Lombard, C. W. and Schollmeyer, M. (1981) Permanent pacemaker implantation in the dog. *J. Am. Anim. Hosp. Assoc.,* **17,** 746–750

EDWARD J. HALL

Primary treatment of small intestinal diseases

INTRODUCTION

THE TREATMENT of small intestinal diseases can be divided into three categories: primary or specific, supportive and symptomatic.

Supportive treatment of diarrhoea consists of replacing fluid and electrolye loss by parenteral fluid therapy and/or oral glucose–electrolyte solution administration. In addition, dietary restriction allows restoration of epithelial integrity, reduction of continuing fluid loss from osmotic diarrhoea, and elimination of possible irritants in ingested foodstuffs.

Symptomatic treatment involves the use of drugs such as:
1. Motility modifiers, e.g. diphenoxylate, loperamide.
2. Adsorbents/protectants (efficacy unproven), e.g. kaolin-pectin, aluminium hydroxide, magnesium trisilicate, bismuth, activated charcoal.
3. Antimicrobials. There is no indication for the routine use of antimicrobials.
4. Antiprostaglandins, e.g. flunixin meglumine.
5. Small, bland, low-fat meals, e.g. boiled rice and cottage cheese, prescription diets.

Treatment of acute diarrhoea usually requires only supportive and symptomatic therapy. Most animals that die with acute diarrhoea do so as a result of dehydration, acidosis and shock following fluid and electrolyte depletion and not as a result of the inciting cause, which is usually self-limiting. Indeed, for such common causes of acute diarrhoea as dietary indiscretion and viral enteritis there are no specific therapies available.

Primary or specific therapy is aimed at treating the underlying causes of intestinal disease. It is most appropriate in the treatment of chronic diarrhoea because this is rarely self-limiting. However, it is necessary to establish an accurate diagnosis in order to be able to prescribe appropriate and specific therapy for effective treatment. The limitations of routine screening procedures, the relative inaccessibility of the small intestine to biopsy and, in many cases, the absence of distinct histological changes in the mucosa have made accurate diagnosis difficult. Thus there has been a tendency to rely on the results of empirical treatment.

New procedures have been introduced in order to help overcome some of these problems. Firstly, assay of serum trypsin-like immunoreactivity has been established as a sensitive and specific test for exocrine pancreatic insufficiency (Williams and Batt, 1988), eliminating its erroneous diagnosis in many cases of small intestinal disease. Secondly, assays of serum folate and cobalamin concentrations can provide

226

valuable information to assist the identification of small intestinal disease in the dog (Batt and Morgan, 1982). Thirdly, a peroral biopsy procedure has been introduced (Batt, 1979) and predominantly biochemical criteria have been applied to the objective assessment of intestinal damage in addition to the examination of histological changes in the mucosa in order to characterize the disease more accurately (Batt, 1986a).

This chapter reviews specific medical therapy of the most clearly defined small intestinal diseases in the dog and cat.

INTESTINAL PARASITISM

HELMINTHS

Intestinal parasitism is extremely common in companion animals. Helminth infections, especially hookworms and whipworms, can be a serious cause of diarrhoea. The investigation of any chronic intestinal disease should rule out parasitism by appropriate faecal examination before further diagnostic procedures are performed. There is a wide range of anthelminthics available for treatment. The more common ones are listed in Table 1.

Table 1 ANTHELMINTHIC COMPOUNDS FOR SMALL ANIMALS

Generic drug	Spectrum	Species	Dosage (mg/kg)	Remarks
Bunamidine	*Taenia* *Dipylidium*	Canine Feline	22–51	Irritating; fasting required
Dichlorvos	Ascarids Hookworms Whipworms	Canine Feline	11–22	Organophosphate toxicity
Fenbendazole	Ascarids Hookworms Whipworms *Taenia*	Canine Feline	20 100	Five days Single dose
Mebendazole	Ascarids Hookworms Whipworms *Taenia*	Canine Feline	22	2 days for ascarids; 5 days for all worm species hepatotoxicity?
Niclosamide	*Taenia* *Dipylidium*	Canine Feline	125	Fasting required
Nitroscanate	*Ascarids* Hookworms *Taenia* *Dipylidium*	Canine	50	Tablet given whole with small amount of food
Piperazine	Ascarids	Canine Feline	110	Intestinal hypomotility
Praziquantel	Cestodes	Canine Feline	5	Oral or injectable; superior efficacy

PROTOZOA

Infections with coccidia may be a significant cause of diarrhoea in young and immunocompromised animals (Greene and Prestwood, 1984). Diagnosis by faecal examination should be followed by treatment of symptomatic animals with sulphonamides (50–60 mg/kg sid or divided bid for 5-21 days.

Giardia spp. can also be a significant cause of diarrhoea, although confirmation of the diagnosis by faecal examination can be difficult (Hall *et al.*, 1988). Quinacrine, metronidazole and furazolidone are the most widely recommended drugs in the treatment of giardiasis but their relative merits are controversial (Kirkpatrick, 1984, 1986). Quinacrine hydrochloride has been used at a variety of dosages (In dogs: 50–300 mg per animal divided bid or tid for 5–6 days, or 9 mg/kg sid for 6 days; in cats: 11 mg/kg sid for 12 days). However it can cause toxicity if its use is prolonged and it may fail to eliminate the infection. Metronidazole, given orally at the rate of 25 mg/kg bid for 5 days is usually adequate, although a variable efficacy in dogs has been reported. Furazolidone (4 mg/kg bid for 5 days) has been shown to be effective in cats (Kirkpatrick, 1986), and has been used successfully by the author in dogs when *Giardia* infection was not eliminated by metronidazole therapy.

BACTERIAL ENTERITIS

The use of antibacterials in intestinal disease should be limited to specific infective causes and bacterial overgrowth. Antibacterial therapy is not indicated as a routine treatment for non-specific, acute or chronic diarrhoea. This general guideline is compromised by the finding of mixed microbial infections of *Campylobacter* and *Salmonella* spp. infections in parvovirus infection, and the apparent efficacy of tylosin, tetracycline, ampicillin and chloramphenicol in some dogs with chronic non-specific diarrhoea (Van Kruiningen, 1976; Dillon, 1984). This emphasizes the danger of failing to make an accurate diagnosis.

The irrational use of antibiotics can result in modifications of the intestinal ecosystem. The changes in bacterial interactions may allow one species to become dominant and attack and invade the mucosa, thereby causing diarrhoea. Nevertheless, when severe damage to the mucosa is suspected, because of the presence of haemorrhagic diarrhoea or leucocytosis, antibacterial therapy may be indicated because normal luminal bacteria may penetrate into the circulation.

SPECIFIC INFECTION

The isolation of a known pathogen, such as *Salmonella* spp. may indicate the need for specific antibacterial therapy with potentiated sulphonamides, gentamicin, or even chloramphenicol, although public health risks should be considered. The evidence for *Campylobacter* as a primary pathogen is controversial (Fox *et al.*, 1983). Treatment with erythromycin (40 mg/kg/day for 5–10 days) may only be indicated when infection is associated with clinical disease. The role of *Escherichia coli* in the aetiology of diarrhoea in dogs and cats is unclear. However, the existence of pathogenic strains in other species suggests that they may be an important cause of diarrhoea which requires antibacterial therapy.

BACTERIAL OVERGROWTH

This condition occurs when the normal bacterial population proliferates within the proximal intestinal lumen. The clinical signs and diagnosis have been reviewed (Batt, 1986b). Specific therapy with oral broad-spectrum antibiotic, e.g. oxytetracycline (10 mg/kg tid) for periods of between 7 and 28 days, has been effective. Alternative antibiotics are metronidazole (10 mg/kg bid) or tylosin (10 mg/kg tid). Because it seems likely that the underlying reason for the bacterial colonization may not resolve, repeated treatment with antibiotics may be necesssary. In addition, parenteral vitamin B_{12} (500 μg a month) should be administered because a deficiency of this vitamin caused by binding by luminal bacteria could contribute to the mucosal lesions and may also have deleterious systemic consequences.

DIETARY-INDUCED DISEASE

Dietary indiscretion is undoubtedly a common cause of acute diarrhoea but is a self-limiting condition requiring only supportive and symptomatic therapy. Dietary sensitivity, causing chronic diarrhoea, may also be common. Accurate diagnosis and specific treatment with elimination diets has rarely been documented in the veterinary literature. Largely anecdotal evidence of gluten-sensitivity exists (Strombeck, 1979; Henderson, 1985). However, a wheat sensitive enteropathy in Irish setter dogs has been reported (Batt *et al.*, 1987). This condition has now been demonstrated to represent a gluten-sensitive enteropathy that responds to treatment with a gluten-free diet (Hall and Batt, 1988). Sensitivity to other dietary components, such as beef, fish, soya, egg and milk antigens is often suspected in chronic diarrhoea but definitive diagnosis is usually lacking. Cutaneous manifestations of dietary hypersensitivity have been reported (August, 1985; Medleau *et al.*, 1986), perhaps because clinical responses are easier to observe. However, cessation of diarrhoea after feeding a hypoallergenic diet (e.g. mutton and rice, prescription diet) cannot alone be accepted as irrefutable evidence of dietary sensitivity because other factors such as the fat content of the diet are altered simultaneously. Only by the demonstration of a consistent response to a specific dietary challenge can the diagnosis be verified and an appropriate elimination diet fed.

INFLAMMATORY BOWEL DISEASES

These are diseases of unknown aetiology and are characterized by diffuse infiltration of the mucosa with inflammatory cells. Morphological classification of lymphocytic-plasmacytic, eosinophilic and granulomatous enteritis are based on the predominant cell type present (Sherding, 1983). An immune pathogenesis is suspected, and these conditions may represent final common pathways in the intestinal response to a variety of dietary and/or bacterial antigens. Hypoallergenic diets are rarely effective therapy alone but, in general, these conditions are steroid-responsive. Prednisolone (2–4 mg/kg/day for 2–4 weeks, then gradually decreasing) is the usual recommendation, although the response is variable and the prognosis guarded (Sherding, 1983). A few cases of eosinophilic enteritis have been associated with *Toxocara canis* visceral larva migrans (Hayden and Van Kruiningen, 1973). Larvicidal therapy may be indicated. Lymphocytic-plasmacytic enteritis has been associated with bacterial overgrowth. Treatment with oxytetracycline produced marked improvement (Rutgers *et al.*, 1988).

LYMPHANGIECTASIA

Lymphangiectasia, an obstructive disorder of the intestinal lymphatics, is of unknown aetiology although congenital and acquired forms probably occur (Sherding, 1983). Some animals respond to empirical doses of corticosteroids of antibiotics. Treatment should also include a diet low in long-chain triglycerides (e.g. cottage cheese and rice, prescription diet), with medium-chain triglyceride oil added as a source of lipid calories. The prognosisis is very guarded.

INTESTINAL NEOPLASIA

Intestinal neoplasms generally are managed surgically but alimentary lymphosarcoma may be treated medically with combination chemotherapy. Drugs used include cyclophosphamide, vincristine, methotrexate and prednisolone (Jeglum, 1983). However, the prognosis is more guarded than for some other manifestations of lymphosarcoma.

REFERENCES

August, J. R. (1985) Dietary hypersensitivity in dogs: cutaneous manifestations, diagnosis, and management. *Compendium Contin. Educ. Pract. Vet.*, **7**, 469–477

Batt, R. M. (1979) Techniques for single and multiple peroral jejunal biopsy in the dog. *J. Small Animal Pract.*, **20**, 259–268

Batt, R. M. (1986a) New approaches to malabsorption in the dog. *Compendium Cont. Educ. Pract. Vet.*, **8**, 783–796

Batt, R. M. (1986b) The effects of small intestinal bacterial overgrowth on mucosal enzymes and absorption in the dog. In *The Veterinary Annual (27th issue)* (eds. C. S. G. Grunsell., F. W. G. Hill and M. E. Raw) Wright, Bristol, pp. 188–195

Batt, R. M., McLean, L. and Carter, M. W. (1987) Sequential morphologic and biochemical studies of naturally occurring wheat-sensitive enteropathy in Irish setter dogs. *Digestive Diseases and Sciences*, **32**, 184–194

Batt, R. M. and Morgan, J. O. (1982) Role of serum folate and vitamin B_{12} concentrations in the differentiation of small intestinal abnormalities in the dog. *Res. Vet. Sci.*, **32**, 17–22

Dillon, R. (1984) Bacterial enteritis. In *Modern Concepts and Therapy of Gastrointestinal Disease, Proceedings of the 8th Kal Kan Symposium* (Vernon, California) pp. 65–72

Fox, J. G., Moore, R. and Ackermann, J. I. (1983) Canine and feline campylobacteriosis: epizootiology and clinical and public health features. *J. Am. Vet. Med. Assoc.*, **183**, 1420–1424

Greene, C. E. and Prestwood, A. K. (1984) Coccidial infections. In *Clinical Microbiology and Infectious Diseases of the Dog and Cat* (ed. C. E. Greene) W. B. Saunders, Philadelphia, pp. 824–858

Hall, E. J. and Batt, R. M. (1988) Challenge studies demonstrate gluten sensitivity of a naturally occurring enteropathy in Irish setter dogs. *Gastroenterology*, **94**, A167

Hall, E. J., Rutgers, H. C. and Batt, R. M. (1988) Evaluation of the peroral string test in the diagnosis of canine giardiasis. *J. Small Animal Pract.*, **29**, 177–183

Hayden, D. W. and Van Kruiningen, H. J. (1973) Eosinophilic gastroenteritis in German Shepherd dogs and its relationship to visceral larva migrans. *J. Am. Vet. Med. Assoc.*, **162**, 379–384

Henderson, A. J. (1985) Weight loss in Samoyeds. *Vet. Rec.*, **116**, 167

Jeglum, K. A. (1983) Treatment of lymphosarcoma. In: *Current Veterinary Therapy VIII.* (ed. R. W. Kirk) W. B. Saunders, Philadelphia, pp. 435–438

Kirkpatrick, C. E. (1984) Enteric protozoal infections. In *Clinical Microbiology and Infectious Diseases of the Dog and Cat.* (ed. C. E. Greene) W B. Saunders, Philadelphia, pp. 806–823

Kirkpatrick, C. E. (1986) Feline giardiasis: a review. *J. Small Animal Pract.*, **27**, 69–80

Medleau, L., Latimer, K. S. and Duncan, J. R. (1986) Food hypersensitivity in a cat. *J. Am. Vet. Med. Assoc.*, **189**, 692–693

Rutgers, H. C., Batt, R. M. and Kelly, D. F. (1988) Lymphocytic–plasmacytic enteritis associated with bacterial overgrowth in a dog. *J. Am. Vet. Med. Assoc.*, (in press)

Sherding, R. G. (1983) Disease of the small bowel. In *Textbook of Veterinary Internal Medicine,* 2nd edn. (ed. S. J. Ettinger) W. B. Saunders, Philadelphia, pp. 1278–1346

Strombeck, D. R. (1979) *Small Animal Gastroenterology.* Stonegate Publishing, Davis, California, pp. 234–239

Van Kruiningen, H. J. (1976) Clinical efficacy of tylosin in canine inflammatory bowel disease. *J. Am. Animal Hospital Assoc.*, **12**, 498–501

Williams, D. A. and Batt, R. M. (1988) Sensitivity and specificity of serum trypsin-like immunoreacitivity for the diagnosis of canine exocrine pancreatic insufficiency. *J. Am. Vet. Med. Assoc.*, **192**, 195–201

T. K. DUNN

Canine hypothyroidism

INTRODUCTION

MOST CASES of hypothyroidism in the dog are due to the progressive destruction of the thyroid gland (primary hypothyroidism) resulting in impaired production and secretion of thyroxine (T_4) and triiodothyronine (T_3). Two forms of primary hypothyroidism, lymphocytic thyroiditis and idiopathic atrophy of the thyroid gland, have been identified. Lymphocytic thyroiditis is generally regarded as an immune-mediated disorder.

Approximately 50% of hypothyroid dogs have circulating antibody titres to thyroglobulin (Gosselin *et al.*, 1980; Haines *et al.*, 1984). Secondary hypothyroidism, due to a deficiency of thyrotropin, and tertiary hypothyroidism, due to deficiency of thyrotropin releasing hormone (TRH), are rarer forms of hypothyroidism associated with congenital defects or acquired destructive lesions involving the anterior pituitary and hypothalamus, respectively. Clinical signs of hypothyroidism occasionally develop following destruction of normal thyroid gland by an expanding, non-functional thyroid tumour.

NORMAL THYROID PHYSIOLOGY

The thyroid gland secretes T_4 and smaller amounts of T_3 and reverse triodothyronine (reverse T_3, rT_3). More than 99% of circulating T_4 is bound to plasma proteins. Only the small, unbound fraction, free T_4 (FT_4), is metabolically active and enters target cells to bind with nuclear receptors. A large percentage of T_3 and rT_3 is derived from the peripheral deiodination of T_4. Whereas T_3 is approximately three to five times more potent than T_4, rT_3 is metabolically inactive and is produced in increased amounts during periods of illness or starvation.

The release of thyroid hormones is dependent on the release of TRH from the hypothalamus, which in turn stimulates the release of thyrotropin (thyroid stimulating hormone, TSH) and prolactin from the anterior pituitary. The plasma concentrations of free T_3 and T_4 control TSH secretion via a negative feedback mechanism.

CLINICAL SIGNS

Hypothyroidism occurs more frequently in pure bred, middle-aged (4–6 year old) dogs. A higher incidence has been reported in Golden Retrievers, Doberman Pinschers, Dachshunds, Irish Setters, Miniature Schnauzers, Great Danes, Boxers and Poodles. (Nesbitt *et al.*, 1980).

232

Subjective signs of hypothyroidism are variable and relate to decreased metabolic rate, e.g. mental dullness, lethargy, weight gain, exercise intolerance or reluctance to exercise and heat-seeking behaviour. Common dermatological findings include a bilaterally symmetrical, non-pruritic alopecia of the trunk, flanks and tail (Figure 1). The hair coat is frequently dull, brittle and easily epilated and regrowth of hair from clipped areas is poor. Dryness and scaling of the skin with mild hyperkeratosis and a variable degree of hyperpigmentation may be evident. In severe cases the skin folds around the face are visibly thickened (myxoedematous) resulting in a 'tragic' expression. Secondary seborrhoeic changes and concurrent pyodermas (due to impaired immune function) are common and may result in mild pruritis. Some of the less common reproductive, cardiac, ocular and neuromuscular manifestations of hypothyroidism are listed in Table 1. It is important to note that dogs with secondary or tertiary hypothyroidism due to an expanding pituitary or hypothalamic neoplasm may show central nervous system signs or behavioural changes in addition to signs consistent with other endocrinopathies such as hypo- or hyperadrenocorticism and diabetes insipidus.

Congenital hypothyroidism (cretinism) is a rare disorder characterized by disproportionate dwarfism, bisymmetrical alopecia, retention of the puppy hair coat,

Table 1 CLINICAL SIGNS OF HYPOTHYROIDISM IN THE DOG

Common clinical signs	Mental dullness
	Lethargy
	Exercise intolerance
	Weight gain
	Heat-seeking behaviour
Skin	Bilaterally symmetrical alopecia (trunk, flanks, tail)
Symptoms	Dry, flaky skin
	Hair coat dull and brittle
	Hyperkeratosis
	Seborrhoea
	Hyperpigmentation
	Myxoedema
	Pruritic (secondary bacterial infection)
	Poor wound healing
Less common clinical signs	
Reproductive:	Infertility, lack of libido, prolonged anoestrus, anoestral galactorrhoea, abortion, testicular atrophy, gynecomastia
Ocular:	Corneal lipid deposits, indolent corneal ulcers (especially Boxers), keratoconjunctivitis sicca, uveitis
Cardiac:	Bradycardia
ECG:	Sinus bradycardia, decreased amplitude of R waves, arrhythmias
Neuromuscular dysfunction:	Polyneuropathy or polymyopathy, e.g. paresis, stiffness, muscle wasting, knuckling or dragging of paws, decreased tendon reflexes, laryngeal or facial nerve paralysis
Central nervous system signs or behavioural changes:	Consistent with a space-occupying lesion involving pituitary and/or hypothalamus (secondary or tertiary hypothyroidism)
Gastrointestinal:	Diarrhoea

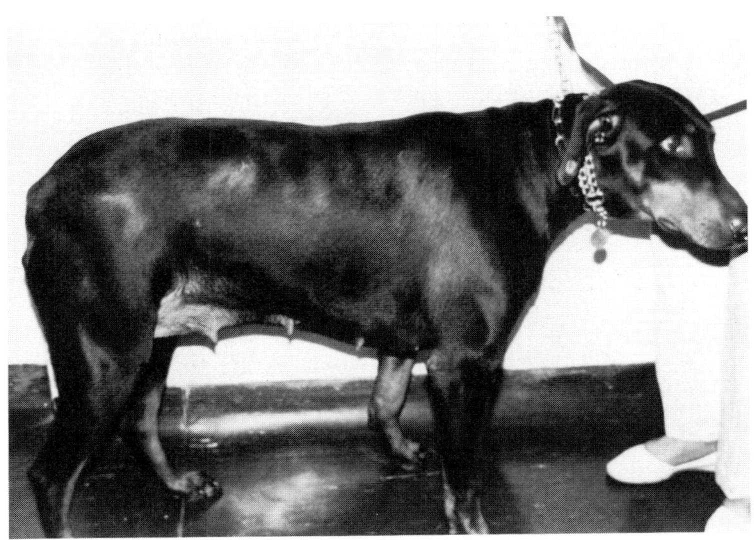

Fig. 1. A 4-year old intact Doberman Pinscher bitch with hypothyroidism showing bilateral alopecia of the trunk and flanks.

myxoedema, lethargy and mental dullness (Figure 2). Goitre may be present depending on the cause (thyroid dysgenesis or abnormal thyroid hormone synthesis). Radiographically, cretinism is characterized by a lack of epiphyseal ossification (epiphyseal dysplasia) (Chastain *et al.*, 1983; Medleau *et al.*, 1985; Jezyk, 1985). A more detailed account of the radiographic changes is given in Dennis (this volume).

DIAGNOSIS

Confirmation of hypothyroidism is based on clinical signs, non-specific haematological and biochemical abnormalities and specific tests of thyroid function. A diagnosis on the basis of clinical signs alone or response to thyroid supplementation is not advocated.

Hypercholestrolaemia occurs in two-thirds of all hypothyroid dogs and approximately 25%–30% have a mild, non-regenerative, normocytic, normochromic anaemia (Chastain, 1982). Elevations in triglycerides, alanine aminotransferase, alkaline phophatase and creatinine phosphokinase are less common. Skin biopsies are not a useful diagnostic aid because the histopathological changes are not specific and may be associated with other endocrinopathies (Scott, 1982) or are a reflection of secondary bacterial infection.

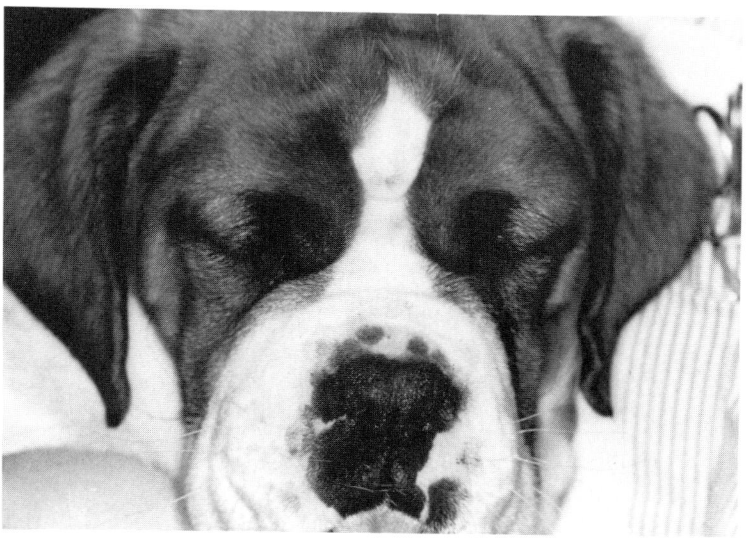

Fig. 2. A 7-month old female Boxer pup with congenital hypothyroidism (cretinism). Note the 'tragic' facial expression and protruding tongue. (photograph courtesy of M. E. Herrtage)

TESTS OF THYROID FUNCTION

BASAL T_4

A basal T_4 concentration is a measurement of total hormone (bound and free fractions). In most commercial laboratories T_4 is measured using a radioimmunoassay (RIA) technique and the normal reference values will vary depending on the laboratory performing the test. Normal values are approximately 18–46 nmol/1 (Larsson, 1988). Pups up to three months of age have basal T_4 concentrations which are two to five times higher than normal adult values (Chastain and Ganjam, 1986). A low basal T_4 concentration, if associated with appropriate clinical signs and biochemical results, is suggestive of hypothyroidism. Unfortunately, there is considerable overlapping of basal T_4 levels between euthyroid and early hypothyroid dogs. Just as T_4 levels may fluctuate below normal in healthy euthyroid dogs, one single normal T_4 value does not indicate normal thyroid reserve. Furthermore basal T_4 may be lowered by non-thyroidal illness (sick euthyroid syndrome), starvation or drug administration (e.g. propylthiouracil, glucocorticoids, phenytoin, phenobarbitol, orthopara' DDD (Mitotane), salicylates and diazepam).

SICK EUTHYROID SYNDROME

Low basal concentrations of T_3 and T_4 have been reported in dogs with chronic renal insufficiency and diabetes mellitus, especially those that are poorly regulated or ketoacidotic (Ferguson, 1984; Feldman and Nelson, 1987). Sick euthyroid animals remain responsive to TSH. Dogs with spontaneous hyperadrenocorticism frequently have low basal T_3 and T_4 levels although again they remain responsive to TSH (Peterson *et al.*, 1984).

BASAL T_3

The failing gland preferentially secretes T_3. Therefore, T_4 may decrease before T_3 (Ferguson, 1984). Because 90% of T_3 is stored intracellularly, circulating T_3 levels may not accurately reflect thyroid function. T_3 concentrations are affected by the same factors which lower T_4 (particularly severe non-thyroidal illness). Therefore, if used alone, basal T_3 provides little additional information over T_4. The normal range of values is approximately 0.7 – 1.81 nmol/l (Larsson, 1988) although the figures will vary slightly depending on the laboratory performing the test.

REVERSE T_3 (rT_3)

Specific assays for rT_3 are not routinely available. Preliminary investigations have shown that rT_3 levels may differentiate hypothyroid dogs from those with low T_3 and T_4 due to a sick euthyroid syndrome.

FREE T_4 (FT_4)

FT_4 should, in theory, permit better separation between euthyroid and hypothyroid dogs because the levels should be less influenced by variables which affect the total T_4 concentration. However, differentiation from a sick euthyroid syndrome may not be as clear cut because low FT_4 concentrations have been reported in dogs with diabetes mellitus and hyperadrenocorticism (Feldman and Nelson, 1987). FT_4 assays are as yet not routinely available and require more critical evaluation. Using human RIA kits, normal values of 6.7–34.0 pmol/l (Larsson, 1988) and 7.5–50 pmol/l (Eckersall and Williams, 1983) have been reported.

T_3 RESIN UPTAKE (T_3RU) TEST

The T_3RU test is an indirect method of estimating changes in the plasma binding of T_3. It is generally regarded as an insensitive indicator of thyroid function in the dog because there is no high affinity plasma binding protein similar to thyroid binding globulin (TBG) in humans. Normal T_3 uptake is 40–60% (Chastain and Ganjam, 1986).

TSH ASSAYS

TSH is a species-specific molecule and as yet a specific and reliable RIA for use in the dog is not commercially available.

TSH STIMULATION

The TSH stimulation test remains the most practical and reliable method of differentiating normal and sick euthyroid dogs from hypothyroid ones. Numerous protocols have been described and interpretation varies with the dose of TSH, the route of administration (i.v. or i.m.) and the post-stimulation sampling time. Following the injection of 5 iu of bovine TSH intravenously, baseline T_4 values double or nearly double within 3 hours with a peak response between 5 and 7 hours. A post-stimulation sample taken at 4 hours with an optional one at 6 hours is a reliable method of assessing thyroid function and is a convenient protocol for the busy small animal practitioner (Oliver and Waldrop, 1983). Dogs with primary hypothyroidism fail to respond to TSH. A low T_4 which doubles but remains below the reference range or a low normal T_4 which fails to double but remains within the normal range of values are difficult results to interpret. Animals in the latter group are generally non-responsive to thyroid supplementation, i.e. are probably not hypothyroid. The response to TSH in cases of secondary or tertiary hypothyroidism is variable.

A more reliable indicator of thyroid function may be the measurement of the absolute difference between post and pre- stimulation T_4. Larsson (1988) reported post-T_4: pre-T_4 ratios of 1.3–3.2 in euthyroid dogs with T_4 increasing by at least 18 nmol/l 4 hours after the intravenous injection of 10 iu of TSH.

Recent administration of thyroxin decreases but does not abolish the response to TSH. To avoid equivocal results it is best if medication is discontinued for at least 4–6 weeks before a TSH stimulation test is performed to reestablish a 'normal' pituitary–thyroid axis.

The recent withdrawal of bovine TSH (Thytropar; Armour Pharmaceutical Co.) from the UK market means that, in the absence of a suitable replacement, the diagnosis of hypothyroidism must be based on either a TRH response test or low basal T_3 and T_4 in association with appropriate clinical signs.

TRH STIMULATION TEST

Having ruled out primary hypothyroidism by demonstrating thyroidal responsiveness to TSH, the TRH stimulation test is the method of choice to differentiate between the secondary and tertiary forms of hypothyroidism. Because valid TSH assays are not available the results are interpretated on the basis of changes in basal T_4 concentration.

Two protocols have been described:
1. TRH intravenously (TRH Roche) (0.1 mg/kg) measuring basal T_4 and post-TRH T_4 at 6 hours. A normal response is a 50% increase in T_4 6 hours post-stimulation with an increase of at least 5 ng/ml (6.5 nmol/1) (Lothrop *et al.*, 1984).
2. TRH (0.2 mg per dog) intravenously measuring basal T_4 and post-TRH T_4 at 4 hours. An increase of at least 12.8 nmol/l indicates a normal pituitary – thyroid axis (Evinger *et al.*, 1985; Chastain and Ganjam, 1986). An absent response is indicative of primary or secondary hypothyroidism. Dogs with hypothalamic dysfunction (tertiary hypothyroidism) would be expected to respond to TRH. Thus the TRH response test may represent an alternative to TSH stimulation if TSH remains unavailable commercially.

The thyroidal uptake of radioiodine and thyroid scintography are useful tests of thyroid function which are not generally available to most veterinary practitioners.

THERAPY

Lifelong therapy with synthetic thyroid preparations is generally necessary. Crude thyroid preparations of animal origin (e.g. dessicated thyroid extract) are not recommended because they have a variable shelf-life and hormonal potency. Thyroid supplementation should be continued for a minimum of three months before its effectiveness is evaluated.

SODIUM LEVOTHYROXINE (T_4) (ELTROXIN; GLAXO)

T_4 is readily converted to T_3 by peripheral tissues. An initial dosage of 20 μg/kg body weight twice daily has been recommended (Feldman and Nelson, 1987). If a favourable clinical response is observed a once-daily maintenance dose of 20 μg/kg may be sufficient to prevent the recurrence of clinical signs. Alternatively, dogs may be dosed on a body surface area basis (0.5 mg/m^2 daily; Table 2) to account for differences in metabolic rate between large and small breed dogs (Chastain, 1982). The drug has a large therapeutic index and iatrogenic thyrotoxicosis is uncommon. An improvement in the dog's general demeanour (increased alertness, activity and appetite) may be noted within the first week. Regrowth of hair and weight loss may not be apparent for 4–6 weeks.

Table 2 DOSAGE OF SODIUM LEVOTHYROXINE BASED ON BODY SURFACE AREA (0.5 mg/m^2 ONCE DAILY). ADAPTED FROM CHASTAIN (1982) AND THEILEN (1975).

Bodyweight (kg)	Approximate body surface area (m^2)	Dose (mg/day)
0–1	0–0.10	0.05
2–3	0.15–0.20	0.10
4–5	0.25–0.29	0.15
6–8	0.33–0.40	0.20
9–11	0.43–0.49	0.25
12–15	0.52–0.60	0.30
16–19	0.63–0.71	0.35
20–23	0.74–0.81	0.40
24–27	0.83–0.90	0.45
28–31	0.92–0.99	0.50
32–36	1.01–1.09	0.55
37–41	1.11–1.19	0.60
42–47	1.21–1.30	0.65
48–53	1.32–1.40	0.70

SODIUM LIOTHYRONINE (T$_3$) (TERTROXIN; GLAXO)

The administration of synthetic T$_3$ or preparations containing a mixture of T$_3$ and T$_4$ offers no advantages over synthetic T$_4$. It is indicated only when T$_4$ therapy alone has failed in a dog with confirmed hypothyroidism or if basal T$_3$ and T$_4$ levels remain low *after* T$_4$ supplementation. Confirmed cases of impaired conversion of T$_4$ to T$_3$ have not been documented in the dog (Feldman and Nelson, 1987). A dose rate of 4–6 µg/kg body weight every eight hours has been suggested (Feldman and Nelson, 1987).

MONITORING

Therapeutic monitoring is rarely necessary. A complete lack of response after 6–8 weeks suggests misdiagnosis and basal T$_3$ and T$_4$ values should be re-evaluated. With levothyroxine, blood samples for T$_4$ should be taken immediately before and 6 hours after administration if dosing twice daily, or before and 8 hours after administration if dosing once daily. With liothyronine, blood for T$_3$ should be taken before and 2–4 hours after administration.

REFERENCES

Chastain, C. B. (1982) Canine hypothyroidism. *J. Am. Vet. Med. Assoc.*, **181**, 349

Chastain, C. B., McNeel, S. V., Graham, C. L. and Pezzanite, S. C. (1983) Congenital hypothyroidism in a dog due to an iodide organification defect. *Am. J. Vet. Res.*, **44**, 1257

Chastain, C. B. and Ganjam, V. K. (1986) The normal thyroid and clinical tests of its function. In *Clinical Endocrinology of Companion Animals* Lea and Febiger, Philadelphia, pp. 113

Eckersall, P. D. and Williams, M. E. (1983) Thyroid function tests in dogs using radioimmunoassay kits. *J. Small Animal Pract.*, **24**, 525

Evinger, J. V., Nelson, R. W. and Bottoms, G. D. (1985) Thyrotropin-releasing hormone stimulation testing in healthy dogs. *Am. J. Vet. Res.*, **46**, 1323

Feldman, E. C. and Nelson, R. W. (1987) Hypothyroidism. In *Canine and Feline Endocrinology and Reproduction*, W. B. Saunders, Philadelphia p. 55

Ferguson, D. C. (1984) Thyroid function tests in the dog. *Vet. Clinics of North America*, **14**, 783

Gosselin, S. J., Capen, C. C., Martin, S. L. *et al.*, (1980) Biochemical and immunological investigations on hypothyroidism in dogs. *Can. J. Comp. Med.*, **44**, 158

Haines, D. M., Lording, P. M. and Penhale, W. J. (1984) The detection of canine autoantibodies to thyroid antigens by enzyme-linked immunosorbent assay, haemagglutination and indirect immunofluorescence. *Can. J. Comp. Med.*, **48**, 262

Jezyk, P. F. (1985) Constitutional disorders of the skeleton in dogs and cats. In *Textbook of Small Animal Orthopaedics* (eds. C. D. Newton and D. M. Nunamaker). J. P. Lippincott, Philadelphia pp. 637

Larsson, M. G. (1988) Determination of free thyroxin and cholestrol as a new screening test for canine hypothyroidism *J. Am. Animal Hospital Assoc.*, **24**, 209

Lothrop, C. D., Tamas, P. M., Fadok, V. A. (1984) Canine and feline thyroid function assessment with the thyrotropin-releasing hormone response test. *Am. J. Vet. Res.*, **45**, 2310

Medleau, L., Eigenmann, J. E., Saunders, H. M. and Goldschmidt, M. H. (1985) Congenital hypothyroidism in a dog. *J. Am. Animal Hospital Assoc.*, **21**, 341

Nesbitt, G. H., Izzo, J., Peterson, L., Wilkins, R. J. (1980) Canine hypothyroidism: a retrospective study of 108 cases. *J. Am. Vet. Med. Assoc.*, **177**, 1117

Oliver, J. W. and Waldrop, V. (1983) Sampling protocol for thyrotropin stimulation test in the dog. *J. Am. Vet. Med. Assoc.*, **182**, 486

Peterson, M. E., Ferguson, D. C., Kintzer, P. P. and Drucker, W. D. (1984) Effects of spontaneous hyperadrenocorticism on serum thyroid hormone concentrations. *Am. J. Vet. Res.*, **45**, 2034

Scott, D. W. (1982) Histopathological findings in endocrine skin disorders of the dog. *J. Am. Animal Hospital, Assoc.*, **18**, 173

Theilen, G. H. (1975). In *Textbook of Veterinary Internal Medicine, Vol. 1* (ed. S. J. Ettinger), W. B. Saunders, Philadelphia, p. 146

POLLY M. TAYLOR

Intensive care of small animals

INTRODUCTION

INTENSIVE CARE is employed in the care of a critically ill animal which would not survive without regular treatment to maintain body function. It may be required for acute trauma cases, after major surgery and for some medical cases.

EQUIPMENT

The main requirement of intensive care is constant nursing attention. This can be achieved in many veterinary practices with little more than some experience and plenty of dedication.

A suitable place must be provided that does not disrupt the running of the clinic but is not tucked out of the way and easily ignored. Space in the anaesthetic recovery area is usually most suitable, although bigger institutions may have a separate intensive care room.

Good lighting, heating and ventilation are essential. Access to drugs, infusion equipment, catheters and the like must be easy. The critically ill animal is best cared for on a table which provides all round access. As its condition improves it can be moved to a kennel. Any kennel used for intensive care must, however, still allow good access to the patient and should be at table height. The debilitated animal is susceptible to infection and a high standard of cleanliness and asepsis must be maintained. A rota for the nursing and veterinary care should be drawn up along with written instructions for treatment and monitoring.

Specific equipment required includes the normal tools of the trade used in any clinical examination such as a stethoscope and thermometer. In addition an oxygen supply and emergency resuscitation kit are essential. The resuscitation kit should contain endotracheal tubes, means of providing intermittent positive pressure ventilation (IPPV) with oxygen and drugs suitable for treating cardiac arrest. Sterile equipment for placing intravenous and urinary catheters, chest drains and tracheo-stomy tubes is also required. Analgesics, intravenous fluids, sedatives, antibiotics, diuretics and steroids are the most likely drugs to be needed. Suitable bedding, heating pads and insulation should be available. Access to basic laboratory facilities is essential for rational treatment of many cases, and regular radiography will be required in the management of all chest cases.

Other more sophisticated equipment such as a blood pressure monitor, an electrocardiograph, laboratory facilities enabling measurement of blood gases and electrolytes and an automatic infusion pump enable improved care and will allow treatment of the most critically ill. However, there is an enormous amount that can be done with standard practice equipment, and lack of exotic equipment should not preclude success in many cases encountered in general veterinary practice.

GENERAL NURSING CARE

General comfort should be assured with regular grooming, prevention or removal of any staining from urine or faeces, washing out the mouth, cleaning the nose and eyes, and comfortable, easily cleaned bedding. Vetbed is ideal for the animal to lie on. Normal temperature must be maintained by ensuring a relatively high ambient temperature and good insulation. Heat pads are less effective than good insulation. Insulation with plastic bubble packing material is effective and enables the animal to be seen easily. Heavy blankets over the animal make nursing far more difficult.

All catheters, chest drains and tracheostomy tubes must be maintained under aseptic conditions. Patency is maintained with regular cleaning and flushing, and hands must be scrubbed meticulously before any line is handled. Chest drains and tracheostomy tubes require particular care because these can cause rapid death if mismanaged. Patency of the tracheostomy tube must be ensured *at all times*. A chest drain, inserted into the pleural cavity in order to drain air or fluid, must be either sealed when not in use or be connected to a one-way valve. On no account must air be allowed to leak back into the pleural cavity.

Many animals in intensive care will be in pain. This should be treated for humanitarian reasons. A pain-free animal is also likely to be relaxed and easier to nurse than a restless, uncomfortable one. Recovery may be more rapid because the animal will begin to eat more readily and take an interest in the environment. A little TLC (tender loving care) also goes a long way towards successful results.

MONITORING

Monitoring is the most important aspect of intensive care. It ensures an early warning system about the animal's condition so that relevant treatment can be given immediately. Written records should be kept to ensure continuity and show any response to treatment. Much information is gained from simple observations and the condition of the animal will suggest how frequently each measurement should be made. Each parameter must be assessed in the light of any other measurements in order to make a full assessment.

The pulse rate and quality should be recorded at frequent and regular intervals. Increased pulse rate may indicate hypovolaemia, hypoxia, pain or sepsis. A weak pulse indicates that the circulation is inadequate.

Respiratory rate and pattern should be recorded regularly, and the chest auscultated. Tachypnoea may indicate pain, hypoxia, sepsis or poor respiratory function. Pulmonary oedema and any sign of respiratory obstruction can be detected. The mucous membranes should be inspected and assessed in the light of the pulse and respiration.

Temperature measurement enables effective maintenance of the body temperature by adjustment of insulation and external heat. Measurement of peripheral and core temperature also provides information about the circulation because peripheral 'shut-down' results in cold extremities. Appropriate thermistors can be placed in the nasopharynx and on the skin. Even palpation of limbs or ears enables crude assessment of peripheral circulation.

Urinary output provides invaluable information about the circulation. In general, if the kidney is producing urine it is adequately perfused. If the kidney is adequately perfused then so is the rest of the body. Approximately 0.5–1.0 ml/kg/h should be produced. Treatment of animals in renal failure will depend on adequate monitoring of both volume and quality of the urine output. The urinary bladder should be catheterized in any case of renal failure and in any animal that cannot be moved so that it can urinate itself. An empty bladder will also make the animal comfortable. Urine should be collected into a bag (e.g. an empty intravenous fluid bag) so that volume can be measured and to prevent soiling of the animal.

Fluid input should be measured so that response to the prescribed treatment can be accurately assessed and adjustments made as necessary. Measurement of central venous pressure (CVP) from a jugular catheter with its tip in the thorax provides a guide to how much fluid should be given. If the CVP is low (negative or less than 5 cm H_2O) more fluid can be given. If the CVP is high and rising it indicates that the heart is unable to pump the venous return adequately and the infusion should be slowed.

The general demeanour of the animal provides much information about its well being and should be regularly assessed. A confused restless animal may be hypoxic, in pain or be developing cerebral oedema.

Additional information can be obtained with more sophisticated equipment. Packed cell volume and plasma protein should be measured several times daily in animals receiving all fluids intravenously. The ECG is often beneficial and is essential for diagnosis and rational treatment or any cardiac dysrhythmia. Measurement of arterial blood pressure, now a practical proposition with Doppler pulse detectors, is valuable after major cardiovascular surgery or trauma. Measurement of arterial blood gases and electrolytes is useful in the critically ill animal, particularly with inadequate respiratory function.

TREATMENT

One of the major requirements of intensive care is the maintenance of fluid balance. Only a brief guide can be given here. Essentially, fluid input is most easily divided into replacement of abnormal losses and provision of daily requirements. As far as possible 'like' should replace 'like'. Thus blood loss should be replaced with blood or plasma replacer and isotonic losses with balanced electrolyte solutions. In general an equal volume to that which has been lost should be given. Daily fluid requirements should be provided by allowing 40 ml/kg/day of a hypotonic solution, e.g. 0.18% NaCl in 4% dextrose. Adjustment of input is made in the light of the information provided by monitoring.

Oxygen may be required in the shocked animal or where respiratory function is compromised. It is best provided by nasal tube or oxygen cage.

Analgesics and sedatives will be required in post surgical or trauma cases. Combinations of one of the benzodiazepams with an opiate provide an excellent synergistic effect. Diazepam up to 1 mg/kg and buprenorphine 0.01 mg/kg can be given intravenously as required, usually every 4 hours.

Broad spectrum antibiotic cover should always be provided. Steroids may be required in the shocked animal or in treatment of cerebral oedema (e.g.

dexamethasone 2–4 mg/kg 4 to 6 hourly). Diuretics may be used in treating renal failure or pulmonary and cerebral oedema (e.g. frusemide 1–2 mg/kg). Vasoactive drugs such as dopamine or dobutamine (1–3 µg/kg/min) may be required where cardiac function is inadequate.

More detailed discussion of all aspects of intensive care in dogs and cats is provided by Burrows (1981) and Houlton and Taylor (1987).

REFERENCES AND FURTHER READING

Burrows, C. F. (1981) Veterinary intensive care. *J. Small Animal Pract.*, **22**, 231–-252
Kirk, R. W. and Bistner, S. I. (1981) *Handbook of Veterinary Procedures and Emergency Treatment*, 3rd edn. W. B. Saunders, Philadelphia
Houlton, J. E. F. and Taylor, P. M. (1987) Intensive Care (Chapter 7), and Techniques (Chapter 8). In *Trauma Management in the Dog and Cat*, Wright, pp. 90–145
Wingfield, W. E. (1981) Emergency medicine. *Veterinary Clinics of North America Small Animal Clinics*, **11** (1)

A. H. M. VAN DEN BROEK

Cutaneous hypersensitivity (allergy) in dogs

INTRODUCTION

HYPERSENSITIVITY REACTIONS are a major cause of skin disease in dogs. They are involved in the genesis of several different conditions with cutaneous manifestations, notably atopy, flea allergic dermatitis (FAD), food and contact allergy, drug hypersensitivity, (endogenous) hormone hypersensitivity, hypersensitivity to intestinal parasites and more controversially, bacterial hypersensitivity. In this review, the pathogenesis, incidence, clinical signs, diagnosis and management of these conditions are considered.

PATHOGENESIS

In all immunologically competent animals repeated or prolonged encounters with the same or cross-reacting, non-self antigen provoke a heightened state immune reactivity. The ensuing antigen–antibody or antigen–immunocompetent cell interaction is normally beneficial and facilitates elimination of antigen from the body. However, in individuals with impaired modulation of the immune response, it may culminate in tissue damage. These injurious interactions, although commonly described as allergic reactions, are properly defined as hypersensitivity reactions.

Four types of hypersensitivity reaction are recognized (Gell and Coombs, 1964). Three types are responsible for the conditions being considered. Each reaction is accompanied by the release of various mediators, enzymes and vaso-active substances. The most important of these in the genesis of cutaneous signs in dogs are histamine, leucotriennes (Willemse, 1987) and proteolytic enzymes (Muller *et al.*, 1983).

Type 1 hypersensitivity is characterized by the interaction of antigen with IgE antibody bound to mast cells or basophils. It is involved in atopy, FAD, food allergy, drug and hormone hypersensitivity and hypersensitivity to intestinal parasites. Type 3 hypersensitivity is distinguished by the combination of antigen with humoral antibody to form microcomplexes which become deposited in the walls of blood vessels. It has been implicated in drug and bacterial hypersensitivity. Type 4 hypersensitivity is mediated by T effector lymphocytes which secrete numerous lymphokines when confronted with the sensitizing antigen. It is responsible for contact allergy, contributes to FAD and has been implicated in drug and hormone hypersensitivity and food allergy. In contact allergy the antigen is often incomplete and must first combine with dermal protein before being processed by Langerhans cells which present it to T lymphocytes.

INCIDENCE

Precise estimates of the incidence of particular conditions vary but FAD and atopy are common and food and contact allergy are relatively uncommon. Hypersensitivity reactions to bacteria, drugs, hormones and intestinal parasites are rare.

BREED INCIDENCE

Although in one study (Walton, 1977a) of contact allergy 20% of the cases were Labrador Retrievers, only atopy has a definite breed predisposition. It occurs most commonly in West Highland white terriers, Cairn terriers, Scottish terriers, Wire-haired fox terriers, Irish Setters, Lhasa Apsos, Miniature Schnauzers, Dalmatians, Labrador Retrievers, Boxers, German Shepherd dogs and Poodles (Halliwell and Schwartzman, 1971; Scott, 1981; Nesbitt, 1983; Willemse and van den Broem, 1983).

AGE INCIDENCE

Irrespective of the condition, the onset of clinical signs rarely occurs before an animal is six months old. It usually occurs between one and three years of age in atopy (Scott, 1981), between three and six years of age in FAD (Kwochka and Bevier, 1987) and after two years of age in food and contact allergy (Walton, 1977a; 1977b).

SEX INCIDENCE

Only in hormone hypersensitivity has a definite sex predilection been reported; 90% of cases were female (Chamberlain, 1974). Reports of sex predisposition in atopy are conflicting (Halliwell and Schwartzman, 1971; Scott, 1981; Nesbitt, 1978; Willemse and van den Broem, 1983).

CLINICAL SIGNS

CUTANEOUS SIGNS

Pruritus is the cardinal sign of cutaneous hypersensitivity and is usually associated with other non-specific signs. Erythema may accompany acute inflammation. Increased thickness, pigmentation and lichenification of the skin may occur with chronic inflammation. Excoriations, broken hair and acute moist dermatitis may result from self-inflicted trauma. Secondary seborrhoea, pyoderma and hair loss may also be present.

Oedematous swellings, urticaria and agioedema, are manifestations of Type 1 hypersensitivity. They may occur in response to atopy, food allergy, hypersensitivity to drugs, hormones, intestinal parasites, insect bites and vaccines. Oedema of the face and pinnae has been associated with food allergy (Walton, 1977b). Pustules and purplish haemorrhagic bullae surrounded by a zone of intense erythema accompany bacterial hypersensitivity (Scott *et al.*, 1978). Fleas and flea dirt may be seen in FAD. Bilateral otitis may occur in atopy and food allergy. Bilateral conjunctivitis is common in atopy.

DISTRIBUTION OF CUTANEOUS SIGNS

Atopic dogs typically exhibit signs of pedal and facial pruritus, notably paw biting or licking and face rubbing. Associated with these there may be evidence of pedal, submandibular, perioral, periorbital and pinna dermatitis. The flexor surfaces of the carpus, extensor surface of the tarsus, the axillae, ventral abdomen and medial thigh are also common sites of inflammation and self-inflicted damage.

FAD classically involves the dorsum, especially the lumbo-sacral region. However, lesions may be more generalized and involve the ventral abdomen, caudo-medial thigh and neck.

Contact allergy usually occurs on the less hairy areas of skin and is localized in areas exposed to the responsible allergen. Contact whilst walking may affect the interdigital web of the paw. Contact whilst sitting may produce lesions on the perineum and ventral aspect of the tail. Contact whilst lying down may involve the ventral abdomen, axillae, medial thigh, pinnae and submandibular area. Contact allergies to food bowls or toys are associated with lesions of the nose, lips and mouth. Contact allergy to shampoos may affect the whole body but allergies to topical medicants are limited to the area of application (Walton, 1977a).

In hormonal hypersensitivity lesions tend to be localized in the perineum, caudo-medial thigh and perigenital areas but many extend to involve the feet, face and ears (Scott, 1978).

Most dogs with food allergies have generalized pruritus. The self-inflicted damage associated with this is often, though not always, localized but has no characteristic distribution (Walton, 1977b).

Hypersensitivity reactions to drugs, bacteria and intestinal parasites produce lesions with a non-specific, generalized distribution.

SYSTEMIC SIGNS

Bitches with hormone hypersensitivity frequently have irregular oestrus cycles and pseudo pregnancies (Scott, 1978). In one study of food allergy (Walton, 1967) vomiting or diarrhoea were recorded in 13% of cases and asthmatic attacks were present in 2% of cases.

Anaphylaxis, serum sickness and petechial haemorrhages may accompany drug hypersensitivity (Wilcke, 1986). Reversed sneezing may occur occasionally in atopy (Willemse, 1987). The presence of hypothyroidism may predispose to bacterial hypersensitivity (Scott *et al.*, 1978).

PERIODICITY OF SIGNS

The pattern of clinical signs reflects exposure to the offending allergen. FAD exhibits a definite seasonal incidence and usually occurs in summer and autumn. Atopy may initially be seasonal, occurring in winter or summer, but often becomes a continuous problem. Contact allergy may also be seasonal. If so, it usually occurs in summer.

The manifestation of hormone hypersensitivity is often associated with, or exacerbated by, the onset of oestrus (Scott, 1978). Contact allergy and drug hypersensitivity may have an intermittent occurrence.

DIAGNOSIS

A definitive diagnosis is based on the history and clinical signs supported by evidence of an allergic reaction obtained from intradermal tests, provocative exposure or response to treatment. Skin histopathology has diagnostic value in bacterial hypersensitivity only.

The importance of intradermal tests, correctly performed and interpreted (Grant, 1986) in the diagnosis of atopy is well established (Reedy, 1980; Nesbitt *et al.*, 1984). However, because some atopic animals fail to give positive reactions, these tests must be seen in the context of the history and clinical signs. A recent proposal (Willemse, 1986) recognizes this and provides a useful basis for reaching a definite diagnosis. It requires the presence of three major and several minor criteria. The major criteria suggested are typical signs and distribution of pruritus, chronic dermatitis and breed or familial predisposition. The minor criteria are: onset before the age of three years, facial erythema and cheilitis, bilateral conjunctivitis, staphylococcal pyoderma, hyperhidrosis, positive intradermal tests and elevated allergen-specific IgE or IgGd.

Intradermal tests are also reported to be of value in the diagnosis of hormone (Scott, 1978) and bacterial hypersensitivity (Scott *et al.*, 1978). A positive, immediate or delayed reaction to oestrogen, progesterone or testosterone supports the diagnosis of hormone hypersensitivity and an Arthus reaction, an erythematous indurated reaction, 24–72 hours after injecting staphylococcal cell wall-toxoid suggests bacterial hypersensitivity. Further evidence for bacterial hypersensitivity may be derived from skin histopathology if vasculitis with leucocytic infiltration is detected. Avoidance followed by provocative exposure is the accepted method of diagnosing food allergy.

Because allergies to more than one food item rarely occur (Walton, 1967), food allergy is readily investigated by feeding two different diets. Each diet must avoid additives and supplements, be fed for three weeks and be composed of only two food items. Examples of suitable diets are: water, boiled rice and chicken and water, boiled potato and mutton. Sustained improvement on either diet supports the diagnosis. That diet is then maintained and each week one food item fed previously is added until the offending allergen is identified. In humans, prick tests provide supportive evidence of food allergy (Lessof *et al.*, 1980). The unreliability of intradermal and prick tests in dogs (Walton, 1977b) suggests that many cases currently diagnosed as food allergy would be more accurately designated food intolerance.

The diagnosis of contact allergy also relies on avoidance and provocative exposure. Avoidance is achieved by phased environmental restriction. Each phase lasts three weeks and excludes exposure to one or a combination of potential contact allergens. Continued clinical improvement during any phase is followed by provocative exposure. A relapse within two to five days supports the diagnosis but, unfortunately, does not distinguish between allergens and irritants. In view of this open (Walton, 1977a) and closed (Scott, 1978) patch testing have been advocated. However, the results are disappointing.

Response to treatment supports the diagnosis of FAD. Intradermal tests may also have supportive value but reports of their reliability are conflicting (Van Winkle, 1981; Halliwell, 1983). Hypersensitivity to intestinal parasites may be suggested by faecal examination and is confirmed by response to treatment.

In suspected drug hypersensitivity improvement following drug withdrawal supports the diagnosis. Theoretically, provocative exposure could confirm the diagnosis but the risk is unacceptable (Wilcke, 1986).

In some cases the history and clinical signs may indicate a tentative diagnosis and the direction of subsequent investigations. However, in many cases they are non-specific. Moreover, they may be mimicked by skin disease caused by external parasites, fungi and folliculitis. In these cases a well ordered approach to diagnosis is essential. First, involvement of external parasites is ruled out by skin scrapings and, if indicated, by treatment. Subsequently, fungal infection is investigated by microscopic examination and culture of hair and scale and involvement of intestinal parasites eliminated by faecal examination. Food and contact allergy are investigated in turn by dietary and environmental restriction. Finally, intradermal tests are carried out to investigate atopy, hormone and bacterial hypersensitivity.

MANAGEMENT

The main methods of long-term management are avoidance of the causative allergen, hyposensitization and glucocorticoid therapy, or a combination of these. Once the offending allergen has been identified avoidance is successful and usually feasible in cases of drug hypersensitivity, food and contact allergy. In cases of hormone hypersensitivity avoidance is achieved by ovariohysterectomy or castration. In FAD, avoidance necessitates instituting and, if indicated, maintaining, a programme of flea eradication. This must include all in contact with the animal and extend to the environment, particularly areas where the animals spend any length of time. Similarly, periodic use of an anthelmintic may be necessary to control hypersensitivity to intestinal parasites.

Hyposensitization is indicated in atopy when avoidance of confirmed allergens is impractical. It significantly benefits approximately 60% of cases (Scott, 1978; Kunkle, 1980). Hyposensitization has also been attempted in FAD. However, a double blind study using commercially available allergens, concluded it was ineffective (Halliwell, 1981).

When strict avoidance is impossible or the response to hyposensitization poor, they may be supplemented with, or replaced by, glucocorticoids. If systemic glucocorticoids are necessary, side effects may be minimized by using alternate-day oral prednisolone therapy. In contact allergy topical glucocorticoids may control the clinical signs.

Recently, dietary supplementation with essential fatty acids combined with appropriate co-factors (EfaVet 1 and 2, Efamol Ltd) has been reported to benefit atopic dogs (Lloyd, 1988). It may also be of benefit in other allergic conditions.

Appropriate systemic antibiotic will control bacterial hypersensitivity. However, this condition may result from underlying hypothyroidism, food allergy or atopy. Long-term management therefore depends on diagnosis and control of the underlying disease (Scott *et al.*, 1978).

REFERENCES

Chamberlain, K. W. (1974) Hormonal hypersensitivity in canines. *Canine Practice*, **1**, 18–25

Gell, P. G. H. and Coombs, R. R. A. (1964) *Clinical Aspects of Immunology.* F. A. Davis, Philadelphia.

Grant, D. I. (1986) Intradermal allergy testing in the dog. In *The Veterinary Annual 26th Issue* (eds. C. S. G. Grunsell, F. W. G. Hill and M.-E. Raw), Scientechnica, Bristol, pp. 283–286

Halliwell, R. E. W. (1981) Hyposensitisation in the treatment of flea bite hypersensitivity. Results of a double blind study. *J. Am. Animal Hospital Assoc.*, **17**, 249–253

Halliwell, R. E. W. (1983) Flea allergy dermatitis. In *Current Veterinary Therapy VIII* (ed. R. W. Kirk), W. B. Saunders, Philadelphia, pp. 496–499

Halliwell, R. F. W. and Schwartzman, R. M. (1971) Atopic disease in the dog. *Vet. Rec.*, **89**, 209–214

Kunkle, G. A. (1980) The treatment of canine atopic disease. In *Current Veterinary Therapy VII* (ed. R. W. Kirk), W. B. Saunders, Philadelphia, pp. 453–458

Kwochka, K. W. and Bevier, D. E. (1987) Flea Dermatitis. In *Contemporary Issues in Small Animal Practice – Dermatology* (ed. G. H. Nesbitt), Churchill Livingstone, New York, pp. 21–55

Lessof, M. H., Wraith, D. G., Merrett, T. G., Merrett, J. and Buisseret, P. D. (1980) Food allergy and intolerance in 100 patients – local and systemic effects. *Q. J. Med.*, **195**, 259–271

Lloyd, D. (1988) Dietary supplementation in the treatment of skin disease. In *Proceedings of the 5th Annual Congress of the European Society of Veterinary Dermatology* (ed. D. Lloyd), pp. 79–81

Muller, G. H., Kirk, R. W. and Scott, D. W. (1983) *Small Animal Dermatology*, 3rd edn, W. B. Saunders, Philadelphia

Nesbitt, G. H. (1978) Canine allergic inhalant dermatitis: a review of 230 cases. *J. Am. Vet. Med. Assoc.*, **172**, 55–60

Nesbitt, G. H. (1983) *Canine and Feline Dermatology,* Lea and Febiger, Philadelphia

Nesbitt, G. H., Kedan, G. S. and Caciolo, P. (1984) Canine Atopy. Part 1. Etiology and Diagnosis. *Compend. Contin. Educ. Pract. Vet.*, **6**, 73–84

Reedy, L. M. (1980) The diagnosis of canine atopic disease. In *Current Veterinary Therapy VII* (ed. R. W. Kirk), W. B. Saunders, Philadelphia, pp. 450–453

Scott, D. W. (1978) Immunological Skin Disorders in the Dog and Cat, *Veterinary Clinics of North America*, **8**, 641–664

Scott, D. W. (1981) Observations on canine atopy. *J. Animal Hospital Assoc.*, **17**, 91–100

Scott, D. W., McDonald, J. M. and Schultz, R. D. (1978) Staphylococcal hypersensitivity in the dog. *J. Am. Animal Hospital Assoc.*, **14**, 766–779

Van Winkle, K. A. (1981) An evaluation of flea antigens used in intradermal skin testing for flea allergy in the canine. *J. Am. Animal Hospital Assoc.*, **17**, 343–354

Walton, G. S. (1967) Skin responses in the dog and cat to ingested allergens. Observations on one hundred confirmed cases. *Vet. Rec.*, **81**, 709–713

Walton, G. S. (1977a) Allergic contact dermatitis. In *Current Veterinary Therapy VI* (ed. R. W. Kirk), W. B. Saunders, Philadelphia, pp. 571–575

Walton, G. S. (1977b) Allergic responses to ingested allergens. In *Current Veterinary Therapy VI* (ed. R. W. Kirk) W. B. Saunders, Philadelphia, pp. 576–579

Wilcke, J. R. (1986) Allergic drug reactions. In *Current Veterinary Therapy IX* (ed. R. W. Kirk), W. B. Saunders, Philadelphia, pp. 444–448

Willemse, T. (1986) Atopic skin disease: a review and reconsideration of diagnostic criteria. *J. Small Animal Pract.*, **27**, 771–778

Willemse, T. A. (1987) In *Contemporary Issues in Small Animal Practice – Dermatology* (ed. G. H. Nesbitt). Churchill Livingstone, New York

Willemse, A. and van den Broem, W. F. (1983) Investigations of the symptomatology and the significance of immediate skin test reactivity in canine atopic dermatitis. *Res. Vet. Sci.*, **34**, 261–265

E. M. MILNE

Insulinoma in the dog

INTRODUCTION

INSULINOMA, (ISLET cell tumour or beta-cell carcinoma) is an uncommon endocrine disorder of dogs which causes episodic weakness and nervous signs resulting from chronic hypoglycaemia. It has also been described in the cat (McMillan *et al.*, 1985).

AETIOLOGY

The endocrine pancreas consists of islets of alpha and beta cells which produce the hormones glucagon and insulin, respectively. Insulin is normally released in response to hyperglycaemia. It facilitates uptake of glucose, amino acids, fatty acids and potassium from the blood. It also stimulates glycogen synthesis and inhibits glucose production by inhibiting glycogenolysis and gluconeogenesis. The net effect of insulin is to decrease blood glucose. Glucagon has an opposing effect and therefore increases blood glucose. Insulin and glucagon are the major hormones of glucose homeostasis although several other hormones, e.g. glucocorticoids, growth hormone, sex hormones and catecholamines, are also antagonistic to the effects of insulin on blood glucose.

Insulinomas are functional (insulin-secreting) adenomas or adenocarcinomas of the beta cells. They are single or multiple firm nodules within the pancreas and range from 5 to 110 mm in diameter. Histopathology reveals cords or groups of cells surrounded by collagenous stroma. The neoplastic cells do not always react positively to specific stains for beta cells (Mattheeuws *et al.*, 1976). Mitotic figures are rarely seen and the degree of invasiveness is a better guide to degree of malignancy. In dogs, 90% are adenocarcinomas whereas in humans, most are adenomas. Metastases occur at an early stage to the regional lymph nodes, liver, omentum, mesentery and occasionally to the lungs (Njoku *et al.*, 1972). Excessive insulin secretion from insulinomas results in hypoglycaemia which is out of the control of the normal negative feedback mechanisms which maintain glucose homeostasis.

OCCURRENCE

Insulinomas are more common in large breeds, especially Irish Setters, Golden Retrievers, Boxers and German Shepherd dogs (Liefer *et al.*, 1986). Middle aged to elderly dogs are most often affected and the age range is 5–14 years (Mehlhaff *et al.*, 1985). There is no sex predilection.

CLINICAL SIGNS

The clinical signs are mainly referable to the effect of fluctuating blood glucose levels on the nervous system. There is usually a history of the gradual onset of several of the following clinical signs: weakness, ataxia, muscle fasciculations, collapse, grand mal seizures, exercise intolerance, polyphagia, weight gain polydipsia and polyuria, hypothermia, visual defects, nervousness and mental confusion. The signs are episodic and their onset may be associated with fasting, excitement or exercise, or may occur after feeding which stimulates insulin release. Initially, affected dogs will be normal between episodes but later the episodes become increasingly frequent and coma or status epilepticus may eventually occur with death resulting from depression of the respiratory centre.

DIFFERENTIAL DIAGNOSIS

The differential diagnosis is that of seizures and episodic weakness which are discussed in detail elsewhere in this volume (Raw, 1989).

DIAGNOSIS

HISTORY AND CLINICAL SIGNS

The history is very important in establishing a tentative diagnosis because the dog may appear normal when presented for clinical examination. Most have a history of showing several of the signs listed above but a few will be presented for a single complaint, e.g. epileptiform seizures. Radiography is unhelpful due to the small size of most lesions (Kruth *et al.*, 1982) and the tentative clinical diagnosis must be confirmed by laboratory investigation.

LABORATORY FINDINGS

Blood glucose and insulin levels

The most accurate means of diagnosis is to demonstrate inappropriately high plasma insulin levels for the level of blood glucose. Insulin and glucose should therefore be measured simultaneously when clinical signs of hypoglycaemia are present or after fasting. Most cases will become hypoglycaemic within 8 hours of fasting but some require fasts of 24 to 72 hours before significant hypoglycaemia develops (Leifer *et al.*, 1986). The aim is to demonstrate a raised blood insulin when blood glucose is low or normal. Blood insulin is likely to exceed normal values and blood glucose will fall below 2 mmol/l during hypoglycaemic episodes. Calculation of the ratio between insulin and glucose may provide confirmation in cases where hypoglycaemia is accompanied by normal plasma insulin levels. This ratio has been expressed as the insulin/glucose ratio (IGR) or the amended insulin/glucose ratio (AIGR). Both are more sensitive diagnostic aids than simply demonstrating a raised fasting blood insulin level. However, they do give more false positive results, particularly the AIGR (Leifer *et al.*, 1986).

They are calculated as follows:

$$IGR = \frac{\text{plasma insulin } (\mu u/ml) \times 100}{\text{plasma glucose } (mg/dl)}$$

$$AIGR = \frac{\text{plasma insulin } (\mu u/ml) \times 100}{\text{plasma glucose } (mg/100ml) - 30}$$

Note that old units are still used for blood glucose when calculating these ratios and SI units (mmol/l) are multiplied by 18.02 to convert them to old units (mg/100 ml) for this purpose. IGR and AIGR values of greater than 30 are said to suggest the presence of an insulinoma. The AIGR is extrapolated from the medical literature and the validity of its use in the dog has been questioned despite its sensitivity and widespread use (Edwards, 1986).

Tolerance tests

A number of tolerance tests have been described for use when blood glucose and insulin results are equivocal. These include glucagon, glucose and tolbutamide tolerance tests. In all these tests, excessive insulin release is stimulated. This carries with it the risk of provoking an acute hypoglycaemic crisis. The glucagon tolerance test has been described in detail by Feldman (1983).

TREATMENT

SURGICAL MANAGEMENT

On confirmation of the diagnosis, surgery should be undertaken as this is likely to enhance survival time (Leifer *et al.*, 1986). Blood glucose levels should first be controlled by feeding small meals high in protein and low in simple sugars, 5 to 6 times daily together with the administration of oral glucocorticoids (0.5–1 mg/kg divided bid) or oral dioxide (10–40 mg/kg divided tid). In addition, intravenous infusion of balanced electrolyte solutions containing 5% glucose will prevent hypoglycaemia if administered before and during surgery. Parasympatholytics before and after surgery reduce the inevitable leakage of pancreatic enzymes (Steinberg, 1982).

Surgery involves removal of all visible and palpable tumours. The drainage lymph nodes should be examined for metastases which should be removed if possible. Even if the tumours are not all resectable or metastases are present, life can be prolonged by medical therapy and euthanasia should not necessarily be carried out at this stage.

Post-operative care involves infusion of intravenous fluids containing 5% glucose and administration of parasympatholytics and antibiotics. Blood glucose levels should be carefully monitored post-operatively. Nothing should be given orally for the first 24–48 hours because exogenous pancreatic secretions will be stimulated, increasing the risk of peritonitis. Other post-operative complications are diabetes mellitus, which is usually transient, and pancreatitis. In most cases treated surgically, signs of hypoglycaemia will eventually return but there may be remission for up to one year.

MEDICAL MANAGEMENT

Dogs presented in an acute hypoglycaemic crisis should be given 2–10 ml of 50% glucose by slow intravenous injection. If acute hypoglycaemia occurs at home, the owner can feed the dog a small meal or smear syrup on the tongue if the dog is unconscious. Oral or intravenous glucose are only emergency measures because they will stimulate further insulin release.

If the owner does not agree to surgery, if surgery only partially controls the hypoglycaemia or where signs recur following remission after surgery, long-term medical treatment is required. Exercise should be limited and dietary control instituted. Diazoxide (Eudemine; Allen and Hanburys), a non-diuretic compound related to the thiazide diuretics, is the drug of choice although it is not licenced for veterinary use. It inhibits insulin secretion, stimulates glucose production from the liver and inhibits tissue utilization of glucose, all of which increase blood glucose. Diazoxide is relatively safe. The major side effect is vomiting but it can occasionally cause diabetes mellitus and bone marrow suppression. The dose required depends on response but a suitable rate is 10–40 mg/kg divided tid. Doses exceeding 100 mg/kg/day have been administered without apparent side-effects (Parker *et al.*, 1982). The cytotoxic agent streptozotocin may result in temporary remission but is also highly nephrotoxic and its use cannot be advocated (Meyer, 1977).

PROGNOSIS

The malignant nature of most insulinomas, resulting in recurrence of the clinical signs for a variable time after surgery. makes the long-term prognosis poor. However, in one survey, the mean survival time of dogs treated by a combination of surgical and medical management was 14 months, (Mehlhaff *et al.*, 1985) so useful prolongation of life can be achieved. This renders treatment well worth attempting.

REFERENCES

Edwards, D. F. (1986) *J. Am. Vet. Med. Assoc.*, **188**, 951–953
Feldman, E. C. (1983) Diseases of the dog and cat. In *Textbook of Veterinary Internal Medicine*, 2nd edn, (ed. S. J. Ettinger) Saunders, Philadelphia, pp. 1644
Kruth, S. A., Feldman, E. C and Kennedy, P. C. (1982) *J. Am. Vet. Med. Assoc.*, **181**, 54–58
Leifer, C. E., Peterson, M. E. and Matus, R. E. (1986) *J. Am. Vet. Med. Assoc.*, **188**, 60–64
Mattheeuws, D., Rottiers, R., Rijcke, J., De Rick, A. and De Schepper, J. (1976) *J. Small Animal Pract.*, **17**, 313–318
McMillan, F. D., Barr, B. and Feldman, E. C. (1985) *J. Am. Animal Hospital Assoc.*, **21**, 741–746
Mehlhaff, C. J., Peterson, M. E., Patnaik, A. K. and Carrillo, J. M. (1985) *J. Am. Animal Hospital Assoc.*, **21**, 607–618
Meyer, D. J. (1977) *Am. J. Vet. Res.*, **38**, 1201–1204
Njoku, C. O., Strafuss, A. C. and Dennis, S. M. (1972) *J. Am. Animal Hospital Assoc.*, **8**, 284–290
Parker, A. J., O'Brien, D. and Musselman, E. E. (1982) *J. Am. Animal Hospital Assoc.*, **18**, 315–318
Raw, M.-E. (1989) Episodic weakness. In *The Veterinary Annual, 29th Issue* (eds. C.S.G. Grunsell, M.-E. Raw and F. W. G. Hill) Butterworth, London, pp. 255–260
Steinberg, H. S. (1982) *J. Am. Animal Hospital Assoc.*, **16**, 695–698

MARY-ELIZABETH RAW

Episodic weakness

EPISODIC WEAKNESS

EPISODIC WEAKNESS can be defined as occuring when an animal experiences periods of weakness but is essentially normal between these periods. The main causes are neurological, cardiovascular and metabolic (Table 1). The weakness may manifest itself as anything from mild ataxia to complete collapse. Episodic weakness may be the first sign of serious progressive conditions.

Table 1 CONDITIONS SHOWING EPISODIC WEAKNESS

Neurological:	Myasthenia gravis
	Cataplexy
	Polymyositis
	Mitochondrial myopathy
	Psycomotor epilepsy
Cardiovascular:	Arrhythmias
	Sick sinus syndrome
	Heart worm disease
	Other cardiac defects
Metabolic:	Hypoglycaemia
	Insulinoma
	Hunting dogs hypoglycaemia
	Glycogen storage disease
	Transient juvenile hypoglycaemia
	Non-pancreatic neoplasia
	Other causes, e.g. pregnancy
	Adrenal insufficiency
	Other electrolyte imbalances
Miscellaneous:	Anaemia
	Idiopathic weakness

NEUROLOGICAL

MYASTHENIA GRAVIS

Myasthenia gravis occurs when there is a defect at the neuromuscular junction caused by a reduction in the numbers of acetyl choline receptors. It is seen in both adult and young dogs. In the acquired adult form antibodies against the acetyl choline receptors are present but this is not so with the congenital form (Palmer, 1980).

Myasthenia gravis manifests itself as tiredness and reduced exercise tolerance. There is muscular weakness. The fore limbs are usually affected first. Megoesophagus is commonly seen in affected dogs. The animal may become so weak that it is only able to take two or three steps before collapsing. Diagnosis is by intravenous injection of edrophonium chloride (Palmer, 1980). If the animal is myasthenic, instant recovery will occur after the injection. This will usually last for a few minutes before the dog reverts to a collapsed state.

Treatment is by oral pyridostigmine bromide, 2.0 mg/kg two or three times a day, to control signs. Steroids may be added if the pyridostigmine does not lead to an improvement (Oliver and Lorenz, 1983). Spontaneous recovery can occur. If the animal has a large megoesophagus, difficulty may be experienced in using tablets for treatment. Medication must be given when the dog has enough muscular strength to swallow the tablets properly. Cold can increase myasthenic signs so the animal must be kept warm (Palmer, 1980).

The congenital form has been reported in Jack Russell terriers and related breeds. Weakness is noted from six weeks of age. Signs are similar to the adult form, except that the hind legs are usually affected first (Palmer, 1980).

CATAPLEXY

Cataplexy is a condition associated with narcolepsy. Narcolepsy has been reviewed elsewhere (Foutz *et al.*, 1980). Affected dogs have sudden episodes of flaccid paralysis, lasting from a few seconds to several minutes. The animal may be playing, eating or exercising when either all the skeletal muscles (complete attack) or certain selected muscle groups (partial attacks) are involved (Foutz *et al.*, 1980a). During a complete attack the dog can lie in any position. The eyes are usually open and can track movements. If a piece of food is in the mouth, the tongue may move and there may be chewing movements. These attacks can usually be reversed by stroking the animal or making a noise (Foutz *et al.*, 1980).

Attacks can be frequent. Severely affected individuals may have over a hundred a day. In milder cases episodes may occur daily or even weekly. Severity of the signs can be assessed by the food-elicited cataplexy test, details of which are to be found in Foutz *et al.*, (1980).

Diagnosis is by exclusion of myasthenia gravis and epilepsy and by the use of the food-elicited cataplexy test. Treatment is by imipramine, given orally, at 0.5 mg to 1 mg/kg (Foutz *et al.*, 1980). This will not stop all the attacks but should reduce them. Unusual excitement should be avoided.

POLYMYOSITIS

Polymyositis can manifest itself as episodic weakness, especially when its course is insidious. In addition to the weakness there may be muscle stiffness and pain. The oesophageal muscle can be affected, resulting in the regurgitation of food due to the formation of megoesophagus.

Increased levels of serum enzymes of muscle origin, especially creatine phosphokinase (CPK), are demonstrated in the blood. A definitive diagnosis is provided by biopsy of an affected muscle. Treatment is by high doses of corticosteroids over two weeks, with gradually decreasing amounts over a further two weeks. More than one course of treatment may be necessary (Griffiths, 1980).

MITOCHONDRIAL MYOPATHY

Mitochondrial myopathy has been reported in Clumber and Sussex spaniels which collapse on exercise but recover after resting (Herrtage and Houlton, 1979; Houlton and Herrtage, 1980). Raised levels of lactate and pyruvate are found in the blood because the muscle mitochondria are unable to oxidize pyruvate. This condition should be differentiated from myasthesia gravis.

PSYCHOMOTOR EPILEPSY

Psychomotor epilepsy has been observed in dogs (Parker, 1980). In most cases of epilepsy there is a definite seizure pattern, with grand mal seizures that are easily recognized (Barker, 1973; Raw and Gaskell, 1985). In psychomotor epilepsy the seizures can be manifested as episodic weakness, including sudden collapse.

Diagnosis depends on the elimination of other causes of episodic weakness, especially myasthenia gravis and cataplexy and the response to treatment by anticonvulsant drugs such as phenobarbitone or primidone.

CARDIOVASCULAR

CARDIAC ARRHYTHMIAS

Cardiac arrhythmias can reduce the cerebral and coronary blood flow sufficiently to produce weakness. Weakness is often episodic, especially in the early stages (Ettinger, 1983). The arrhythmias may not always be detected on auscultation (Farrow, 1983). An ECG examination is always necessary to pinpoint the exact nature of the disturbance so that the correct treatment can be given.

Details of treatment can be found in Bonagura (1983) and Darke (1986).

SICK SINUS SYNDROME

This causes sudden weakness at any time of the day. It can range from staggering to total collapse with transient unconsciousness. These episodes last between two and 10 seconds (Parker, 1983). This condition is particularly seen in middle-aged Miniature Schnauzers and Boxers.

Diagnosis is by ECG monitoring, which shows abnormally long (2–6 s) intervals of sinus arrest (Parker, 1983). The monitoring may have to be prolonged to establish a diagnosis in some cases. If the diagnosis is in doubt, intravenous chlorpromazine (at up to 1 mg/kg) may be given to enhance the ECG abnormality (Parker, 1983).

No drug treatment is entirely satisfactory but a combination of atropine-like derivatives, digitalis and frusemide has been found helpful (Ettinger, 1983). Insertion of a pacemaker is the ideal method of treatment, but the overall prognosis is not good.

HEART WORM DISEASE

Heart worm disease can present as episodic weakness with no other clinical signs (Farrow, 1983; Ettinger, 1983). This is especially so in the early course of the disease. Clinical examination is often unrewarding and diagnosis depends on demonstating microfilariae in the blood. Thoracic radiographs may show characteristic changes (Kealy, 1987).

Further details of diagnosis and treatment of canine heart worm disease can be found from Calvert and Rawlings (1983).

CONGENITAL HEART DISEASE, VALVULAR HEART DISEASE AND CONGESTIVE HEART FAILURE

These may also be the cause of episodic weakness (Farrow, 1983; Ettinger, 1983). Auscultation, radiology and ultrasound and ECG examination confirm the diagnosis.

METABOLIC DISEASE

HYPOGLYCAEMIA

Hypoglycaemia is the commonest metabolic cause of episodic weakness (Farrow, 1983). Signs, which vary from mild weakness to grand mal seizures, depend on the rate of decrease of the plasma glucose levels and the degree of hypoglycaemia. Blood glucose levels may be normal at the time of presentation and it may be necessary to sample after starvation for 24 to 48 hours to get a positive result (Farrow, 1983).

There are a number of causes of hypoglycaemia in dogs:
1. Pancreatic beta-cell neoplasia (Insulinoma): this is discussed by Milne (this volume).
2. Hunting dog hypoglycaemia. This is seen in certain dogs, often of nervous temperament, after an hour or two's work. The problem can be overcome or minimized by frequent feeding of high protein/high energy food throughout the day (Turnwald and Troy, 1984)
3. Glycogen storage disease (GlySD). Type I (von Gierke's disease) is caused by a lack of glucose-6-phosphate. Administration of glucagon causes virtually no response (Turnwald and Troy, 1984). A Type III GlySD has been described in German Shepherd dog puppies (Rafiquazzaman *et al.*, 1976). This was due to a glycogen de-brancher enzyme deficiency. Weakness was seen especially after exercise. The prognosis is grave to hopeless depending on the type of GlySD.
4. Transient juvenile hypoglycaemia. This is seen especially in toy and miniature breeds. Cold and starvation are precipitating factors.
5. Non-pancreatic tissue tumours. Hypoglycaemia has been reported associated with primary liver carcinoma (Strombeck, 1978) and lymphatic leukaemia (De Schepper *et al.*, 1974)
6. Other causes include pregnancy in the bitch (Jackson *et al.*, 1980). Neonatal hypoglycaemia can occur in puppies under six weeks old, especially in small breeds (Turnwald and Troy, 1984).

ADRENOCORTICAL INSUFFICIENCY

Adrenocortical insufficiency can cause episodic weakness, especially during the early stages. This due to the fluctuation of electrolyte levels, which may be severe, and to the changes in blood pressure. There is often a history of gastrointestinal problems. Bradycardia may be detected on auscultation. If there is hyperkalaemia present at the time of ECG there should be the characteristic signs of peaked T-waves and flattened P-waves (Farrow, 1983). Biochemical examination of blood can reveal hyperkalaemia and hyponatraemia but may not do so in the early stages. Definative diagnosis is by assay of plasma cortisol levels before and after ACTH administration (Darke, 1986). Treatment is by hormone replacement therapy.

OTHER METABOLIC DISTURBANCES

Other metabolic disturbances such as hypokalaemia and hyperkalaemia may cause episodic weakness (Ettinger, 1983).

MISCELLANEOUS CAUSES

ANAEMIA

Anaemia may be the cause of episodic weakness. Signs are rarely seen until haemoglobin levels are below 7 to 8 mg% and the PCV is less than 22 to 25% (Ettinger, 1983).

The underlying cause of the anaemia must be investigated and the appropriate treatment given (Darke, 1986).

IDIOPATHIC WEAKNESS

Idiopathic weakness can occur in some dogs. They collapse or 'faint' for no apparent reason. These attacks are rarely fatal (Darke, 1986).

ACKNOWLEDGEMENTS

The advice and criticism of Dr P. E. Holt is gratefully acknowledged.

REFERENCES

Barker, J. (1973) Comparative aspects of canine epilepsy. *J. Small Animal Pract.*, **14**, 281

Bonagura, J. (1983) Therapy of cardiac arrhythmias In *Current Veterinary Therapy VIII* (ed. R. W. Kirk) W. B. Saunders, Philadelphia

Calvert, C. A. and Rawlings, C. A. (1983) Diagnosis and management of canine heart worm disease In *Current Veterinary Therapy VIII* (ed. R. W. Kirk) W. B. Saunders, Philadelphia

Darke, P. G. G. (1986) *Notes on Canine Internal Medicine*, 2nd edn, Wright Scientechnica, Bristol

De Schepper, J., van de Stock, J., De Rick, A. (1974) Hypercalcaemia and hypoglycaemia in a case of lymphatic leukaemia in the dog. *Vet. Rec.*, **94**, 602–603

Ettinger, S. J. (1983) *Veterinary Internal Medicine*, W. B. Saunders, Philadelphia

Farrow, B. R. H. (1983) Episodic weakness In *Current Veterinary Therapy VII* (ed. R. W. Kirk) W. B. Saunders, Philadelphia

Foutz, A. S., Mitler, M. M. and Dement, W. C. (1980) Narcolepsy. In *Veterinary Clinics of North America*, **10**, 65; Advances in Veterinary Neurology (ed. C. Chrisman) W. B. Sanders, Philadelphia

Griffiths, I. R. (1980) Review of Canine Muscle Disease. In *The Veterinary Annual* (20th Issue) (eds. C. S. G. Grunsell and F. W. G. Hill), Wright Scientechnia, Bristol, pp. 117

Herrtage, M. E. and Houlton, J. E. F. (1979) *Vet. Rec.*, **105**, 334

Houlton, J. E. F. and Herrtage, M. E. (1980) *Vet. Rec.*, **106**, 206

Jackson, R. F., Brus, M. L., Growney, P. J., Seymour, W. G. (1980) Hypoglycaemia-ketonuria in a pregnant bitch. *J. Am. Vet. Med. Assoc.*, **177**, 1123–1127

Kealy, J. K. (1987) Diagnostic Radiology of the Dog and Cat, 2nd edn, W. B. Saunders, Philadelphia, p. 292

Milne, E. M. (1989) Insulinoma in the dog. This volume

Oliver, J. E. and Lorenz, M. D. (1983) *Handbook of Veterinary Neurological Diagnosis*, W. B. Saunders, Philadelphia, pp. 213

Palmer, A. C. (1980) Myasthenia gravis. In *Veterinary Clinics of North America*, **10**, 212; Advances in Veterinary Neurology (ed. C. Chrisman) W. B. Sanders, Philadelphia

Parker, A. J. (1980) In *Epilepsy in Current Veterinary Therapy VII*, (ed. R. W. Kirk) W. B. Saunders, Philadelphia

Parker, A. J. (1983) Differential diagnosis of peripheral nerve disease: episodic weakness. *Mod. Vet. Pract.*, **4**, 819–824

Raw, M.-E. and Gaskell, C. J. (1985) A review of one hundred cases of presumed canine epilepsy. *J. Small Animal Pract.*, **26**, 645–652

Rafiquazzaman, M., Svenkerud, R., Strande, A. *et al.*, (1976) Glyconeogenosis. *Vet. Scand.*, **17**, 196–209

Strombeck, D. R. (1978) Clinicopathological features of primary and metastatic neoplastic disease of the liver in dogs. *J. Am. Vet. Med. Assoc.*, **173**, 267–269

Turnwald, G. H. and Troy, G. C. (1984) Hypoglycaemia: Clinical Aspects. *Comp. Cont. Edn.*, **6**, 115–122

P. LIEVESLEY and T. J. GRUFFYDD-JONES

Episodic collapse and weakness in cats

INTRODUCTION

EPISODIC COLLAPSE is recognized as an important presenting clinical sign in dogs but is less commonly encountered in cats. Nevertheless, there are several conditions in cats which can lead to episodic collapse, or more commonly, weakness. Some of these have only recently been reported. Those more recently reported syndromes are not well understood and are not yet widely recognized. Some, such as 'spasticity', appear to affect specific breeds. This breed predilection strongly suggests an hereditary basis for these conditions although no definitive evidence of this is available. Even though these conditions are not common, their recognition is important in view of the implications for subsequent breeding programmes. Other well characterized conditions which cause episodic collapse in cats, although not common, may be underdiagnosed due to difficulties in confirming a diagnosis in practice.

This chapter will focus on the more recently recognized causes of episodic collapse in cats and provide a brief outline of other conditions. It is important to appreciate that none of these conditions are common.

MYASTHENIA GRAVIS

Several cases of myasthenia gravis have now been reported in cats (Dawson, 1970; Mason, 1976; Indrieri *et al.*, 1986). Two forms of the disease appear to occur. A congenital form is seen in young cats, usually under six months of age, and an acquired form occurs in older individuals. Antibodies directed against acetylcholine (ACh) receptors have been detected in the acquired myasthenia gravis but not in the congenital form (Indrieri *et al.*, 1983). Congenital myasthenia gravis has been reported in several breeds of dog and is generally considered to be inherited as an autosomal recessive trait. No data are available to assess the possibility heritability of the condition in cats.

The main sign is muscle weakness which is exaggerated by exercise. Cats with myasthenia gravis tend to sleep excessively and are reluctant to exercise. They tire easily and may show muscle tremors. The weakness may involve all four limbs simultaneously or may first affect either the front or hind legs. The muscle weakness may induce collapse after taking only a few steps. Characteristically, the cat shows a crouching gait, then flops onto one side, with the head resting on the front paws. There may be megoesophagus and some affected cats will show dysphagia. Dysphonia may also be noted, typically with either a low or barely audible miaow. In severe cases there may be involvement of the intercostal muscles leading to respiratory distress.

Affected cats are usually in good bodily condition and no abnormalities are found on routine blood examination except for perhaps a slight increase in creatine phosphokinaes (CPK) concentrations. Radiography will identify megoesophagus if this is present. A diagnosis of myasthenia gravis is confirmed by demonstrating an improvement following administration of a cholinesterase inhibitor. Atropine is given first to block the unwanted muscarinic effects. Edrophonium chloride (Tensilon; Roche) is then administered intravenously at a dosage of 0.2–0.5 mg. An improvement in muscular strength will be seen within a minute but is only short-lived. It will subside within five minutes. Electromyography shows reduced amplitude of the potential induced by repetitive muscle stimulation which improves after administration of cholinesterase inhibitors.

Longer acting cholinesterase inhibitors are used for treatment. Neostigmine (Prostigmine) has been used at a dosage of 0.2–0.25 mg. However, it may be necessary to repeat the treatment every six hours to maintain its effect. Pyridostigmine (Mestinon; Roche) has a longer duration of action and can be administered orally. There is a wide dosage range of 0.5–3.0 mg/kg and it is necessary to assess the optimal dosage by trial and error.

Corticosteroids may also be indicated. These drugs are only likely to be beneficial in acquired cases in which there is evidence of antibody production against ACh receptors. Prednisolone is the preferred corticosteroid in view of its potent immunosuppressive activity. It is given at an initial dosage of 2–4 mg/kg daily with a gradual reduction over a period of six to eight weeks. There is limited experience of the likely prognosis. However, congenital cases may maintain improvement after withdrawal of the cholinesterase inhibitors and, in acquired cases, prednisolone alone may prevent recurrence.

'SPASTICITY' IN DEVON REX CATS

We have recognized a specific syndrome of muscle weakness in Devon Rex cats in the UK (Gruffydd-Jones and Evans, unpublished data) and have received reports of a similar condition in Rex cats from Australia, New Zealand, The Netherlands and North America. The syndrome has been termed 'spasticity' by breeders. However, this may be inappropriate because there is no evidence of any central nervous system (CNS) defect. It appears to be a congenital condition although in mild cases signs may be overlooked initially and may not be recognized until the kitten is several months of age. We have seen the condition exclusively in Devon Rex cats. This breed predisposition, together with its occurrence in closely related cats, strongly suggests hereditary involvement.

The condition appears to vary in clinical severity. Affected cats develop a peculiar posture with flexion of the neck causing the chin to be tucked into the sternum. Severely affected individuals show evidence of generalized muscle weakness and may tire easily. They flop down after only a few steps, with the head resting on one side on the front paws. The episodic muscle weakness may be exacerbated by stress such as moving to an unfamiliar environment. There may also be some stiffness of the legs leading to a slightly high stepping gait. Some affected cats adopt a peculiar 'dog-begging' position with the front legs resting on a convenient object (Figure 1). A

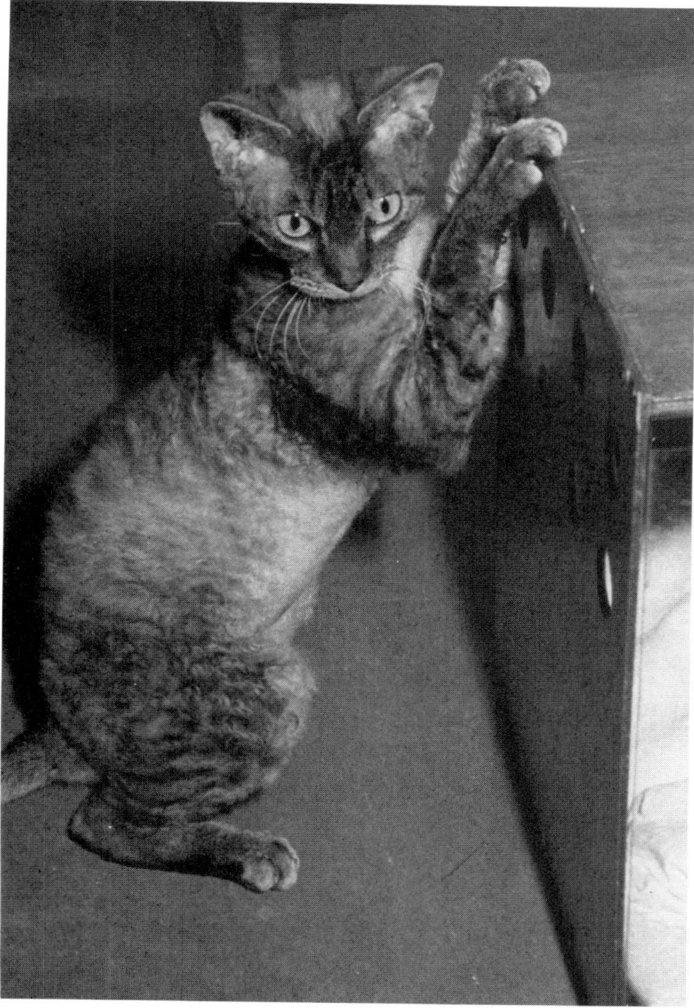

Fig. 1. Devon Rex cat with 'spasticity' showing the characteristic posture sometimes adopted whilst resting

peculiar action may also be shown whilst eating. The head remains 'bent over' with the chin tucked on the sternum and the cat may walk backwards chewing a morsel of food obtained from its food bowl whilst maintaining this posture. The extreme neck flexion may impede swallowing. We have encountered several cases of death in affected cats due to obstruction of the larynx by food material.

The cause of this syndrome is not known. We have found abnormalities on electromyography but have been unable to demonstrate any lesions in muscle biopsies on light or electron microscopy although there have been unsubstantiated reports from the USA of electron micrographic changes indicative of a myopathy.

Table 1 OTHER CONDITIONS TO CONSIDER IN CATS WITH EPISODIC
COLLAPSE OR WEAKNESS

CNS hypoxia:	Arteriovenous anomalies
	Airway obstruction
	Anaemia
	Haemoglobinopathies
Primary CNS disorders:	Epilepsy
	Neoplasia
	Lentivirus infection
	FIP
	Meningitis
	Trauma
	Congenital disease, hydrocephalus, storage diseases, cerebellar hypoplasia
Metabolic disorders:	Terminal uraemia
	Hepatic encephalopathy
	Addison's disease
Peripheral nerve disorders:	Neuropathies
Orthopaedic disorders:	Patellar luxation
	Hip dysplasia
	Spinal diseases
Other diseases:	Poisons
	Thiamine deficiency

Routine blood tests are normal and we have not found any changes in CPK, pyruvate
or lactate as described in brief reports in lay articles in the USA.

No treatment is effective for this condition. Whilst mildly affected cats may have a
reasonable quality of life, euthanasia may be necessary for severe cases.

CONN'S SYNDROME

Conn's syndrome is caused by an aldosterone producing tumour of the adrenal gland.
The inappropriate production of aldosterone leads to excessive urinary potassium
excretion, hypokalaemia and eventually muscle weakness. There is a single,
well-documented report of Conn's syndrome in an aged D.S.H. cat (Eger *et al.*,
1983) but a similar syndrome has also been seen in cats presented to our clinic.
These cats have had high plasma aldosterone concentrations which strongly
suggested Conn's syndrome. However, because the owners have declined surgery
and post-mortem examination there has been no opportunity to confirm the presence
of a tumour.

The condition initially causes intermittent muscle weakness and collapse which
becomes progressively more severe. Affected cats lose weight and have a poor coat.
Blood examination reveals hypokalaemia with high CPK. This can be confirmed by
demonstrating raised aldosterone concentrations, although aldosterone assays are
not widely available. Monitoring urinary potassium levels will confirm excessive
excretion.

Dietary supplementation with potassium and administration of spironolactone at a
dosage of 10–100 mg, which reduces potassium excretion by blocking the action of
aldosterone, may produce some temporary improvement.

POLYMYOPATHY ASSOCIATED WITH HYPOKALAEMIA

There have been several recent reports of polymyopathy syndromes in cats. Although it is not clear whether these represent the same condition. The signs associated with the muscle weakness are similar in all cases. The earliest indication of the syndrome may be reluctance to jump up. This progresses to involve a generalized muscle weakness. All four limbs will usually be involved although the fore-limbs or hind-limbs may be more noticeably affected initially. The limbs become stiff and the cat develops a stilted gait. There is also ventroflexion of the neck leading to the adoption of a peculiar posture with the chin tucked into the sternum. Severely affected cats may show a reluctance to walk.

We have recognized this syndrome in a number of distinct groups of cats.

YOUNG BURMESE CATS

A specific syndrome of periodic muscle weakness associated with intermittent hypokalaemia and high serum levels of CPK in Burmese kittens was first reported from our clinic (Blaxter *et al.*, 1986). A similar syndrome of muscle weakness in two Burmese kittens associated with hypokalaemia was briefly mentioned in the Australian report of a cat with Conn's syndrome. There have been further recent reports of a similar syndrome in Australia (Church, personal communication) including a description of episodic weakness in seven Burmese cats (Mason, 1988). This latter report cannot be adequately evaluated due to the paucity of data provided. No blood biochemical findings were reported and it was suggested that the condition might be caused by a thiamine deficiency on the basis of a poorly documented response to thiamine supplementation.

We now have data based on 14 affected Burmese kittens. There has been no noticeable sex predisposition. Clinical signs have first become evident between two and six months of age. Breeders report that the signs may be precipitated by stress or vigorous exercise. Our experience has shown that clinical signs may resolve if affected individuals are hospitalized. This may be due to restricted opportunity for exercise. In addition to the clinical signs described above, some kittens have shown a very distinctive peculiar knuckling of the carpus which is persistent during clinical phases of the disease. They tend to sink on their hocks and may sit with stifles abducted.

Serum CPK concentrations may be extraordinarily high in these cases, frequently above 50 000 iu/l and the increase in CPK may not always appear to be related to the hypokalaemia.

The cause of this syndrome is not clear. The absence of any detectable abnormalities on electromyography as well as light and electron microscopic examination of muscle biopsies suggests that this is unlikely to be a primary myopathy. Inadequate dietary intake of potassium is unlikely to have been responsible for the hypokalaemia because all affected cats have received varied diets based mainly on standard canned foods. Neither does excessive loss of potassium appear to be a factor because urinary potassium levels were normal.

This syndrome bears some similarities to periodic hypokalaemic paralysis in man. In this condition, there is a sudden shift of potassium from the extracellular to the intracellular compartment leading to hypokalaemia. The condition first becomes apparent around the time of adulthood and is thought to be hereditary. The occurrence of the syndrome in Burmese kittens, some of which have been closely related, strongly suggests that the condition in cats is also hereditary. Periodic hypokalaemic paralysis in man can be precipitated by a number of factors including stress, vigorous exercise, a high carbohydrate meal and insulin therapy. However, administration of glucose and insulin to affected cats has failed to provoke clinical signs.

Supplementation with oral potassium chloride at a dosage of 150–160 mg daily has been used to manage affected kittens. However, it is uncertain how effective this treatment is because some kittens have improved after a period of time with or without treatment and have not subsequently shown any further episodes. Other cats have shown recurrent bouts and owners have reported some apparent improvement with potassium supplementation.

OLD CATS

The occasional older cat with episodic muscle weakness and typical signs of polymyopathy associated with hypokalaemia has been seen in our clinic. Conn's syndrome has been discounted in these cases by demonstration of normal plasma aldosterone concentrations.

Similar cases have been reported in the USA by Schunk (1984) and more fully by Dow, LeCounter et al., (1987). There is no particular breed disposition. In contrast to the syndrome seen in young cats, which do not show other signs, affected individuals are usually thin with a poor coat. CPK concentrations are raised but not to the same extent as in the Burmese kittens. Dow, Feltman et al., (1987) have also reported raised creatinine concentrations with increased urinary potassium loss in older cats with the syndrome and suggested that the underlying cause is renal dysfunction. However, no evidence of excessive urinary potassium loss was found in younger cats with polymyopathy and hypokalaemia. The diets of some affected cats were found to be deficient in potassium and this was considered to be an additional contributory factor. Correction of the dietary deficiency of potassium led to resolution of the polymyopathy.

ASSOCIATED WITH HYPERTHYROIDISM

Typical signs of polymyopathy associated with hypokalaemia have been noted in two hyperthyroid cats at our clinic shortly after surgical thyroidectomy had been performed. One of the elderly cats with polymyopathy in the series of cases described by Dow et al., (1987) was reported to have become hyperthyroid six months later. Periodic paralysis associated with hypokalaemia is also recognized as a feature of some humans with hyperthyroidism (Ferreiro et al., 1986). The pathophysiology of thyrotoxic periodic paralysis is not clear but it is suggested that the hyperadrenergic state in hyperthyroidism enhances insulin release which may lead to a shift in potassium into the intracellular compartment.

HYPOGLYCAEMIA

Clinical signs attributable to hypoglycaemia are rare in cats. Although this may lead to episodic collapse, from the few reported cases of hypoglycaemia in cats, it is more likely to result in seizures.

There is one well-documented case report of a functional pancreatic islet cell tumour in a twelve year old Siamese cat (McMillan *et al.*, 1985). The cat showed intermittent seizures which began as twitching of the skin and progressed to muscle tremors. Each seizure lasted one to two hours during which the cat appeared disorientated although consciousness was retained. The seizures were ameliorated by feeding glucose. Blood examination revealed hypoglycaemia and leucopenia. A single tumour was present in the right pancreatic lobe. This was excised but the cat developed seizures associated with hypoglycaemia soon afterwards and died.

Hypoglycaemia has also been reported as a complication of chronic renal failure in a cat (Edwards *et al.*, 1987). However, other clinical signs indicative of the underlying renal failure are likely to be evident some time before hypoglycaemia occurs.

HYPERNATRAEMIA

Muscle weakness with ventral flexion of the neck has been reported in a cat with hypernatraemia (Dow, Feltman and LeCouteur, 1987). The primary disorder in this cat was diagnosed as hypodipsia associated with a defect in the osmoreceptors. Hydrocephalus was demonstrated and there was evidence of temporary pituitary hypofunction. The mechanism by which the hypernatraemia caused muscle weakness was not clear.

HYPOCALCAEMIA

Hypocalcaemia may lead to tetanic spasms of the limbs and episodic weakness. Although a number of disorders have been reported to cause hypocalcaemia in other species, such as pancreatitis and Addison's disease, only iatrogenic hypoparathyroidism secondary to thyroidectomy and inability to meet the extra demands for calcium arising during pregnancy or lactation are of importance in cats.

CARDIOVASCULAR DISEASE

Episodic collapse due to CNS hypoxia may occasionally result from cardiovascular disease. In immature cats this is most likely to be associated with congenital heart disease. Episodic collapse has been the main reason for the referral of several cats with congenital cardiac disease to our clinic. Occasionally clinical signs have not arisen until the cat is at least 1-year old. The most likely congenital cardiac diseases to cause collapse are aortic stenosis, ventricular septic defects or complex defects such as the Tetralogy of Fallot. A murmur is likely to be audible on auscultation and there may be a palpable thrill. Cats with the Tetralogy of Fallot may be cyanotic. Acquired cardiac disease in the form of cardiomyopathy may result in episodic collapse in the older cat. This may be associated with dysrhythmias or conduction disturbances. Thromboembolism is recognized as a common complication of cardiomyopathy in cats and it is possible that cerebral vascular occlusion may occur although the collapse in such cases is unlikely to be intermittent in nature.

NARCOLEPSY

Narcolepsy is a CNS disorder which leads to sudden inappropriate episodes of sleep. The precise mechanism for the disorder is not clear. A tentative diagnosis of narcolepsy in a young Siamese cat has been reported (Knecht *et al.*, 1973). The episodes began as bouts of salivation which progressed to periods of loss of consciousness. Severe depression with apparent blindness and deafness were evident between the episodes of collapse. The diagnosis was based primarily on the clinical signs and not on EEG findings. Some improvement in response to dextroamphetamine treatment was reported. Catalepsy involving loss of muscular activity is recognized in dogs but has not been reported in cats.

MYOTONIA

Myotonia has not been reported in cats although one case has been seen in our clinic. Clinical signs were first noted when the cat was a few months of age and the condition was presumed to be congenital although no information about the cat's relations was available. The cat showed stiffness of all limbs which was most noticeable after periods of inactivity. The stiffness appeared to be exacerbated by cold weather, but improved with activity. If the cat was startled she would become rigid and fall to one side with prolapse of the nictitating membranes. Her claws were usually protruded and would catch in carpets. After yawning the cat was unable to close her mouth for a few seconds. Clinical examination revealed striking muscle hypertrophy. The diagnosis was confirmed by demonstration of myotonic discharges on electromyography. Treatment with procainamide was attempted but no significant improvement was noted.

REFERENCES

Blaxter, A. C., Lievesley, P., Gruffydd-Jones, T. J. and Wotton, P. R. (1986) Periodic muscle weakness in Burmese kittens. *Vet. Rec.*, **118**, 619–620

Dawson, J. R. B. (1970) Myasthenia gravis in a cat. *Vet. Rec.*, **86**, 562–563

Dow, S. W., LeCouteur, R. A., Feltman, M. J. and Spurgeon, T. L. (1987) Potassium depletion in cats: hypokalemic polymyopathy. *J. Am. Vet. Med. Assoc.*, **191**, 1563–1568

Dow, S. W., Feltman, M. J., LeCouteur, R. A. and Hamar, D. W. (1987) Potassium depletion in cats: renal and dietary influences. *J. Am. Vet. Med. Assoc.*, **191**, 1569–1575

Dow, S. W., Feltman, M. J. and LeCouteur, R. A. (1987) Hypodipsic hypernatremia and associated myopathy in a hydrocephalic cat with transient hypopituitarism. *J. Am. Vet. Med. Assoc.*, **191**, 217–221

Edwards, D. F., Legendre, A. M. and McCracken, M. D. (1987) Hypoglycaemia and chronic renal failure in a cat. *J. Am. Vet. Med. Assoc.*, **190**, 435–436

Eger, C. E., Robinson, W. F. and Huxtable, C. R. R. (1983) Primary aldosteronism (Conn's syndrome) in a cat: a case report and review of comparative aspects. *J. Small Animal Pract.*, **24**, 293–307

Ferreiro, J. E., Arguelles, D. J. and Rams, H. (1986) Thyrotoxic periodic paralysis. *Am. J. Med.,* **80,** 146–150

Indrieri, R. J., Creighton, S. R., Lambert, E. H. and Lennon, V. A. (1983) Myasthenia gravis in two cats. *J. Am. Vet. Med. Assoc.,* **182,** 57–60

Knecht, C. D., Oliver, J. E., Redding, R., Selcer, R. and Johnson, G. (1973) Narcolepsy in a dog and a cat. *J. Am. Vet. Med. Assoc.,* **162,** 1052–1053

Mason, K. V. (1976) A case of myasthenia gravis in a cat. *J. Small Animal Pract.,* **17,** 467–472

Mason, K. (1988) A hereditary disease in Burmese cats manifested as an episodic weakness with head nodding and neck ventroflexion. *J. Am. Animal Hospital Assoc.,* **24,** 147–151

McMillan, F. D., Barr, B. and Feldman, E. C. (1985) Functional pancreatic islet cell tumour in a cat. *J. Am. Animal Hospital Assoc.,* **21,** 741–746

Schunk, K. L. (1984) Feline myopathy. In *Proceedings 2nd Annual Forum Am. Coll. Vet. Intern. Med.* pp. 197–200

SIMON J. WHEELER

Spinal tumours in cats

INTRODUCTION

IN CONSIDERING the clinical aspects of spinal tumours in cats, a number of significant questions arise. These include:
How prevalent are spinal tumours in cats compared with other spinal disorders?
What presenting signs will alert the clinician to the presence of a spinal tumour?
What differential diagnosis should be considered in such a case?
How is the diagnosis made?
What pathological changes underlie the clinical picture?
What treatment is feasible?
What is the prognosis?
This chapter considers these questions and provides the clinician with information related to the management of spinal tumours in cats.

THE PREVALENCE OF SPINAL TUMOURS

Whilst it is asserted that neoplasms account for a higher proportion of spinal cases in cats compared with dogs, there have been no studies which enumerate the relative incidence of feline spinal diseases. One study of cats in which myelograms were performed showed a 50% incidence of tumours (Wheeler *et al.*, 1985) This study comprised a selected population and no trauma cases were included. However, this level of incidence is clearly higher than that which is seen in dogs. Thus, the index of suspicion for neoplasia must always be higher in a cat with spinal cord diseases than in a similarly affected dog. There are a number of published descriptions of the pathological features of spinal tumours and the relative incidence of different tumour types.
A series of 50 cats seen at the Royal Veterinary College and the Veterinary Teaching Hospital of North Carolina State University indicated the following incidence of spinal diseases (Wheeler and Kornegay, unpublished data):
Neoplasia 21 (42%)
Trauma 6 (12%)
Intervertebral disc protrusion 4 (8%)
Degenerative spinal disease 3 (6%)
Congenital deformity/malformation 2 (4%)
Toxoplasmosis 2 (4%)
Vascular disease 2 (4%)
Chronic inflammatory mass 2 (4%)

270

Aortic embolus, cryptococcus, toxicity, poliomyelitis 1 (each) (2%)
No diagnosis 4 (8%)

This confirms that tumours are the most common cause of spinal cord disease in cats in a referral situation. However, this finding is biased because it reflects a selected population in which spinal cord trauma is undoubtedly under-represented. Most cases are diagnosed without need for referral.

CLINICAL SIGNS OF SPINAL TUMOURS

The clinical signs, which include neurological deficits in the limbs, visceral dysfunction and spinal hyperaesthesia, are an indication of the degree of spinal cord damage. The neurological deficit present is largely governed by the level of the spine at which the tumour lies (Figure 1). The severity of the neurological deficit also varies depending on the degree of spinal cord involvement. Whilst some cats have mild deficits, such as ataxia and proprioceptive deficits, others have significant weakness or even paraplegia. Clinical signs progress through these stages in some cases as the effect of the tumour becomes more pronounced. Spinal hyperaesthesia is also a frequent feature in affected cats.

Whilst the clinical picture in most cats is somewhat chronic, a relatively acute case does not preclude the possibility of a tumour being present. The spinal cord apparently accommodates slowly growing progressive compression to a certain point, after which there may be a precipitous decline in the neurological status.

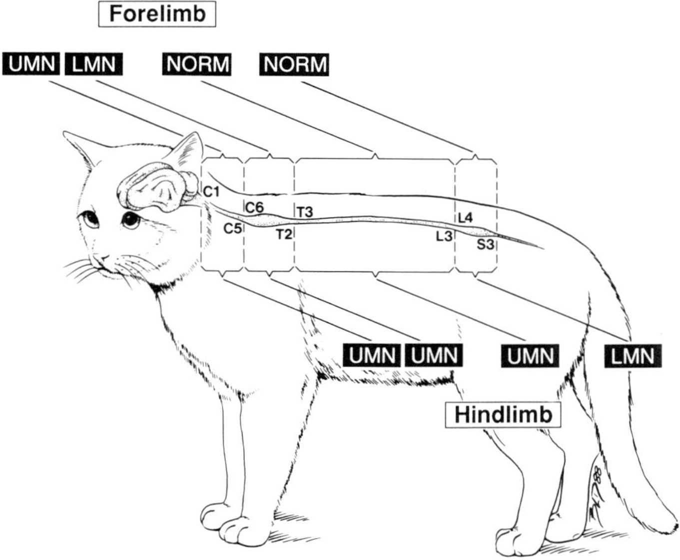

Fig. 1. Neurological signs seen with lesions at different levels of spine, categorized by type of deficit seen in forelimbs and hindlimbs. UMN, upper motor neurone type deficit; LMN, lower motor neurone type deficit; Norm, normal.

Involvement of other body systems may lead to additional signs of systemic disease. Thus, the general health of the cat should always be evaluated when a spinal tumour is suspected. The mean age of the cats with tumours described above was 6 years, with a range of 6 months to 10 years. Thus, age is not a factor which can be used to exclude the possibility of a spinal tumour being present.

DIFFERENTIAL DIAGNOSIS

The differential diagnosis for a cat with signs of spinal cord disease includes disc protrusions, inflammatory conditions, metabolic disorders and intoxications. However, none of these is particularly common.

Trauma, usually as a result of a road traffic accident, is a significant cause of feline spinal dysfunction. Clearly, an acute onset of signs is usual but a definite history of trauma is less commonly reported in cats than in dogs. This is possibly due to the more independent life style of the feline species. Radiography will confirm the diagnosis where a fracture is present.

In the paraplegic cat, the possibility of ischaemic neuromyopathy (aortic thrombo-embolism) should always be considered. An acute history and the typical clinical signs of absent femoral pulse, cold limbs, firm, painful muscles and absent deep pain sensation should provide the diagnosis.

The relatively chronic clinical course seen in most spinal tumours may be mimicked by changes in the spinal column due to hypervitaminosis A. Affected cats are typically lethargic, reluctant to move and hyperaesthetic. They have been exposed exclusively to a vitamin A rich diet. The diagnosis will be apparent by the typical changes seen radiographically.

DIAGNOSIS

The diagnosis of spinal neoplasia is made largely by radiography. Some extradural tumours may affect the vertebral bodies thus causing bony changes (Figures 2 and 3). However, this is not typical because there are usually no bony abnormalities apparent with most tumours. Thus, myelography is required to confirm the diagnosis in most cases. The technique and findings have been described elsewhere (Wheeler *et al.*, 1985). Cisternal puncture and the use of the non-ionic, water soluble contrast medium iohexol (Omnipaque, Nycomed) ensures that the procedure is safe and highly likely to prove diagnostic. The findings in a number of cat myelograms are shown in Figures 2–4.

Other radiographic findings may indicate the possible presence of a spinal tumour. In some cases, an area of soft tissue density is present in the dorsal thorax immediately ventral to the spinal column at the level of the tumour. Soft tissue densities in the anterior thorax may be present where lymphosarcoma affects the mediastinum. Pulmonary metastases may also be present in other cats.

Other diagnostic tests are indicated to confirm the presence of a tumour and to define its nature. Haematological evaluation, FeLV testing, bone marrow aspiration and cerebrospinal fluid analysis will all contribute to the diagnosis. In some instances, biopsy at exploratory surgery may be the only means of making a histological diagnosis.

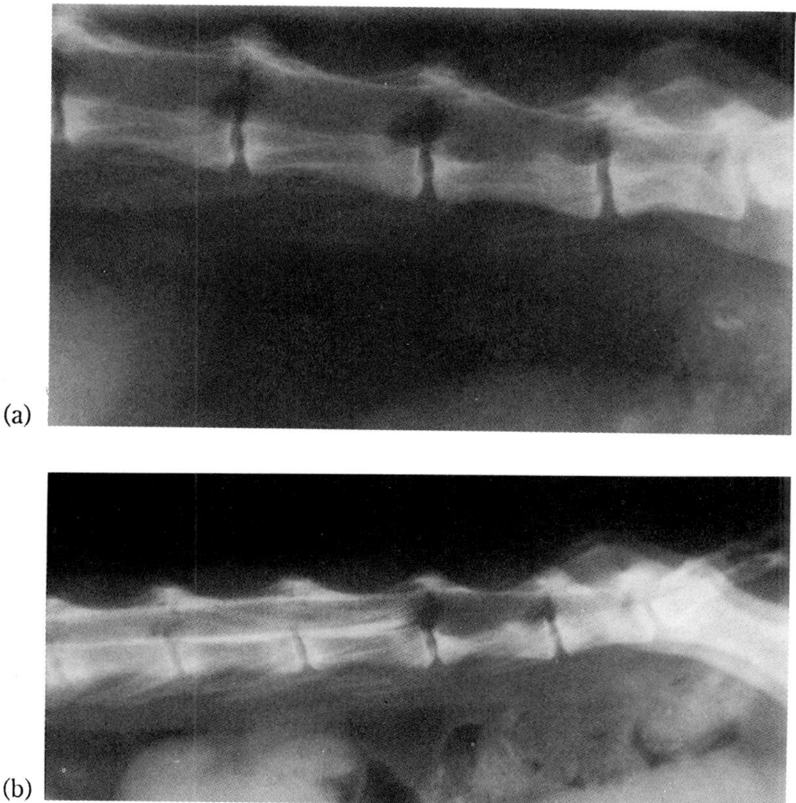

(a)

(b)

Fig. 2. (a) Lateral projection, lumbar spine. Note loss of floor of spinal canal L_6, enlargement of $L_{5/6}$ intervertebral foramen. (b) Following cisternal myelogram, ventral contrast column displaced dorsally at $L_{5/6}$ with accumulation of dye and arrest of flow. The diagnosis is neurofibrosarcoma

PATHOLOGY

A limited number of tumour types have been reported in the feline spine. Lymphosarcoma (LSA) is most common. Neurological signs were seen in 8% of cats with the disease in one series (Meincke, *et al.*, 1972) and 10.9% in another (Kornegay, 1981). Whilst these figures cannot be regarded as absolute, they do give an indication of the number of cats with LSA which have nervous system involvement. Lymphosarcoma of the central nervous system most commonly affects the spine. Zaki and Hurvitz (1976) found that 82% of cats with LSA of the central nervous system had spinal involvement. In these cases the tumours were situated extradurally with a low incidence of invasion of the vertebral bodies, dura or spinal cord itself. However, other authors consider that neoplastic infiltration of these structures is relatively common (Schappert and Geib, 1967; Heavener, 1978; Kornegay, 1981). In Zaki and Hurvitz's study, all cats had LSA in other organs,

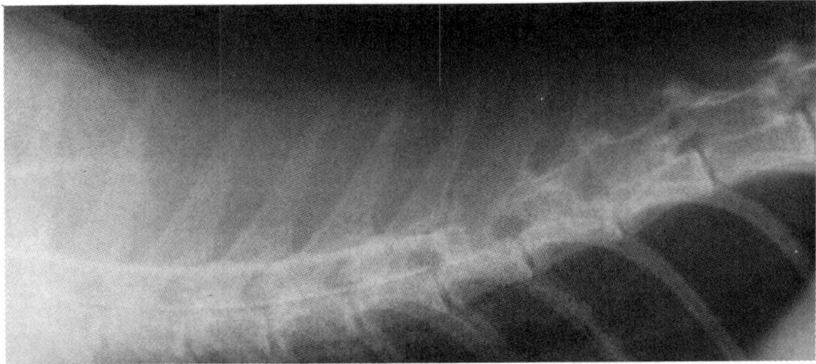

Fig. 3. Lateral projection, thoracic spine following cisternal myelogram. Contrast columns arrested at $T_{7/8}$. Dorsal column tapers and is displaced ventrally suggesting extradural mass. Lucent destructive lesion present in dorsal spine, dorsal arch and pedicles of T_8 vertebra. The diagnosis is atypical osteosarcoma.

suggesting that the spine had become involved secondary to metastatic spread. The bone marrow is involved in approximately 50% of cats with extradural LSA (Cotter, 1976; 1986) and, thus, aspiration of marrow will aid in the diagnosis in these cases.

Other tumour types are far less commonly encountered. Vertebral osteosarcomas (Engle and Brodey, 1969; Dorn, 1976; O'Brien *et al.*, 1980; Wheeler *et al.*, 1985), a plasma cell sarcoma (Mitcham *et al.*, 1985), a glioma (Haynes and Leininger, 1982) and neurofibrosarcoma (Wheeler *et al.*, 1985) have been reported. Meningiomas, whilst occurring commonly in the brain, are rarely seen in the spine (McGrath, 1962; Luginbuhl *et al.*, 1968; Ross and Wyburn, 1969; Jones, 1974; Wheeler *et al.*, 1985; Averill, 1987).

TREATMENT

Treatment of spinal tumours is dependent on a number of factors. The neurological status must be such that recovery is likely following therapy. Thus, absence of deep pain sensation may preclude treatment. With the high likelihood of lymphosarcoma, consideration of systemic involvement also has a bearing.

In the presence of a positive diagnosis of LSA, surgical debulking followed by suitable chemotherapy is probably the treatment of choice because this will lead to the most rapid improvement in neurological function. However, it has been suggested that chemotherapy alone will lead to a similar rate of recovery (Cotter, 1983; 1986). Chemotherapeutic protocols have been discussed elsewhere (Cotter, 1986). Clearly, surgical treatment alone in cases of LSA is not appropriate, due to the multifocal nature of the disease.

Where the presence of LSA has not been confirmed, excisional biopsy is required to make the diagnosis. Once the histological identity of the tumour is known, suitable chemotherapy may be instituted. The ease with which dorsal laminectomy can be performed in the thoraco-lumbar spine of the cat makes surgical exploration a feasible proposition. Radiotherapy may also be of benefit in some cases of LSA, but inaccessibility of facilities precludes its use in most instances.

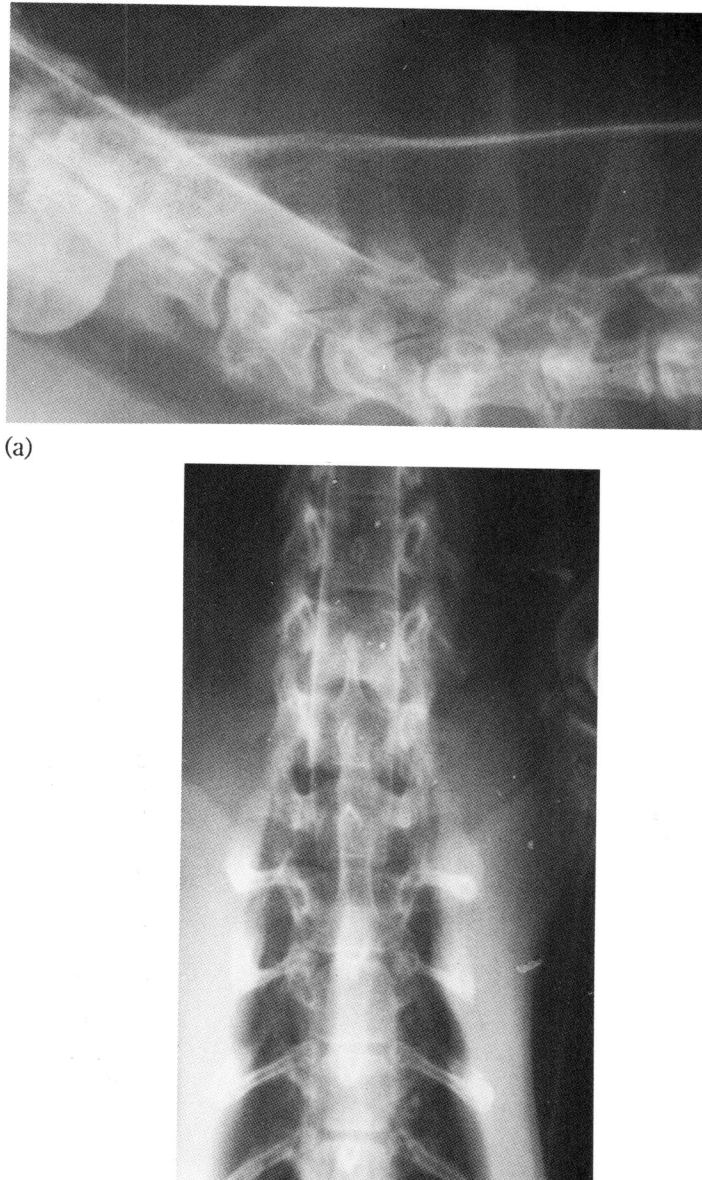

Fig. 4. (a) Lateral projection cervicothoracic spine following cisternal myelogram. Tapering of dorsal column and arrest of flow in C_7. (b) Ventrodorsal projection. Columns converge and taper over C_7 and terminate over T_1, suggesting extradural mass. The diagnosis is extradural lymphosarcoma.

PROGNOSIS

In many cats, initial improvement in the neurological status is likely following surgical excision. This may be maintained for some time with appropriate chemotherapy. However, the long term prognosis is unfavourable due to the propensity for multifocal involvement or local recurrence.

CONCLUSION

The diagnosis of spinal tumours in cats is well within the capabilities of most clinicians. Treatment, which may very well prolong the useful life of the patient, is also possible. However, because of the behaviour of neoplastic diseases, the long term prognosis is often poor.

ACKNOWLEDGEMENTS

The author is grateful to Dr Joe N. Kornegay for reading the manuscript and to Barbara Davidson for the illustrative work. Figures 2–4 appeared in *Journal of Small Animal Practice* (1985) **26**, 143–152 and are reproduced by permission.

REFERENCES

Averill, D. R. (1987) Tumours of the nervous system. In *Feline Diseases* (ed. J. Holzworth) W. B. Saunders Co., Philadelphia

Cotter, S. M. (1976) Feline leukemia virus induced disorders in the cat. *Veterinary Clinics of North America*, **6**, 367–378

Cotter, S. M. (1983) Treatment of lymphoma and leukaemia with cyclophosphamide, vincrisine and prednisolone, 2: Treatment of cats. *J. Am. Animal Hospital Assoc.*, **19**, 166

Cotter, S. M. (1986) Clinical management of lymphoproliferative, myeloproliferative and plasma call neoplasia. In *Oncology* (ed. N. T. Gorman) Churchill Livingstone, New York

Dorn, C. R. (1976) Epidemiology of canine and feline tumours. *J. Am. Animal Hospital Assoc.*, **12**, 307–312

Engle, G. C. and Brodey, R. S. (1969) A retrospective study of 395 feline neoplasms. *J. Am. Animal Hospital Assoc.*, **5**, 21–31

Haynes, J. S. and Leininger, J. R. (1982) A glioma in the spinal cord of a cat. *Vet. Pathol.*, **19**, 713–715

Heavener, J. M. (1978) Neural lymphomatosis in cats. *Mod. Vet. Pract.*, **59**, 122–124

Jones, B. R. (1974) Spinal meningioma in a cat. *Aust. Vet. J.*, **50**, 229–231

Kornegay, J. N. (1981) Feline neurology. *Compendium on Continuing Education*, **3**, 203–213

Luginbuhl, H., Fankhauser, R. and McGrath, J. T. (1968) Spontaneous neoplasms of the nervous system of animals. *Prog. Neurol. Surg.*, **2**, 85–164

McGrath, J. T. (1962) Meningiomas in animals. *J. Neuropathol. Experim. Neurol.*, **21**, 327–328

Meincke, J. E., Hobbie, W. V. and Hardy, W. D. (1972) Lymphoreticular malignancies in the cat: clinical findings. *J. Am. Vet. Med. Assoc.*, **160**, 1093–1099

Mitcham, S. A., McGillivray, S. R. and Haines, D. M. (1985) Plasma cell sarcoma in a cat. *Can. Vet. J.*, **26**, 98–100

O'Brien, D., Parker, A. J. and Tarvin, G. (1980) Osteosarcoma of the vertebra causing compression of the thoracic spinal cord in a cat. *J. Am. Animal Hospital Assoc.*, **16**, 497–499

Ross, J. and Wyburn, R. S. (1969) A report on the clinical investigation of a paraplegic cat. *N.Z. Vet. J.*, **17**, 251–253

Schappert, H. R. and Geib, L. W. (1967) Reticuloendothelial neoplasms involving the spinal canal of cats. *J. Am. Vet. Med. Assoc.*, **150**, 753–757

Wheeler, S. J., Clayton-Jones, D. G. and Wright, J. A. (1985) Myelography in the cat. *J. Small Animal Pract.*, **26**, 143–152

Zaki, F. A. and Hurvitz, A. L. (1976) Spontaneous neoplasms of the CNS of the cat. *J. Small Animal Pract.*, **17**, 773–782

C. D. HOPPER and D. A. HARBOUR

Feline T-lymphotropioc lentivirus – a new disease

INTRODUCTION

THE RECOGNITION of the acquired immunodeficiency syndrome (AIDS) in man has led to an increased awareness of similar immunodeficiencies in animals. As a consequence, a new feline virus has been discovered, namely feline T-lymphotropic lentivirus (FTLV), which is associated with an AIDS-like syndrome in cats.

Pedersen and workers at the University of California first isolated FTLV whilst investigating the outbreak of an immunodeficiency-like syndrome in a colony of cats in Northern California (Pedersen *et al.*, 1987). This household of rescue cats was screened regularly for feline leukaemia virus and had no serious disease problems prior to the introduction of a young female cat which became ill soon after arrival. The cat developed a variety of chronic illnesses over a period of three years. During this time other cats also became ill and showed similar signs. Several cats, including the cat thought to have introduced the disease, eventually died.

Feline T-lymphotropic lentivirus is placed in the same family (Retroviridae) as feline leukaemia virus (FeLV), feline sarcoma virus (FeSV) and feline syncytium forming virus (FeSFV). All are enveloped RNA viruses which utilize the enzyme reverse transcriptase during replication. However, the viruses belong to different subfamilies (Figure 1), and have very different properties.

FeLV and FeSV are oncornaviruses, or cancer-forming viruses, whereas FeSFV is a spumavirus (foamy agent) and is generally considered to be apathogenic. FTLV is a lentivirus or slow virus. Infection is characterized by a long incubation period and

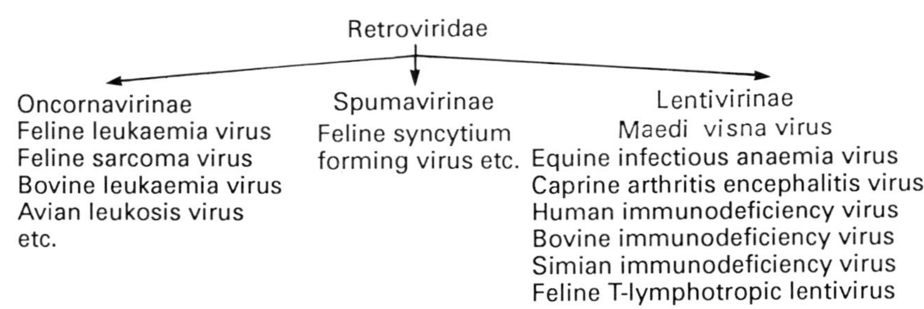

Fig. 1. Classification of retroviruses

slow development of disease. There are likely to be many antigenic variants of FTLV because mutation of envelope glycoproteins is common in lentiviruses. The genomic structure of FTLV has not been determined, so its exact relationship to other lentiviruses is still unknown. However, in clinical terms, FTLV most closely resembles the other lymphotropic lentiviruses: bovine immunodeficiency virus (BIV), human immunodeficiency virus (HIV) and simian immunodeficiency virus (SIV), which, like FTLV, preferentially infect T-lymphocytes.

There has been much speculation as to the origin of FTLV. No antigenic relationship to HIV or to the animal lentiviruses has yet been demonstrated. FTLV is thought to be a highly species-adapted virus which evolved in cats some time ago (Pedersen *et al.*, 1987). Evidence for this comes from reports of FTLV infection in cats in Japan (Ishida *et al.*, 1988) North America (Pedersen *et al.*, 1987; Horzinek, 1987) Holland, Switzerland and France (Lutz, 1988) and the UK (Harbour *et al.*, 1988; Lutz, 1988). Given that there is very little international movement of cats, it is unlikely that a recently evolved virus could be so widespread. There is no evidence to suggest that FTLV originated from HIV (or vice versa). Antibodies to FTLV have been found in stored serum samples taken from cats in the UK in the early 1970s (Gruffydd-Jones, personal communication), which is well before the emergence of HIV infection in countries outside Africa.

PATHOGENESIS

Much work is required before the pathogenesis of feline lentivirus infection is established, particularly because it is though that different isolates of FTLV vary in their pathogenicity. The route by which the virus enters the body is undetermined but dissemination throughout the body is likely to occur through the circulation of infected lymphocytes.

In humans HIV has been shown to infect the subset of thymus-derived lymphocytes known as T-helper (T_H) cells. Other cells reported to be infected are monocytes and macrophages and their precursors, astrocytes and oligodendrocytes in the brain (Levy *et al.*, 1987) and enterochromaffin cells in the colonic mucosa (Nelson *et al.*, 1988). In the cat, although FTLV infects T-lymphocytes, it is not yet possible to differentiate between the T-cell subsets in order to determine whether T_H cells are the main target cells for infection. Because neurological signs and chronic diarrhoea are seen in some FTLV infected cats, it is possible that FTLV may also infect neural tissue and gut mucosal cells. Indeed, we have isolated FTLV from the brain of a cat with neurological signs although the infected cell type is not known.

The feline immune system is poorly characterized and consequently it is difficult to assess the ways in which FTLV might cause immunosuppression. It remains to be seen whether FTLV, like its human counterpart, HIV, can cause T_H cell depletion, reduced responses to antigenic stimuli and polyclonal activation of B-lymphocytes. The latter give rise to increased production of non-specific antibodies and a subsequent hypergammaglobulinaemia. Interestingly, we have seen hypergammaglobulinaemia in some cases of FTLV infection.

Humans infected with HIV are found to have free viral antigen in the blood in the acute stages of infection. With time, viral antigen disappears from the blood stream or occurs intermittently in low levels. During this period the patient is asymptomatic. The re-emergence of antigen is associated with the development of clinical signs, i.e.

AIDS related complex, which often leads to full-blown AIDS. The relationship between antigenaemia and clinical signs may be similar to FTLV infected cats. Further comparison of FTLV and HIV infection shows that in both cases the development of viral antibodies does not appear to be protective and, consequently, persistent infection will occur. In humans, it may be weeks or months post-infection before antibodies to HIV are present. We have found that there is a much shorter delay before antibody development occurs in FTLV infected cats.

The mortality of FTLV infection in cats is not known. Ishida *et al.*, (1988) reported that 5/86 FTLV positive cats died but the period of follow-up was 6 months or less. In California, 10 of 26 cats died over a four year interval (Pedersen *et al.*, 1987). This suggests that the mortality rate may increase with time. However, long-term follow-up of a large number of infected cats will be necessary to confirm this.

CLINICAL SIGNS

A wide range of clinical signs is seen in cats infected with FTLV. Experimental infection of two young kittens with FTLV caused generalized lymphadenopathy four weeks post inoculation, followed by low-grade pyrexia with a concurrent drop in leucocyte count two weeks later (Pedersen *et al.*, 1987). During this period, one kitten developed a bacterial skin infection with marked pyrexia but responded well to antibiotic treatment. Signs in both kittens disappeared after two to four weeks although the lymphadenopathy remained. It is likely that similar non-specific illness can occur soon after natural infection with FTLV and these symptoms may be sufficiently severe to lead to the death or euthanasia of the cat. However, it is thought that most cats recover after the initial stage of infection and that a proportion, as yet unknown, go on to develop one or more chronic illnesses as a result of immunosuppression caused by FTLV. Individuals frequently have a history of recurrent bouts of illness with gradual deterioration over a long period of time. However, some cats with no previous history of illness show acute onset of symptoms such as severe diarrhoea or necrotic stomatitis with rapid deterioration and death. A list of signs commonly seen in FTLV infection is given in Table 1. In general, non-specific signs, haematological changes and secondary problems such as gingivitis, diarrhoea and upper respiratory tract infection occur most often. Diagnosis of FTLV infection cannot be made from clinical signs alone.

Table 1 CLINICAL SIGNS OF FTLV INFECTION (HARBOUR *ET AL.*, 1988; ISHIDA *ET AL.*, 1988; PEDERSEN *ET AL.*, 1987; HOPPER, UNPUBLISHED DATA)

General signs	Lethargy, inappetence, weight loss, lymphadenopathy, pyrexia, poor coat
Secondary infections	Gingivitis, periodontitis, stomatitis pustular dermatitis, chronic dermatitis, ear infections, chronic rhinitis, chronic conjunctivitis, chronic keratitis, chronic diarrhoea
Other signs	Vomiting, renal disease, abortion, vague neurological abnormalities, neoplasia
Haematological changes	Anaemia, leucopenia, lymphopenia, myeloproliferative disorders

PATHOLOGY

There has been little work to investigate the pathological changes caused by FTLV or to identify the sites where it is harboured in the body. In future, the cloning of FTLV and development of monoclonal antibodies to viral antigen will enable the use of sophisticated immunohistochemical techniques to study the presence of FTLV in various tissues. Findings at post-mortem are usually few and correlate with the clinical signs seen in the patient, e.g. colitis found in cases of diarrhoea, reactive lymph nodes where lymphadenopathy was present.

EPIZOOTIOLOGY

The natural modes of infection of FTLV have still to be determined but it is thought that the virus is spread directly from cat to cat via saliva (Hardy, 1988). It is not known whether the virus must be introduced by a wound or bite. However, biting is thought to be important in transmission of infection (Pedersen, personal communication). Pedersen also suggests that FTLV is not spread during sexual contact, nor vertically from mother to offspring (Connor, 1987). The effect of individual factors such as age, breed, sex, lifestyle and concurrent infections on the infectivity of FTLV is not fully understood.

It has been suggested that cats in the older age range are more commonly infected with FTLV (Horzinek, 1987) but the survey in Japan (Ishida *et al.*, 1988) showed that over half the cats with antibody to FTLV were under five years of age. The same survey revealed that amongst infected individuals the ratio of male to female was 2:1. The authors suggested that, because male cats tend to roam further afield and fight more frequently than females, they have greater contact with other cats and thus an increased exposure to FTLV. Pedersen has also found an increased incidence of infection among male cats (Pedersen, personal communication). It has been suggested that these free-roaming cats could play an important role in transmitting the infection in areas with a high cat population. FTLV infection in closed breeding catteries appears to be very rare.

Several surveys have been carried out to determine the incidence of FTLV infection in various countries. The findings are summarized in Table 2. The incidence of infection is high when the sample tested is drawn from an area with a high cat population, e.g. Tokyo or Paris. However, Pedersen reports that most infected cats in California come from rural areas (Pedersen, personal communication).

DIAGNOSIS

The available methods for diagnosis of FTLV infection are summarized in Table 3. The simplest and most rapid method of diagnosis is the detection of viral antibody in serum or plasma. Immunofluorescence is reasonably accurate but false positives may occur if antibody to FeSFV is present (Lutz, 1988). The more complex method of Western blotting is much more accurate. This technique involves the separation of viral proteins by gel electrophoresis, blotting the bands of protein onto nitrocellulose paper and incubating a strip of nitrocellulose with test serum to identify the proteins to which antibody is present. The newly developed ELISA is also very accurate. It

Table 2 THE INCIDENCE OF FTLV INFECTION IN VARIOUS COUNTRIES

Country		FTLV Ab positive (%)	Number tested	Reference
USA	(California)	Approx. 50		Horzinek, 1987
Switzerland	(sick)	3.7	775	Lutz, 1988
	(healthy)	2.8	178	Lutz, 1988
France (Paris)	(sick)	22.1	208	Lutz, 1988
UK	(sick)	12.8	431	Lutz, 1988
	(healthy)	0	98	Lutz, 1988
Netherlands	(sick)	3	98	Lutz, 1988
	(healthy)	1	123	Lutz, 1988
Japan (Tokyo)	(sick)	22.7	260	Ishida *et al.*, 1988
	(healthy)	3.6	55	Ishida *et al.*, 1988

Table 3 METHODS OF FTLV DIAGNOSIS

Detection of antibodies:	Immunofluorescence (IFA)
	Western blotting
	Enzyme linked immunosorbent assay (ELISA)
Virus isolation:	Cytopathic effects in lymphocyte culture
	Electron microscopy (EM) of lymphocyte culture
	Reverse transcriptase assay (RTA) of culture supernatant

has excellent sensitivity and specificity and has the advantage of being simple and rapid to use. A CITE (concentration immunoassay technology) test for FTLV has also been developed.

The disadvantage of diagnosis by detection of antibody is that some FTLV-infected cats do not have antibody to the virus. (Conversely, it seems that virus can be isolated from all cats with antibody to FTLV). This discrepancy also occurs in humans with HIV infection, although the incidence is low. Until the proportion of FTLV-infected cats which lack antibody is determined it would be unwise to base a control policy purely on serological results.

The definitive test for FTLV is by virus isolation. It is thought that infection with FTLV is lifelong. Consequently, if a cat has become infected with FTLV it should always be possible to isolate the virus, although this may be easier in some individuals than others. The technique of virus isolation involves the separation of lymphocytes from a heparinized blood sample, culture of lymphocytes with mitogens and lymphokines to promote proliferation, followed by co-culture with similarly activated lymphocytes from a specific-pathogen-free (SPF) donor cat to stimulate viral replication. Cytopathic effects, consisting of ballooning degeneration (Figure 2) and syncytium formation, are seen if the lymphocytes are infected with FTLV. The presence of FTLV can be confirmed by electron microscopy, RTA and IFA. Unfortunately, virus isolation is a lengthy and labour intensive procedure and is dependent on a supply of SPF lymphocytes. Therefore, it is not ideal for screening purposes.

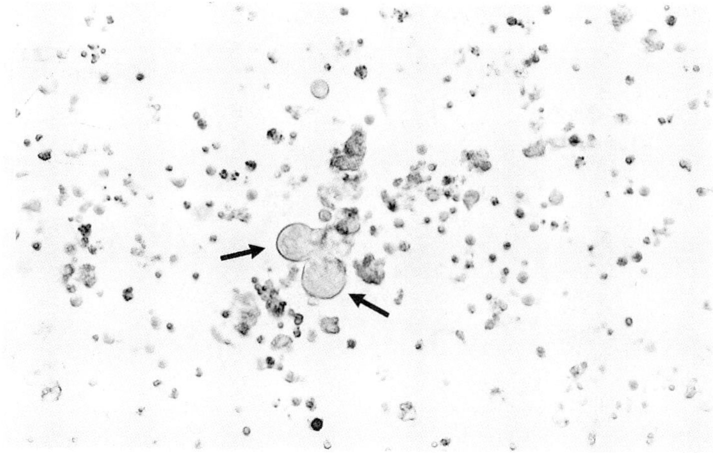

Fig. 2. Colonies of lymphocytes free-floating in culture medium. There is ballooning degeneration (arrows) of two cells in the central colony. Magnification × 112.

Further work is needed to develop a technique which can identify virus-infected lymphocytes, for example the use of a DNA probe specific for FTLV.

TREATMENT AND CONTROL

As yet there is no specific therapy to combat FTLV infection. Clinicians are restricted to the use of symptomatic treatment. This usually involves support with antibiotics and anabolics. Occasionally, corticosteroids have been helpful in alleviating symptoms such as diarrhoea or erythema but they should be used with caution because their immunosuppressive properties may potentiate the effects of FTLV. Great efforts are being made to develop specific antiviral drugs and to develop a vaccine.

Advice regarding control of FTLV infection is not straightforward because very little is known of the epizootiology. Because FTLV is an enveloped virus, it is readily destroyed by disinfectants. However, infection is thought to pass directly from cat to cat and not via the environment, so disinfection procedures are unlikely to halt the spread of the virus. It would be wise to ensure that infected cats have minimal contact with other cats, or are kept in isolation. Similarly, owners of uninfected cats would be sensible to discourage their cat from roaming in order to minimize contact with potentially infected cats.

More radical measures such as test and removal programmes have been suggested (Hardy, 1988) but such measures would be inadvisable until much more is known about the incidence, spread and pathogenesis of feline lentivirus infection.

ACKNOWLEDGEMENTS

The authors would like to thank Mr A. H. Sparkes and Dr T. J. Gruffydd-Jones for their help in supplying clinical information. C. D. Hopper is currently supported by Duphar Veterinary Ltd.

REFERENCES

Connor, S. (1987) *New Scientist,* **1585,** 20
Harbour, D. A. *et al.,* (1988) *Vet. Rec.,* **122,** 84–86
Hardy, W. D. (1988) *J. Am. Animal Hospital Assoc.* **24,** 241–243
Horzinek, M. C. (1987) In *Virus Infections of Carnivores* (ed. M. J. Appel) Elsevier, Amsterdam, pp. 337–338
Ishida, T. *et al.,* (1988) *Jpn. J. Vet. Sci.,* **50,** 39–44
Levy, J. A. *et al.,* (1987) *Ann. Inst. Pasteur,* **138,** 101–111
Lutz, H. (1988) *FAB Bull.* **25,**(2):20
Nelson, J. A. *et al.,* (1988) *Lancet i,* 259–262
Pedersen, N. C. *et al.,* (1987) *Science* **235,** 790–793

D. WHITTAKER

Pasteurellosis in the laboratory rabbit: a review

INTRODUCTION

THE RABBIT is an important species in research laboratories. However, its disease profile is poorly understood and consequently poorly controlled by comparison with other laboratory animals such as rodents. Morbidity and mortality are often much higher than in other laboratory maintained animals. This has an obvious impact on breeding, research and not least of all, welfare.

The two major health problems of rabbits are enteropathies of multiple aetiology and respiratory disease. *Pasteurella multocida* plays a significant role in respiratory disease and associated conditions of the rabbit. The term Pasteurellosis includes a broad spectrum of these conditions ranging from sub-clinical rhinitis through to otitis media, pneumonia, septicaemia and death.

THE ORGANISM

Pasteurella multocida is a small ovoid Gram-negative rod. Brogden (1980), reviewed the characteristics of 48 *P. multocida* cultures from rabbits and described appearances varying from uniform arrangements of Gram-negative short coccobacillary-shaped rods occurring singly, in pairs and short chains to Gram-negative rods of varying lengths. In carefully stained preparations the organism has a distinct bipolar appearance. The organism is easily grown on blood agar but will not grow on MacConkeys.

Serotyping is based on capsular and cell wall (somatic) antigens. The most common serotype isolated from rabbits is 12:A (Carter, 1967; Lu *et al.*, 1978; Chengappa *et al.*, 1982; Lu *et al.*, 1983 and Manning, 1984).

OCCURRENCE AND INCIDENCE

Pasteurella multocida has been isolated from rabbits in many parts of the world. No reliable information is available on the incidence within the UK but it is probable that most colonies, excepting a few caesarean re-derived and barrier maintained units, have some degree of infection. It has been demonstrated that a large proportion of clinically normal rabbits within an endemically infected colony may be carriers, (Hagen, 1967; Lu *et al.*, 1978; Weisbroth and Scher, 1969; Webster, 1924). Post-mortem surveys show that respiratory disease and related conditions may account for between 5 and 26% of all deaths (Whitney *et al.*, 1976; Hinton, 1977; 1979; Ostler, 1961). Finally Flatt and Dungworth (1971) showed that sub-clinical enzootic pneumonia may be present at a significant level in apparently normal rabbits.

TRANSMISSION

Horizontal transfer is the common mode of transmission both by direct nose to nose contact and by the aerosol route (Llelkes and Corbett, 1983). Rabbits can not effectively sneeze beyond six feet and therefore spread between rabbits separated by this distance will be controlled (Llelkes, 1985, personal communication).

DiGiacomo *et al.*, (1983) studied infection and disease caused by *P. multocida* from birth to maturity and found that the earliest nasal infection occurred around 12 weeks. Indirect horizontal transmission via fomites and mechanical transmission during coitus appears to be possible but not common (Smith, 1927; McKennedy and Shillinger, 1938). Holmes *et al.*, (1983) however, suggest that spread via contaminated water supplies may be common. Successful elimination of the organism by caesarean re-derivation is strong evidence that there is no vertical transmission (Pleasants, 1959; Wostman and Pleasants, 1959; Scher *et al.*, 1969).

COLONIZATION AND DISSEMINATION

When sufficient numbers of bacteria are transmitted a sub-clinical infection is established in the rabbit's upper respiratory tract. Bacteria become abundant in the mucous film covering the mucous membrane but are scarce in the sinuses. In a few cases organisms disappear from the nares. In most cases however, a balance is achieved between bacterial proliferation and mucocillary clearance. Once this balance is established sub-clinical infections become chronic. When in this state *P. multocida* appears to behave as a commensal. The pathogenic potential is only realized when the balance between bacterial growth and clearance is disrupted. The disrupting factors are as yet unclear.

Although infection of the upper respiratory tract (snuffles) is the most common form of infection and diseases, the organism may also disseminate to other parts of the body. The most common variants are pneumonia, via the blood stream, (Webster, 1926), otitis media, via the Eustachian tube, (Flatt *et al.*, 1977) and septicaemia. Possible routes of spread are shown in Figure 1.

FACTORS AFFECTING DISEASE

Although the horizontal mode of transmission is relatively well understood the factors involved in the progression from commensal infection to clinically significant disease are far from clear. They include virulence of the organism, host genotype and factors affecting host resistance such as environmental stress and host immunity.

The virulence of the organism may be a significant factor in disease (Heddleston, 1976). The strain of rabbit may also be as important a factor as the strain of organism in determining the outcome of infection (Webster, 1927).

Stressing influences on infections of *P. multocida* include normal biological functions such as pregnancy, parturition and lactation (Paterson, 1956). Other

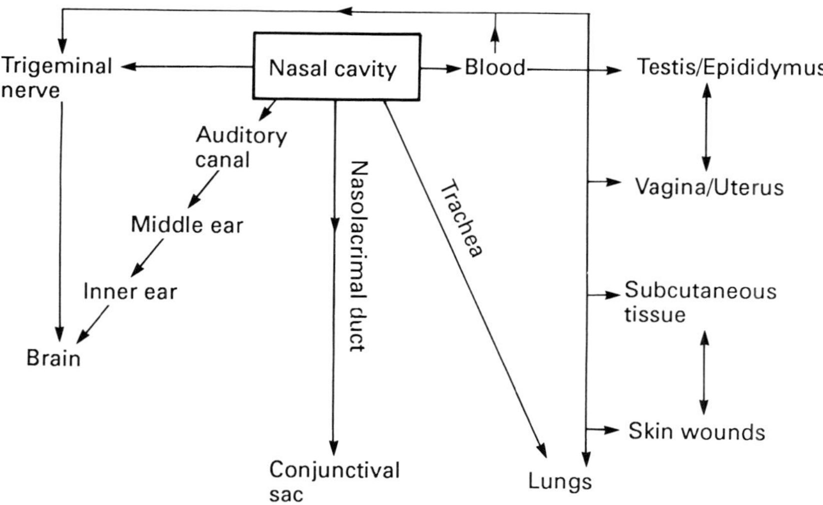

Fig. 1. Possible routes of spread within the body (adapted from Flatt, 1974).

stresses include poor environmental conditions, nutritional state, season and experimental procedures. Cowie-Whitney (1977) emphasized that poor management and inadequate nutrition are often associated with respiratory disease.

Immunological aspects of host resistance are gaining interest because vaccination is one potential means of control. In summary, the rabbit produces a humoral response to *P. multocida* which may or may not give local and/or systemic protection. Cellular response to infection appears to be lacking or defective resulting in chronic infections, though mechanisms of this fault have yet to be elucidated. Infected dams pass on passive immunity to their young via the placenta which is thought to protect them from infection until its disappearance at around 8 weeks (Llelkes, 1985 (personal communication); Corbeil *et al.*, 1983; Mushin and Schoenbaum, 1980; DiGiacomo *et al.*, 1983; Collins, 1977).

SPECIFIC CLINICAL CONDITIONS

Pasteurella multocida is implicated in a number of clinical conditions, most of which stem from dissemination of the organism from the upper respiratory tract. The factors causing this dissemination and clinical signs are many fold. Table 1 lists the clinical manifestations together with a comment on each state. Figures 2, 3 and 4 show mild and moderate forms of snuffles and a case of otitis media respectively.

TREATMENT OF *P. MULTOCIDA* INFECTIONS

In vitro sensitivity testing of isolates from rabbits indicates a wide spectrum of antibiotic sensitivity. However, experience shows that treatment of most *P. multocida* infections in the rabbit is futile.

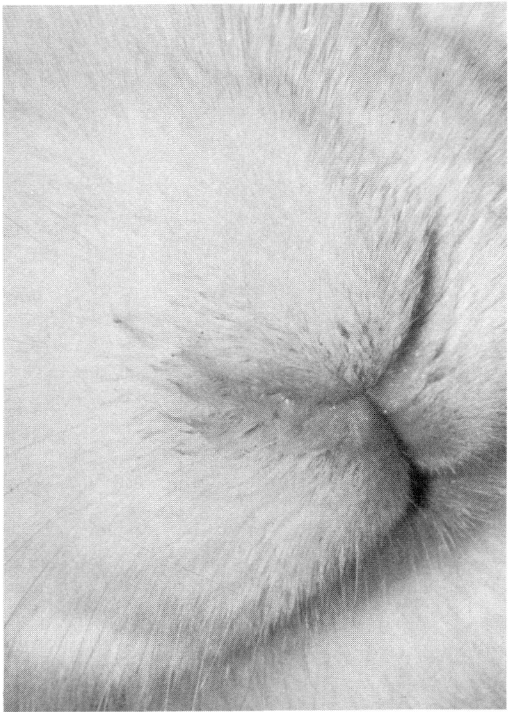

Fig. 2. A case of mild snuffles with serious nasal discharge.

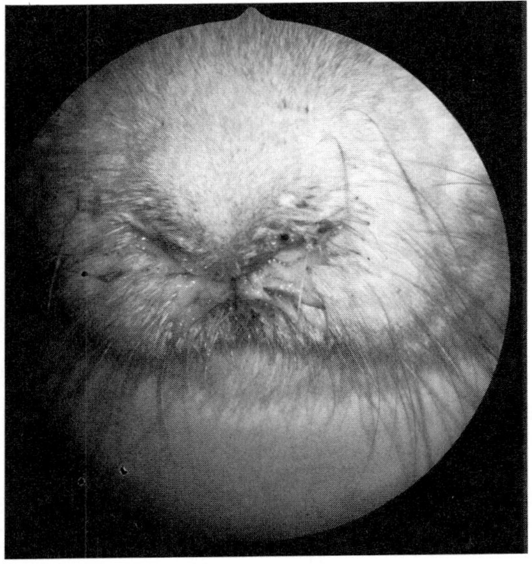

Fig. 3. A case of moderate snuffles with mucopurulent nasal discharge.

Table 1 CLINICAL MANIFESTATIONS OF *P. MULTOCIDA* IN RABBITS

Condition	*Comment*
1. Snuffles	Commonest and earliest form of infection. Infections of *B. bronchiseptica* will cause similar disease. Antibiotic treatment will bring about remission of signs but not cure.
2. Septicaemia	Commonest cause of sudden death. Few preceeding clinical signs. Usually follows a stressful experience.
3. Pneumonia	Common sequelae to snuffles. Fibrinous pleurisy a common post-mortem finding. Usually unresponsive to treatment.
4. Otitis media	Acute onset torticollis, animal usually remains otherwise well. Treatment usually futile.
5. Conjunctivitis	Although often implicated, *P. multocida* rarely isolated from cases of conjunctivitis.
6. Genital tract infection	Testicular abscesses in males. Endometritis and pyometra in does.
7. Abscess	In addition to sites already mentioned, abscesses are common in the subcutis.
8. Osteomyelitis	Most common site is the mandible. Treatment is futile.
9. Meningo-encephalitis	Probably results from progression of otitis media or via the haematogenous route.

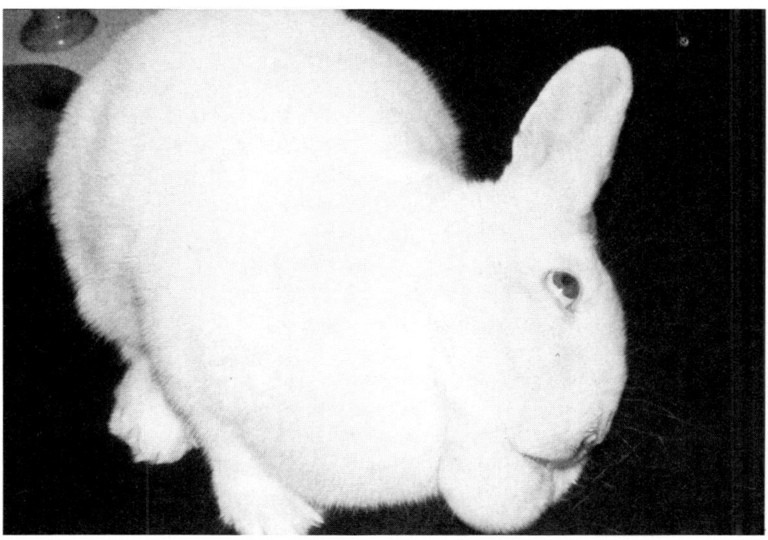

Fig. 4. A case of otitis media (courtesy of Dr. Flecknell, Newcastle University).

Septicaemia and pneumonias are acute diseases with no time available for therapy. Conditions such as osteomyelitis, otitis media and genital infections although slow in advancement, are usually too far advanced on clinical recognition for treatment to be effective.

There is no doubt that antibiotic treatment of snuffles will bring about remission of the clinical signs but there is general agreement that even prolonged regimes will not eliminate the bacteria (Flatt, 1974; Llelkes, 1985, personal communication).

CONTROL AND PREVENTION

It is because the treatment of Pasteurella infections is unrewarding that control and prevention is so important. Even so, little progress has yet been made in successful containment and elimination of the organism from production colonies.

VACCINATION

Pasteurella multocida vaccines are successfully used to prevent and control disease in many species, such as fowl and sheep. From the literature it would seem that they have a role to play in control of the disease in rabbits. Whilst clinical success is clearly achievable in certain circumstances (Ferry and Hoskins, 1920; Alexander *et al.*, 1951; Chengappa *et al.* 1980; Lu and Pakes, 1981) much work remains to be done both on the immunological mechanisms of the rabbit and on the antigenic components of the organism before consistently reliable vaccination of rabbits can be achieved (Manning, 1982; Hofing *et al.*, 1979).

HUSBANDRY PRACTICES

Removal of weaning animals to a physically separate area from infected adults should provide a very effective method of control if reports by DiGiacomo *et al.*, (1983) and Llelkes (1985, personal communication) are correct and young animals remain immune or, at least, uninfected until around 12 weeks of age. It must be remembered however, that this is a very stressful period for rabbits and such movements and mixing may bring about enteric disease with equally devastating results. In endemically infected colonies cross-infection can also be reduced by increasing the distance between animals, although in most instances this will not be a realistically economical proposition. Of course, normal hygiene practices must be operated in terms of keeping units clean together with disinfection or sterilization of as much equipment as possible, especially watering systems.

Clinical disease can be minimized in endemically infected units and colonies by paying attention to the environmental conditions and stress factors. The actual temperature at which the animals are held is less important than avoiding large temperature fluctuations. The optimum temperature range aimed for in most UK laboratories is 18± 2°C. Clough (1982) states that control of relative humidity is important in the control and management of airborne disease and, generally speaking, should be maintained between 50–70%. In addition to maintaining favourable environmental conditions attention must also be paid to the actual volume of air circulating in the unit. Most UK laboratories now aim for a circulation rate of around 20 air changes per hour. Ideally, to obtain maximum dilution of airborne organisms, total fresh air systems or efficient filtering systems should be incorporated.

Finally, it can not be over-emphasized that any stress factor may bring on a clinical outbreak of disease.

Foundation of a *P. multocida*-free colony is best achieved by a caesarean re-derivation programme (Pleasants, 1959; Wostman and Pleasants, 1959; Scher, Collins and Weisbroth, 1969; Ward 1973). Llelkes (1985, personal communication) suggests that feeding antibiotics to weaning animals from infected colonies may increase the chance of getting a *Pasteurella* free colony. He recommends tetracycline at 1 mg/ml of drinking water of sulphonamides at the rate of 4 ml of a 12.5% solution per pint of water. Chemoprophylaxis however, is generally considered inappropriate in most laboratory situations.

CONCLUDING REMARKS

Like many infectious diseases of animals *P. multicoda* is a condition of the intensively reared and maintained rabbit. *P. multicoda* infection of wild rabbits is not a recognized problem, nor is respiratory disease in general (Ross, 1985, personal communication).

Pasteurella multocida is undoubtedly the single most important bacterial pathogen of the rabbit. It has enormous impact on their welfare, economic production and use as an experimental model. Whilst the condition has now been recognized as a clinical entity for around 100 years effective prevention, control and treatment regimes have still to be elucidated and applied on a wide scale.

REFERENCES

Alexander, M. M., Swain, P. B. and Roehm, D. A. (1951) Respiratory infection in the rabbit: an enzootic caused by *Pasteurella lepiseptica* and attempts to control it by vaccination. *J. Infect. Dis.*, **90**, 30–33

Brogden, K. A. (1980) Physiological and serological characteristics of 48 *Pasteurella multocida* cultures from rabbits. *J. Clin. Microbiol.*, **11**, 646–649

Carter, G. R. (1967) Pasteurellosis: *Pasteurella multocida* and *Pasteurella haemolytica*. *Adv. Vet. Sci.*, **11**, 321–379

Chengappa, M. M., Myers, R. C. and Carter, G. R. (1980) A streptomycin dependent live *Pasteurella multocida* vaccine for the prevention of rabbit Pasteurellosis. *Lab. Anim Sci.*, **30**, 515–518

Chengappa, M. M., Myers, R. C. and Carter, G. R. (1982) Capsular and somatic types of *Pasteurella multocida* from rabbits. *Can. J. Comp. Med.*, **46**, 437–439

Clough, G. (1982) Environmental effects on animals used in biomedical research. *Biol. Rev.*, **57**, 487–523

Collins, F. M. (1977) Mechanisms of acquired resistance to *Pasteurella multocida* infection. *Cornell Vet.*, **67**, 103–138

Corbeil, L. B., Strayer, D. S., Skaletsky, E., Wunderlich, A., Sell, S. (1983) Immunity to pasteurellosis in compromised rabbits. *Am. J. Vet. Res.*, **44**, 845–850

Cowie-Whitney, J. (1977) Disease of the commerical rabbit. *Vet. Rec.*, **101**, 299–303

DiGiacomo, R. F., Garlinghouse, L. E., Van Hoosier, G. L. (1983) Natural history of infection with *Pasteurella multocida* in rabbits. *J. Am. Vet. Med. Assoc.*, **183**, 1172–1175

Ferry, N. S. and Hoskins, H. P. (1920) Bacteriology and control of contagious nasal catarrh (snuffles) of rabbits. *J. Lab. Clin. Med.*, **5**, 311–318

Flatt, R. E. and Dungworth, D. L. (1971) Enzootic pneumonia in rabbits: Naturally occurring lesions in lungs of apparently healthy young rabbits. *Am. J. Vet. Res.*, **32**, 621–626

Flatt, R. E. (1974) Chapter 9 In *The Biology of the Laboratory Rabbit* 1st edn. (eds. S. H. Weisbroth, R. E. Flatt and Kraus), Academic Press, London, pp 194–205

Flatt, R. E., Deyoung, D. W. and Hogle, R. M. (1977) Suppurative otitis media in the rabbit: Prevalence, pathology, and microbiology. *Lab. Anim. Sci.*, **27**, 343–347

Hagen, K. W. (1967) Effect of antibiotic-sulphonamide therapy on certain micro-organisms in the nasal turbinates of domestic rabbits. *Lab. Anim. Care*, **17**, 77–80

Heddleston, K. L. (1976) Physiologic characteristics of 1268 cultures of *Pasteurella multocida*. *Am. J. Vet. Res.*, **27**, 493–497

Hinton, M. (1977) Disease in adult rabbits: An analysis of the post-mortem findings in 180 rabbits. *Vet. Med. Rev.*, **2**, 183–192

Hinton, M. (1979). Post-mortem survey of diseases in young rabbits. *Vet. Rec.*, **104**, 53–54

Hofing, G. L., Rush, H. G., Petkus, A. R. and Glorioso, J. C. (1979) *In vitro* killing of *Pasteurella multocida*: The effect of rabbit granulocyte and specific antibody source. *Am. J. Vet. Res.*, **40**, 679–683

Holmes, H. T., Patton, N. M. and Cheeke, P. R. (1983) Pasteurella contaminated watering valves: Its incidence and implication. *J. Appl. Rabbit Research*, **6**, 123–124

Llelkes, L. and Corbett, M. J. (1983) A preliminary study of the transmission of *Pasteurella multocida* infection in rabbits. *J. Appl. Rabbit Research*, **6**, 125–126

Lu, Y. S., Ringler, D. H. and Park, J. S. (1978) Characterization of *Pasteurella multocida* isolates from the nares of healthy rabbits and rabbits with pneumonia. *Lab. Anim. Sci.*, **28**, 691–697

Lu, Y. S. and Pakes, S. P. (1981) Protection of rabbits against experimental pasteurellosis by a streptomycin-dependent *Pasteurella multocida* serotype 3: A live mutant vaccine. *Infect. Immun.*, **34**, 1018–1024

Lu, Y. S., Pakes, S. P. and Stefanu, C. (1983) Capsular and somatic serotypes of *Pasteurella multocida* isolates recovered from healthy and diseased rabbits in Texas. *J. Clin. Microbiol.*, **18**, 292–295

Manning, P. J. (1982) Serology of *Pasteurella multocida* in laboratory rabbits: A review. *Lab. Anim. Sci.*, **32**, 666–671

Manning, P. J. (1984) Naturally occuring Pasteurellosis in laboratory rabbits: Chemical and serological studies of whole cells and lipopolysaccharides of Pasteurella multocida. *Infect. Immun.*, **44**, 502–507

McKennedy, F. D. and Shillinger, J. E. (1938) Transmission of *Pasteurella cuniculicida* in rabbits by breeding. *J. Am. Vet. Med. Assoc.*, **93**, 161–164

Mushin, R. and Schoenbaum, M. (1980) A strain of *Pasteurella multocida* associated with infections in rabbit colonies. *Lab. Anim.*, **14**, 353–356

Ostler, D. C. (1961) The diseases of broiler rabbits. *Vet. Rec.*, **73**, 1237–1252

Paterson, J. S. (1956) *Bull. Pap. Lab. Animal Bureau.* **4**, 37

Pleasants, J. R. (1959) Rearing germ-free caesarian born rats, mice and rabbits through weaning. *Ann. N. Y. Acad. Sci.*, **78**, 116–126

Scher, S., Collins, G. R. and Weisbroth, S. H. (1969). The establishment of a specific pathogen free rabbit breeding colony. I. Procedures for establishment and maintenance. *Lab. Anim. Care*, **19**, 610–616

Smith, D. T. (1927) Epidemiological studies on respiratory infections of the rabbit. X. A spontaneous epidemic of pneumonia and snuffles caused by *Bacterium lepisepticum* among a stock of rabbits at Saranac Lake N.Y. *J. Exp. Med.*, **45**, 553–559

Ward, G. M. (1973) Development of a *Pasteurella*-free colony. *Lab. Anim. Sci.*, **23**, 671–674

Webster, L. T. (1924) The epidemiology of a rabbit respiratory infection III. Nasal flora of laboratory rabbits. *J. Exp. Med.*, **39**, 857–877

Webster, L. T. (1926) Epidemiological studies of respiratory infections of the rabbit. VII Pneumonias associated with *Bacterium lepisepticum. J. Exp. Med.,* **43,** 555–572

Webster, L. T. (1927) Epidemiological studies on respiratory infection of the rabbit IX. The spread of *Bacterium lepisepticum* infection at a rabbit farm in New City N.Y. An epidemiological study. *J. Exp. Med.,* **45,** 529–551

Weisbroth, S. H. and Scher, S. (1969) The establishment of a specific-pathogen-free rabbit breeding colony II. Monitoring for disease and health statistics. *Lab. Anim. Care,* **19,** 795–799

Whitney, J. C., Blackmore, D. K., Townsend, G. H., Parkin, R. J., Hugh-Jones, M. E., Crossman, P. J., Graham-Marr, T., Rowland, A. C., Festing, M. F. W. and Krzysiak, D. (1976) Rabbit mortality survey. *Lab. Anim.,* **10,** 203–207

Wostman, B. S. and Pleasants, J. R. (1959) Rearing of germ free rabbits. *Proc. Anim. Care Panel,* **9,** 47–54

S. JONES and P. J. LLEWELLYN

Precepts for the successful husbandry of lizards and snakes: how best to avoid disease

INTRODUCTION

WITH THE universal appearance of jet airlines offering rapid freighting services, the late 1960s saw a boom in the commercial trans-shipment of wild animals for the pet trade. Initially reptiles of almost any species could be collected *en masse* from virtually any chosen country and shipped to importers in Europe, North America and Japan as pets. Increasing local awareness of the value of resource protection saw a rapid proliferation of protective legislation from most former exporter nations through the 1970s and 1980s. To date, only a small minority of states permit the collection and exportation of native fauna and flora for trade.

Because the demand for wild animals seems fairly constant, to supply this demand, importers respond by importing almost any available species from the few exporters available. This has resulted in the current situation whereby virtually all wild reptiles offered by retailers in the UK are wholly unsuited to maintenance in captivity. The ecologies of most species offered are almost entirely unknown, even to experienced herpetologists.

Perhaps the majority of species are imported from rain forest environments such as those of Thailand, Southern Mexico and Guyana. Such species typically occupy highly specialized ecological niches which is reflected in their diets. Many of the snakes imported will feed only on particular genera of chameleons, geckoes, frogs, toads or other snakes. Relatively few will adapt easily to the captive staple diet of laboratory rodents.

Many reptiles may feed apparently well but are virtually impossible to maintain, let alone breed, in captivity. These include all chameleons, horned toads (*Phrynosoma* sp.) and agamas. These animals should simply never be imported or purchased.

In fact, perhaps 90% of wild reptiles available in the UK are 'those obtainable' rather than 'those suitable' as captive subjects. Even such species as the legions of skinks, *Mabuya* sp.; Tokay geckoes, *Gecko gecko*; Wall lizards, *Podarcis* sp., Curly-tailed lizards, *Liocephalus*; Spiny lizards or swifts, *Sceloporus*; Iguanas, *Iguana iguana*; Water Dragons, *Physignathus coccinus*; Basiliscs, *Basiliscus* sp.; Monitor lizards, *Varanus* sp., Asian ratsnakes, *Elaphe* sp. and Garter snakes, *Thamnophis sirtalis* which are amongst the most commonly available reptiles, typically survive for only a few months to a year before dying. The truth is that whilst some lizards and snakes live, breed and can be seen to thrive in captivity, such races are only a small minority of those available. They are rarely available from importers.

294

Intentionally or otherwise, most reptiles collected from the wild provide dealers with a ready source of high volume, low unit cost merchandise which will survive in the hands of the private buyer perhaps 1–24 months, often without ever feeding. Even small reptiles can last relatively long periods without feeding. This is a function of environmental stress. Their death tends to occur such a long time after purchase that it is no longer immediately attributable to the supplier. Death often occurs after a sufficiently lengthy period as to provide at least some return for their cost and the hope that the next animal might fare 'even better'. Most wild-collected lizards and snakes cost the keeper only approximately £0.50–£2.00 per month, even assuming a captive lifespan of approximately 6–12 months. This is calculated as the cost of an average priced wild lizard or snake plus food costs, if any, divided by longevity in months.

The cheapness of the animals is one factor which discourages many keepers from seeking professional help with their animals' ailments. Other factors include a lack of concern or a pessimistic prognoses developed by conditioning as well as the often deeply entrenched belief of many hobbyists that veterinary surgeons are not very competent in dealing with reptile subjects.

PROBLEMS OF CAPTURE AND MAINTENANCE

Imported wild reptiles, even those of species capable of performing well in captivity, are severely prejudiced by their conditions of capture and maintenance in the country of origin, the cost-conscious details of freighting and the management practices of importers, retailers and hobbyists. Both authors have been involved with the receipt and care of entire commercial shipments of reptiles after official seizure by HM Customs and Excise at various UK airports. Typically between 5–20% of animals examined were found to be dead on arrival (DOA). Some were apparently already dead when consigned. Many of the dead were heavily gravid females of the larger species such as royal python (*Python regius*) and Savannah or Bosc's monitor lizard (*Varanus excanthematicus*).

Virtually all reptiles examined have borne large ectoparasite burdens of several tick and mite genera (e.g. *Aponoma* sp., *Ophionyssus* sp. and *Ornithodorus* sp.). These vectors of disease are omnipresent in wild-collected reptiles in trade and can transmit an enormous array of pathogens. One UK importer himself is known to have enjoyed a two week stay in hospital after contracting Q-fever from a West African snake tick. It seems reasonable that more cases of this difficult to diagnose, flu-like disorder may have been transmitted undetected.

Unfortunately, whilst acarines may be treated quite easily with Ivermectin, Neguvan or small dichlorvos strips, the rapid turnover of high volume, low unit cost has so far precluded even such basic quarantine procedures by UK importers. All importers and the vast majority of retailers may be regarded as being perpetually infested with an array of acarines and their pathogens. Many pathogens isolated from wild animals in trade have proved virtually impossible to identify and therefore specifically treat (L. Greenham and M. G. R. Varma, personal communication).

PROBLEMS OF MANAGEMENT AND HYGIENE

Dehydration, trauma and large-scale dermal lesion as a result of poor management and hygiene by exporters and importers are very common problems. Because importers trade in animals of more than one continent, disease problems are made worse when diseases endemic to one region are transmitted to more animals from different regions or continents. Quarantining might help but because the animals would almost certainly die in a short space of time regardless, through starvation, stress-induced disorders and mismanagement, its deployment seems of cosmetic value.

Often enormous numbers of animals are held by importers in wholly inadequate accommodation with animals piled many bodies deep in a cage. Sometimes they are not even transferred from the exporters' freight boxes or bags at all prior to sale. The provision of adequate space, heating, hygiene, food and shelter by importers has yet to be encountered by either author.

REPTILES IN CAPTIVITY

Clinical discussions of the diseases of reptiles are beyond the ability of the authors. Of more importance is the unsurprising information that different species of reptiles perform differently in captivity. The majority of species imported have almost no chance of survival in private (or professional) hands. Stress plays a major role. A large part of the reptilian mid-gut fauna are benign commensals or may even help in mechanical degradation of food material (Iverson, 1982). However, in stressed reptiles, many such organisms, such as nematodes and protists, develop parasitic traits in the increasingly immunodeficient host.

Many of the popular species of reptiles initially seem to adapt reasonably well to captivity. However, with increasing size and maturity they become increasingly stressed by cramped accommodation. Such species as iguanas, monitors, basiliscs and water dragons are only suited to the largest accommodation offered by zoological exhibitions. Even an entire domestic room would not enable a 2 m long lizard to enact a fraction of its normal daily behaviour. Stress and deterioration result.

CAPTIVE-BRED REPTILES

As an alternative, captive-bred reptiles are increasingly widely available. These species are likely to survive and breed in captivity and are, from the start, largely pathogen-free. A list of the lizard and snake species suitable for the attentions of private keepers, including novices, is presented in Table 1. All these species are relatively easily obtainable as captive-bred young animals in the UK. The cost of captive-bred animals is generally a little higher than those caught in the wild and imported but this is offset by incomparable benefits. Purchased as babies, the lizards listed in Table 1 will mature in as little as 6–18 months. The snakes will mature in 1–4 years. It is perfectly possible that some of these animals will enjoy a captive lifespan measured in years or decades rather than months.

Table 1 LIZARD AND SNAKE SPECIES SUITABLE FOR PRIVATE COLLECTORS

Lizards

Eublephorus macularis – Leopard Cecko
Tiliqua gerradi – Pink Tongued Skink
T. gigas – New Guinea Blue-Tongued Skink
T. scincoides – Common Blue Tongued Skink
Chalcides ocellatus – Ocellated Skink
Lacerta viridis – Green Lizard
L. trilineata – Balkan Green Lizard
L. lepida – Eyed Lizard
Anolis carolinensis
Phelsuma madagascariensis – Giant Day Geckc

Snakes

Elpahe guttata – Corn and Great Plains rat snake
E. obsoleta – includes Yellow, Grey, Bairds, Black and Everglades rat snake
E. subocularis – Trans-Pecos rat snake
E. quatorlineata – Four-lined snake
Pituophis melanoleucus – includes Pine, Bull and Gopher snakes
Heterodon nasicus – Plains Hognose
Lampropeltis calligaster – Prairie Kingsnake
L. getulus – includes Chain, Californian, Florida, E. Black, Mexican Black, Desert and
        Speckled Kingsnakes
L. triangularum – includes Sinaloan, Campbells and Honduran Milksnakes
Boaedon fuliginosus – African House Snake
Lichanura roseofusca – Rosy boa
Eryx sp. – Sand Boas
Boa constrictor – Common Boa
Epicrates cenchria – Rainbow Boa
Morelia spilotes – Carpet and Diamond Python
Liasis childreni – Children's Python

HOUSING REQUIREMENTS

Wooden glass-fronted cages with ample ventilation panels are far preferable to the traditional glass aquarium for reptile accommodation. Aquariums are thermally inefficient and glass presents reptiles with a cold incomprehensible material. Wood caging provides a much higher degree of security. This is an important consideration in housing stress-prone animals.

Good ventilation is rarely provided for captive reptiles. This can lead to overheating and is implicated in a number of respiratory complaints especially in boids. Wood shavings are the preferred medium but newspaper, hortag pellets and bark chipping are all used with success. Aquarium gravel is to be discouraged because it is not absorbent, may disguise soiled areas and retains moisture in depth. Whilst occasional misting is beneficial, the cage medium should be kept dry. Even semi-aquatic species are highly prone to develop dermal lesions in the permanently moist cages. Clean water should be provided *ad libitum*.

In the last decade not very much information about reptile husbandry has been published. Amongst the most thorough accounts of how to raise, maintain and breed snakes in captivity is that of Coote (1985). Most of the manuals published for the hobbyists have been poor. Recently several good basic volumes have become available. They deal, to varying extents, with most aspects of reptile husbandry (e.g., Mattison, 1982; Zimmermann, 1986).

COMMON MALPRACTICES

Common malpractices by hobbyists include inadequate temperature and humidity regulation, inadequate provision of secure refugia, failure to provide diurnal lizards with ultra-violet (UV) light and utilizable mineral and vitamin supplements as well as improper mixing of sexes and species, overcrowding and the provision of a too limited a range of foodstuffs for lizards.

HEATING

There is a tendency to forget that reptiles do not maintain a high body temperature continuously. Heating biased towards one end of the cage or towards a small spot will help provide an essential temperature gradient. Reptiles maintained at high temperature permanently will metabolize fat deposits faster than they can digest and assimilate them and so starve (Avery, 1985). Heating should therefore be confined to one area of the cage or reduced by night. Typically, the animals listed in Table 1 will require the ability to raise their body temperature to 25–28°C for snakes and 25–35°C for lizards. By night the ambient temperature of the cage could fall to 21–24°C. Low wattage (10, 16 or 20W) heating plates can now be easily obtained for home-brewing or pet-keeping. They are ideal low cost spot-warmers for reptile accommodation.

REFUGIA

Most reptiles are secretive to some extent. Pieces of easily moved bark or cardboard boxes to hide under confer little security. Heavy clay half-pipe or roof tiles or other heavy material should be used to provide refugia in both warm and cool parts of the cage. Refugia should be long but as narow and low as possible to enable the animal to turn within it. Conferring maximum surface contact, many secretive reptiles will bask increasingly confidently in full view of the keeper when provided with such secure bolt-holes.

OSTEOLOGICAL DISORDERS

Developmental osteological disorders are a common, easily prevented problem with captive lizards (Cooper and Jackson, 1981; Tonge, 1985; Jones, 1987). Kyphosis is easily prevented by providing diurnal lizards with an artificial source of UV light from a fluorescent or similar UV emitting source such as Trulite (see Blatchford, 1987, for review of environmental lighting). Calcium lactate in drinking water or preferably, ground cuttlefish bone to lick from a dish or sprinkled onto foodstuffs should be provided for lizards. Calcium supplements are necessary because most cultured invertebrates offered as food have a poor calcium content. Specific reptile vitamin supplements with a correct Ca:P ratio should also be provided. (Note that Sa37 and Vionate do not meet this requirement).

OVERCROWDING

With few exceptions most snakes are best kept individually and brought together only for mating. At most a pair of the same species should be kept together but watched carefully when fed. Many snakes will feed less satisfactorily and gradually decline if not kept solitarily. Very few male reptiles will tolerate the presence of another male. Lizards are generally the best kept in pairs or trios. However there are a few exceptions, including the popular blue-tongued skinks (*Tiliqua* sp.), which are solitary.

It is also better not to accommodate more than one species per cage. A pair of most snakes of 1 m in length or most of the lizards listed in Table 1 could be housed comfortably in a 60 × 60 × 30 cm tall cage. Generally baby snakes are more secure and grow faster if initially housed in small polypropylene boxes such as those used for ice cream. These are suitable until the snake reaches about 40 cm in length.

FEEDING PROBLEMS

The commonest feeding problem witnessed in captive-bred snakes is overfeeding. Lizards are often provided with too limited a range of foodstuffs. Most young snakes should be offered the number of young mice they can comfortably consume once each week. Many adult snakes will readily gorge themselves if food is offered too regularly or in excessive quantities. This soon leads to obesity.

Once the space available for the enlargement of fat bodies, which are normally small and discrete in wild snakes, is entirely filled in obese animals, fat may even be deposited as discrete round fat bodies under the dermis. Obese snakes may have a couple of dozens of these disfiguring bodies which seem to diminish little even after severe long-term food restriction. Perhaps the majority of captive snakes are clinically obese. This is evident by the loss of their genus-characteristic cross-section. Most snakes should appear straight-sided with a flat or rounded dorsum; very few snakes are actually round in cross-section. However, obese snakes appear more or less cylindrical with bulging, rounded flanks. Most adult snakes of 1 m in length should be fed only 1–2 mice no more than once per week.

Obese reptiles are aesthetically displeasing, less readily bred from, shorter lived, more frequently retain ova and are frequently recorded as prolapsing. Typically, adult captives feed less often live longer, are more active, more fecund and remain healthier than overfed individuals.

STRESS

Most lizards and snakes are easily stressed. The less often they are caught and handled or disturbed the better. Provided with the relatively simple accommodation they require, captive lizards and snakes are amongst the easiest animals to keep and breed in a domestic environment. They can prove to be amongst the longest lived, most fecund and disease-free pets when derived from captive-bred stock.

It is worth noting that even the most successful reptile breeders will only keep a very few species other than those listed in Table 1. The truth is that only a tiny minority of reptile species adapt well to confinement. Most hobbyists buy wild-caught animals of unsuitable species rather than confining their attentions to a possibly less spectacular, more limited selection of suitable captive-bred species. Educating hobbyists to these realities will play a major role in reducing the numbers of wild-caught animals imported. Education of keepers will enable them to increase their husbandry skills. As a result there will be more efficient farming of reptiles as well as increased subject longevity and better breeding results. In addition, the incidence of death and disease of captive reptiles will be greatly reduced.

REFERENCES

Avery, R. A. (1985) Thermoregulatory behaviour of reptiles in the field and in captivity. In *Reptiles: Breeding, Behaviour and Veterinary Aspects.* (eds S. Townson and K. Lawrence), British Herpetological Society, London, pp. 61–72

Blatchford, D. (1987) Environmental lighting. In *Proceedings of the 1986 UK Herpetological Societies Symposium on Captive Breeding.* (ed. J. Coote), British Herpetological Society, London

Cooper, J. E. and Jackson, O. F. (1981) *Diseases of the Reptilia* Academic Press, London

Coote, J. (1985) Breeding colubrid snakes, mainly *Lampropeltis.* In *Reptiles: Breeding, Behaviour and Veterinary Aspects* (eds S. Townson and K. Lawrence) British Herpetological Society, London, pp. 5–18

Iverson, J. B. (1982) Adaptations to herbivory in Iguanine lizards. In *Iguanas of the World* (ed. G. Burghardt) Noyes Publications, New Jersey, pp. 77–83

Jones, S. (1987) A report on a reproducible and sustainable system for the captive propagation of the genus *Tiliqua*, Gray 1825. In *Proceedings of the 1986 UK Herpetological Societies Symposium on Captive Breeding* (ed J. Coote), British Herpetological Society, London

Mattison, C. (1982). *The Care of Reptiles and Amphibians in Captivity* (revised 1987) Butler and Tanner, London

Tonge, S. (1985) The management of juvenile Telfairs skinks, *Leiolopisma telfairii* with particular reference to the role of ultra-violet light. In *Reptiles: Breeding, Behaviour and Veterinary Aspects.* (eds S. Townson and K Lawrence), British Herpetological Society, London, pp. 61—72

Zimmerman, E. (1986) *Breeding Terrarium Animals,* T. F. H. Publications

Index